WL 365

The Clinical Neuropsychiatry of Multiple Sclerosis

Multiple sclerosis (MS) is the most common cause of neurological disability in young and middle-aged adults. This fully updated and revised new edition provides a detailed account of the many neuropsychiatric disorders associated with MS and is relevant to both the research and the clinical setting. Using the latest brain imaging findings and results from treatment trials, the symptoms, assessment, diagnosis and treatment of depression in MS are covered, as are psychosocial factors and the link between depression and magnetic resonance imaging abnormalities. Subsequent chapters focus on cognitive dysfunction in MS, including the natural history of cognitive change, the use of screening instruments and neuropsychological batteries, brain imaging correlations and management strategies. The book concludes with a survey of the behavioral benefits and risks associated with disease-modifying drugs. It will be valuable to all mental health professionals, neurologists and others caring for those affected by MS.

Anthony Feinstein is Professor of Psychiatry at the University of Toronto.

Reviews of the First Edition

"This is a clinically oriented volume, which is well researched, written and edited ... Feinstein should be congratulated for his effort in reviewing and bringing together what is known of the psychiatry of MS ..."

British Journal of Psychiatry

"This readable book is both a comprehensive overview, to be read cover-to-cover, and a reference volume, to be consulted as appropriate ... Feinstein deserves particular commendation for his strong pragmatic and clinical bias ... All in all, I recommend this book to complement any MS library."

The International MS Journal

This volume illustrates the refreshing advantage of a single-authored work, which avoids the redundancy, inconsistency of approach, and lack of balance of multiauthored works. It is a pleasure to read. I recommend it not only for the long list of those who manage MS patients but for general neurologists and residents in neurology and psychiatry as well.

Annals of Neurology

This is a useful, well-written book that would be of interest to anyone concerned about cognitive dysfunction and the utility of neurological illnesses in illuminating the relationships between brain and behavior.

American Journal of Psychiatry

To my parents

The Clinical Neuropsychiatry of Multiple Sclerosis

Second edition

Anthony Feinstein
University of Toronto, Canada

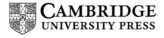
CAMBRIDGE
UNIVERSITY PRESS

CAMBRIDGE UNIVERSITY PRESS

Cambridge, New York, Melbourne, Madrid, Cape Town, Singapore, São Paulo

Cambridge University Press
The Edinburgh Building, Cambridge CB2 8RU, UK

Published in the United States of America by Cambridge University Press, New York

www.cambridge.org
Information on this title: www.cambridge.org/9780521852340

First published 1999
Second edition 2007

Printed in the United Kingdom at the University Press, Cambridge

A catalog record for this publication is available from the British Library

ISBN 978-0-521-85234-0 hardback

Contents

Acknowledgement

I would like to thank Alison Baldock, who kindly provided the cover illustrations.

Foreword

Among neurological disorders, multiple sclerosis has the unfortunate honor of being the most frequent cause of disability in young individuals. With the evolution of the disease, the brain is progressively deprived of sensory inputs and largely loses the ability to produce adequate responses. A combination of inflammation and degeneration causes progressive brain and spinal cord atrophy, which starts very early in the disease course and increases during the disease process. In addition, widespread damage takes place in the surviving gray and white matter. Not surprisingly, the disease often impacts on higher brain functions with neuropsychiatric manifestations. These processes are all admirably reviewed in this book and, for each cognitive and psychiatric disorder, the physiopathological theories are extensively and critically examined, making the book very useful not only for physicians, but also for researchers. The exceptional experience of Anthony Feinstein in this area, demonstrated by many key papers produced in the last decade, emerges clearly, page after page: the analysis of the literature is always combined with the "personal" view and a very useful summary of the main findings.

There are many reasons why neuropsychiatric disorders assume a key role in the management of multiple sclerosis patients: they occur early and affect about half of the patients; they are the most frequent cause of unemployment and a major determinant of a reduced quality of life; moreover, they negatively affect the ability of the patients to adhere to therapeutic protocols and to benefit from the most recent advances in both etiologic and somatic treatment.

This book should be read by all multiple sclerosis physicians because it can contribute to better care for many patients.

Professor Giancarlo Comi, M.D.
Director of the Department of Neurology
and Clinical Neurophysiology
San Raffael Hospital, Milan, Italy

Multiple sclerosis: diagnosis and definitions

Many a chapter, monograph and paper on multiple sclerosis (MS) begins with the observation that the disease is the most common cause of neurological disability in young and middle-aged adults. While the emphasis for much of the nineteenth and twentieth centuries was on the neurological manifestations of the disease, since the mid 1980s clinicians, researchers and patients have become more aware of the associated behavioral changes. A burgeoning literature devoted to the neuropsychiatry of MS attests to this new found interest, although those with knowledge of the medical history of MS may find themselves a little surprised why it took so long for this enthusiasm to re-ignite. Descriptions of altered mentation in MS patients long predate the man credited with naming, describing and making the condition known, the French behavioral neurologist Jean-Martin Charcot (Charcot, 1868; see also Murray, 2005).

One cannot describe the psychiatric and cognitive changes associated with MS without first referring to the neurology and pathology of the disorder. This chapter, therefore, begins with a summary of the pathogenesis, pathology, signs and symptoms, diagnosis and differential diagnosis of MS. With the book's emphasis on mentation, this introduction will by design be brief and those seeking more detailed explanations are encouraged to consult the many texts specifically devoted to these aspects. This chapter will, however, discuss in depth the research guidelines for diagnosing MS and furnish clear definitions for terms that apply directly to the disease. These points are important for they will clarify at the outset many descriptive terms that appear in the MS research literature and are used throughout this book. The chapter will conclude with a discussion on rating disability and how behavioral changes may affect this assessment.

Epidemiology

In the UK, the lifetime risk for multiple sclerosis is 1:800, which translates into approximately 60 000 people with the disease (Compston, 1990). In the USA, the figure is at least four times greater. There is a recognition that some cases of MS go undetected in life, appearing as a chance finding at postmortem (Gilbert and Sadler, 1983). Estimates that up to 20% of cases fall into this category (Mackay and Hirano, 1967) introduces a cautionary note in interpreting the epidemiological data. Generally, MS is seen with greater frequency as the distance from the equator increases in either hemisphere (Gonzalez-Scarano *et al.*, 1986; Skegg *et al.*, 1987). It is twice as common in women and, although it may occur at any age, the onset is typically in early adult life. The etiology is unknown and both genetic and environmental influences are considered important. The 31% monozygotic concordance rate, at six times the dizygotic rate (Sadovnik *et al.*, 1993), attests to the former, while evidence of environmental influences comes from three main sources. Migration studies have demonstrated that those who emigrate during childhood assume the risk of the country of adoption (Dean, 1967); disease epidemics have been reported in isolated communities such as the Faroe Islands (Kurtzke and Hyllested, 1979), and marked variations in prevalence have been found in genetically homogenous populations (Miller *et al.*, 1990).

Clinical features

The disorder may present with diverse neurological signs that vary considerably between patients. Initial symptoms, which reflect the presence and distribution of the plaques, commonly involve numbness or tingling in the limbs or weakness affecting one or more limbs, loss of vision or impaired visual acuity, diplopia, facial numbness, vertigo, dysarthria, ataxia, urinary frequency or urgency and fatigue. Prominent cortical signs (i.e. aphasia, apraxia, recurrent seizures, visual field loss, early dementia and extrapyramidal symptoms such as chorea and rigidity) are unusual and seldom define the clinical presentation (Noseworthy *et al.*, 2000). The course of the disease is variable and initially difficult to predict. Approximately 5–10% of patients show a steady progression of disability from the onset of the disease. The remainder run a relapsing–remitting course of which 20–30% never become seriously disabled and continue to function productively 20–25 years after symptom onset (Sibley, 1990). However, the largest group (almost 60%) enter a phase of progressive deterioration a variable number of years after symptom onset. Even within this group, there is considerable variability, with a patient's condition fluctuating between relapses, periods of stability and progressive deterioration. Recent longitudinal outcome data from a study of 2837 MS patients paints a more optimiztic picture than previously thought, with a median of 27.9 years elapsing before patients require a cane, at least, for walking (Tremlett *et al.*, 2006).

Pathology

Although the exact pathogenesis of MS is uncertain, there is firm evidence of an autoimmune-mediated inflammatory disorder affecting the central nervous system (CNS) (Lisak, 1986; ffrench-Constant, 1994). The target of the inflammatory response is myelin, a lipoprotein made by oligodendrocytes and investing the axons. Along the length of a nerve, the myelin sheaths are separated by gaps, the nodes of Ranvier. Nerve transmission is facilitated by impulses jumping from node to node in a process known as saltatory conduction. With damage to the myelin (i.e. demyelination), the conduction becomes impaired, transmission of nerve impulses is delayed or blocked completely and symptoms ensue.

Postmortem findings have further elucidated the neuropathological changes that occur (Allen, 1991). In patients severely affected by MS and who come to autopsy, the brain shows a mild degree of generalized atrophy with sulcal widening and dilatation of the ventricles. Plaques, which show histological evidence of demyelination, have a striking predilection for a bilateral periventricular distribution, particularly the lateral angles of the lateral ventricles, the floor of the aqueduct and the fourth ventricle. When viewed on sagittal section, the relationship of demyelination to the terminal veins may be seen. In some patients, the cerebrum is relatively spared, the main lesion load involving the optic nerves, brainstem and spinal cord (Allen, 1991). Cortical demyelination (Bruck and Stadelmann, 2005; Kutzelnigg and Lassmann, 2005; Merkler et al., 2006) and cortical atrophy (Carone et al., 2006; Prinster et al., 2006) occur more often than previously thought, with the degree and type of pathological change correlating with the disease type. In a postmortem study of 52 MS patients of differing disease type (acute, relapsing–remitting, primary and secondary progressive; see p. 16), active and focal inflammatory demyelinating lesions in the white matter predominated in patients with acute and relapsing MS, whereas diffuse injury to white matter of normal appearance and cortical demyelination were characteriztic of primary and secondary MS (Kutzelnigg et al., 2005). The latter changes reflected diffuse axonal injury with an underlying global inflammatory response affecting the whole brain and meninges. Significantly, the relationship between the focal white matter lesion load on the one hand and diffuse white matter injury or cortical demyelination, on the other, was either weak or absent. These data point to a clear temporal sequence of pathological events: MS beginning as a focal inflammatory disease with circumscribed white matter plaques giving way over time to a chronic picture of diffuse inflammatory changes, slowly progressive axonal injury and cortical demyelination.

The conventional view of neuropathological changes can be briefly summarized as follows. In the early stages of myelin breakdown, oligodendrocytes are still recognizable. As disease progresses, the myelin becomes progressively attenuated, partially detached from the axon and ultimately phagocytosed by invading macrophages. The early, established lesion shows a characteriztic pattern of increased cells (macrophages, astrocytes), a mixture of intact and disintegrated myelin sheaths, perivascular inflammation (lymphocytes, plasma cells, macrophages), oligodendrocyte loss, relatively preserved axons and, within the gray matter, preservation of cell bodies. In non-acute but active plaques, there is hyperplasia of macrophages and astrocytes and lesions contain myelin lipid degradation products. Perivascular inflammation, although present, is sparse. While the edges of active lesions are hypercellular with evidence of normal and disintegrating myelin sheaths, the core of such lesions may resemble older, inactive plaques. As the lesion evolves from an active to non-active phase, signs of inflammation disappear. Chronic lesions, which generally make up the bulk of the large characteriztic periventricular lesions seen in magnetic resonance imaging (MRI) or at postmortem, are, therefore, hypocellular, demyelinated, gliosed and contain few oligodendrocytes. The small venules are not inflamed, as in acute lesions, but rather show thickened hyalinized walls (Allen, 1991).

More recent data from actively demyelinating lesions, however, suggest a picture of greater complexity. Lucchinetti *et al.* (2000) examined biopsy and autopsy material with an array of immunological and biological markers and found marked lesion heterogeneity. Four different types of demyelination were noted based on the degree of myelin protein loss, the site and size of plaques, the patterns of oligodendrocyte destruction and the immunopathological evidence of complement activation. The four types of lesion (type I, macrophage-mediated demyelination; type II, antibody-mediated demyelination; type III, distal oligodendrogliopathy and apoptosis; and type IV, primary oligodendroglia degeneration) are thought to differ with respect to pathogenesis, as their descriptors indicate (Lucchinetti *et al.*, 2000; Lassmann *et al.*, 2001).

Advances in neuropathology have also challenged the historical view of MS as primarily a demyelinating disease in which axons are relatively spared. Using an antibody against amyloid precursor protein as a proven marker of axonal damage, Ferguson *et al.* (1997) examined paraffin-embedded MS lesions of varying ages. The results revealed the expression of amyloid precursor protein in damaged axons within acute MS lesions and in the active borders of less acute lesions. Confirmatory evidence of early axonal damage was soon provided by Trapp *et al.* (1998). Immunohistochemistry and confocal microscopy revealed that transected axons were a consistent feature in MS brain lesions, correlating with the degree of inflammation within a lesion. Thus, the greatest frequency of transected axons ($11\,236/mm^3$) was found in active lesions, the density falling in the hypocellular edges of chronic active lesions ($3138/mm^3$) and declining still further in the hypocellular center of chronic active lesions ($875/mm^3$).

Irrespective of the stage of the lesion, remyelination may affect the changes observed. Remyelination has been noted in acute MS lesions (Prineas *et al.*, 1993), giving rise to thin myelin sheaths in areas previously noted to be free of myelin. Newly formed as opposed to surviving oligodendrocytes are thought to be the source (Prineas *et al.*, 1989). In chronic lesions where not all the myelin is lost, demyelination and remyelination are thought to be occurring simultaneously. In MS, remyelination is not complete, perhaps because repaired areas are subject to repeated bouts of demyelination, leading to either a reduction in oligodendrocyte precursors (termed 02A progenitor cells) or the creation of an environment that inhibits their migration (ffrench-Constant, 1994).

Imaging studies during an acute attack have shown leakage of contrast-enhancing materials, indicative of a breakdown in the blood–brain barrier. The compromised barrier results in edema and the entry of immune mediators (antibodies and lymphocytes), which may contribute to myelin destruction. The leakage disappears spontaneously over 4–6 weeks (Miller *et al.*, 1988) and may be reversed temporarily by the administration of corticosteroids (Barkhof *et al.*, 1991). Postmortem studies have confirmed that lesions visualized by MRI and axial computed tomography (CT) correspond to MS plaques (Ormerod *et al.*, 1987). Furthermore, an in vivo study of MRI and histological parameters from six biopsy-proven cases of inflammatory demyelination of the CNS has shown that changes observed on MRI correlated with the evolving pattern of lesions (i.e. from acute to less active to chronic; Bruck *et al.*, 1997).

An important observation is that white matter that appears normal to the naked eye will more often than not show histological abnormalities. These include microscopic foci of demyelination; diffuse gliosis; perivascular inflammation; deposits of iron, lipofuscin and calcium; collagenization of small vessels; and axonal loss. Furthermore, this evidence of a more diffuse pathological process may occur in the absence of significant plaque formation. The clinical significance of these findings is that neuroimaging of the brain and spinal cord with standard sequences devised for plaque detection may mislead the observer into thinking the normal appearing white matter was indeed normal. Alternative imaging procedures for probing these more subtle changes have been devised, namely magnetic resonance spectroscopy, diffusion tensor and magnetization transfer imaging.

Diagnosis

The diagnosis of MS carries major implications for patients and their families. Uncertainty over the future, the ability to work, earn a living and live independently are all issues that readily come to mind. It is, therefore, imperative for the clinician to be clear about what symptoms and signs constitute a diagnosis of MS. In addition, making an early, correct diagnosis has assumed added importance because, for the first time, the MS patient is facing a choice of treatment options.

The diagnosis of MS can be made on clinical grounds alone. This requires that a patient have at least two episodes of neurological disturbance implicating different sites in the central white matter. A number of investigations may help the clinician to establish the presence and site of white matter lesions, thereby facilitating a diagnosis. It is, however, important to realise that these investigations (neuroimaging, evoked potentials and cerebrospinal fluid [CSF] electrophoresis) are not specific for MS and should be viewed only as helpful adjuncts to the clinical presentation.

From a research perspective, correctly diagnosing MS is equally important. The need for researchers across sites to talk the same language has prompted serial attempts to develop a set of diagnostic guidelines. For many years those of Schumacher *et al.* (1965) sufficed, but in response to improved laboratory and clinical procedures these gave way to the Poser criteria (Poser *et al.*, 1983).

The Poser Committee's recommendations

The Poser Committee convened in Washington, DC in 1982 and comprehensively reviewed historical and clinical symptomatology in MS; immunological observations; CSF tests; a variety of neurophysiological, psychophysiological and neuropsychological procedures; neuroimaging procedures (CT and MRI); and urological studies of bladder, bowel and sexual function. They concluded that revisions to existing criteria were essential in order to conduct multicenter therapeutic trials, to compare epidemiological data, to evaluate new diagnostic procedures and to estimate disease activity (Poser *et al.*, 1983; Poser, 1984).

>Definitions and guidelines were provided for what constituted an MS attack (synonyms here included bout, episode, exacerbation, relapse), a remission, *clinical* evidence of a lesion, what constituted separate lesions, *paraclinical* evidence of a lesion (i.e. abnormalities on evoked potentials [Fig. 1.1], MRI [Fig. 1.2] and urological assessment) and *laboratory* support indicative of MS (i.e. increased production of immunoglobulin G (IgG) and the presence of CSF oligoclonal bands in the absence of such bands in the serum [Fig. 1.3]. The authors made it clear that MRI and evoked potential abnormalities were not considered *laboratory* evidence, but rather an extension of the *clinical* examination, hence the *paraclinical* label. Bringing together all these strands of evidence enabled the neurologist to arrive at one of four possible diagnoses: clinically definite MS, laboratory supported definite MS, clinically probable MS and laboratory supported probable MS. Of note was the committee's view that neuropsychological evidence of impaired

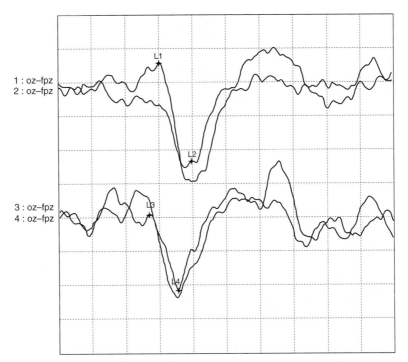

Fig. 1.1.   Visual evoked potentials in a 33-year-old female with multiple sclerosis. Note the mildly delayed conduction in the right optic nerve (top) compared with left nerve (bottom); this is comparable with optic neuritis.

cognition in someone under 50 years, although suggestive of MS, was not specific enough to be considered diagnostic.[1]

In concluding, the committee acknowledged that there would always be patients who defied easy categorization. The experienced neurologist would have to rely on intuition and accumulated clinical skill in arriving at diagnoses for this group. The criteria outlined were primarily for research purposes. Furthermore, there was a recommendation that clinical trials and research protocols should be limited to patients in one of the two *definite* groups. The category of *probable* was designed for the purpose of prospectively evaluating new diagnostic methods. The Poser criteria would hold sway over the MS world for the next 18 years.

The McDonald Committee's recommendations

In 2000, the International Panel on the Diagnosis of MS was convened with the aim of setting out new diagnostic criteria to be used by clinicians and adapted, as necessary,

---

[1] This recommendation, which was made in 1983, predated the plethora of studies from later in the decade that unequivocally demonstrated the presence of clinically significant cognitive dysfunction in approximately 40% of community based MS patients (Rao *et al.*, 1991, McIntosh-Michaelis *et al.*, 1991).

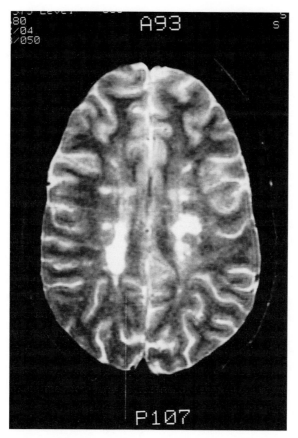

Fig. 1.2.　Axial T_2-weighted (spin echo) scan demonstrating the extensive white matter lesions (multiple sclerosis plaques) in a typical periventricular distribution.

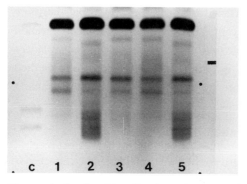

Fig. 1.3.　Abnormal oligoclonal banding in patients 2 and 5, who both have a diagnosis of multiple sclerosis.

for clinical trials (McDonald *et al.*, 2001). Much had changed since the formulation of the Poser criteria, including significant advances in MRI technology, the advent of disease-modifying treatments such as the interferons beta-1a and beta-1b, and the recognition of a new disease course, namely primary progressive (see below).

The committee kept certain sacrosanct principles intact, namely that obtaining objective evidence of dissemination of lesions (typical of MS) in time and place was essential in making a secure diagnosis. Furthermore, while history taking was clearly informative, clinical evidence depended essentially on objectively determined neurological signs. A diagnosis of MS based purely on clinical grounds would, therefore, depend on objective evidence of lesions separated in time and space. Radiological and laboratory investigations retained their utility in the diagnostic process, but with some further caveats; For example, visual evoked potentials were still considered helpful but not somatosensory and brainstem readings, which were thought to contribute little to the diagnosis. Following a diagnostic evaluation, an individual was either deemed to have, or not to have, multiple sclerosis. While a category of *possible MS* was thought necessary (referring to a patient whose evaluation met some, but not all, of the necessary criteria), diagnostic categories such as clinically definite and laboratory supported MS were considered obsolete.

Definitions

Definitions from previous diagnostic criteria were reviewed and where needed refined and clarified.

Attack (exacerbation, relapse)

An attack referred to an episode of neurological disturbance (a subjective report *and* objective evidence) lasting at least 24 hours and not to be confused with a pseudo-attack, as might be caused by infection or change in core body temperature.

Time between attacks

In defining what constituted separate attacks, it was felt that a minimum of 30 days should separate the onset of the first event from the onset of the second.

Paraclinical abnormalities: what are they?

When Poser and his committee set out their criteria in 1982, MRI technology was in its infancy. Two decades later, the technique had substantially evolved and, given its pivotal role in assessing patients with MS, considerable attention was devoted to it by McDonald *et al.* (2001). A more detailed account of MRI abnormalities in MS appears in Chapter 10. Here it is sufficient to note that the McDonald criteria emphasised that MRI can provide evidence of dissemination of lesions in both time and space. A stringent procedure was adopted for determining that MRI abnormalities were indicative of MS (Barkhof *et al.*, 1997; Tintoré *et al.*, 2000).

In keeping with the removal of the laboratory supported diagnostic label, the McDonald criteria incorporated CSF abnormalities under the paraclinical rubric. Analysis of CSF assumes greater importance if imaging results are equivocal or when the clinical presentation is atypical, but information from CSF cannot provide evidence of dissemination in time. As with the Poser definition, CSF significance pertains to the presence of oligoclonal IgG bands (distinct from such bands in the serum) and/or the presence of an elevated IgG index. Lymphocyte pleocytosis should be less than 50/mm^3.

Abnormal visual evoked potentials typical of MS (delayed but with well-preserved waveform) remained a useful adjunct to the clinical examination and could provide evidence of a second lesion providing that the sole clinical manifestation was not limited to the visual pathways.

The McDonald classification criteria revised

Four years after their publication, the McDonald criteria were revised (Polman *et al.*, 2005). New guidelines were provided to define what is meant by the dissemination of lesions in time, to clarify the significance of spinal cord lesions and to simplify the diagnosis of primary progressive MS. In the introduction to the revisions, the authors emphasised that the primary aim of the McDonald criteria was to help clinicians to make a valid and reliable diagnosis. This focussed on balancing the importance of arriving at an early, correct diagnosis with the need to avoid a false-positive diagnosis.

The committee acknowledged that the McDonald criteria had been derived from data largely pertaining to an adult Caucasian population. Therefore, the results from ongoing studies in Asian and South American groups were needed to validate the criteria more widely. Similarly, the applicability of the criteria to children was also questioned, with further work needed here. As with their predecessors, the committee made reference to the challenges posed by diseases that could mimic MS and the uncertainty over how best to classify disorders such as acute disseminated encephalomyelitis and neuromyelitis optica.

Give the central importance of these refined recommendations to any discussion of multiple sclerosis, the salient points are given here in greater detail.

Magnetic resonance imaging criteria to demonstrate brain abnormality and dissemination in space

Three of the following are required.
1. At least one contrast (gadolinium)-enhancing lesion or nine T_2 hyperintense lesions if there is no contrast-enhancing lesion.
2. At least one infratentorial lesion.

3. At least one juxtacortical lesion (i.e. involving the subcortical U fibres)
4. At least three periventricular lesions.

A spinal cord lesion was considered equivalent to a brain, infratentorial lesion; a contrast-enhancing spinal cord lesion was considered equivalent to a brain contrast-enhancing lesion and individual spinal cord lesions could be added to the overall count of lesions to meet the threshold count of nine lesions.[2]

Lesions should ordinarily be more than 3 mm in cross-section.

Magnetic resonance imaging criteria to demonstrate dissemination of lesions in time

This can be done in two ways.

1. Detection of a contrast-enhanced lesion at least three months after the onset of the initial clinical event, if not at the site corresponding to the initial event.
2. Detection of a *new* T_2 lesion if it appears at any time compared with a reference scan done at least 30 days after the onset of the initial clinical event.

Diagnosis of multiple sclerosis in disease with progression from onset

The revised criteria are as follows.

1. One year of disease progression (retrospectively or prospectively determined).
2. Plus two of the following:
   - positive brain MRI (nine T_2 lesions or four or more T_2 lesions with positive visual evoked potentials)
   - positive spinal cord MRI (two focal T_2 lesions)
   - positive CSF (iso-electric focussing evidence of oligoclonal immunoglobulin G (IgG) bands or increased IgG index, or both).

These guidelines have been incorporated into the full diagnostic criteria, which appear in Table 1.1.

The 2005 McDonald criteria revised for multiple sclerosis

To summarize, the revised McDonald criteria for MS (Table 1.1) retained the emphasis on objective clinical findings, repeated the importance for evidence of dissemination of lesions in time and space and clarified the use of confirmatory paraclinical examination to reduce the likelihood of false-positive and false-negative diagnoses (with a focus on specificity rather than sensitivity). In the authors' opinion, the revisions to the original McDonald MRI and CSF criteria, in particular, were of major import and the prediction was that they would have a matching effect on clinical practice.

---

[2] The reader is directed to Polman *et al.* (2005) for a more detailed account of what constitutes MS-related spinal cord pathology.

Table 1.1. The full diagnostic criteria of the revised McDonald classification

Clinical presentation	Additional data needed for MS diagnosis
Two or more attacks; objective evidence of two or more lesions	None
Two or more attacks; objective clinical evidence of one lesion	Dissemination in space, demonstrated by MRI; *or* two or more MRI-detected lesions consistent with MS plus positive CSF; *or* await further clinical attack implicating a different site
One attack; objective clinical evidence of two or more lesions	Dissemination in time, demonstrated by MRI *or* second clinical attack
One attack; objective clinical evidence of one lesion (monosymptomatic presentation; clinically isolated syndrome)	Dissemination in space, demonstrated by MRI *or* two or more MRI-detected lesions consistent with MS plus positive CSF; *and* dissemination in time demonstrated by MRI *or* second clinical attack
Insidious neurological progression suggestive of MS	One year of disease progression (retrospectively or prospectively determined) *and* two of the following demonstrations of dissemination in space: (a) positive brain MRI (nine T_2 lesions or four or more T_2 lesions with positive visual evoked potential) (b) positive spinal cord MRI (two focal T_2 lesions) (c) positive CSF

Note: See Polman *et al.* (2005) for more complete details.

Comparisons between the Poser and McDonald criteria

Comparisons between the Poser and McDonald (pre-revisions) criteria have been undertaken. In a study of 76 patients whose clinical features suggested a new diagnosis of MS, 38% were classified as clinically definite and 46% as laboratory definite MS according to the Poser system whereas 52% were diagnosed with MS by the McDonald criteria with the remaining 48% having 'possible MS' (Fangerau *et al.*, 2004). All patients with clinically definite MS were also diagnosed with MS by the McDonald method, but the same could only be said of 4 out of 35 patients with laboratory supported MS. Overall, using the McDonald criteria led to more diagnoses of MS than Poser's clinically definite criteria. However, when the numbers were combined from Poser's clinically and laboratory definite categories, they exceed those diagnosed with MS by the McDonald system.

A second study assessed the two methods in a heterogenous sample of 41 MS patients (15 relapsing–remitting, two secondary progressive, five primary progressive and 19 clinically isolated syndromes) and three non-MS cases (Zipoli *et al.*, 2003). Four neurologists were asked to make diagnoses according to both sets of criteria. Moderate inter-rater reliabilities were noted for both methods with respect to overall diagnosis (κ values of 0.52 and 0.57 for the McDonald and Poser criteria, respectively). A similar picture emerged for each system when it came to inter-rater agreements for distinct diagnostic categories. Finally, to assess possible sources of diagnostic disagreement, each rater was asked to assess specific factors such as dissemination over time and space, based on clinical and paraclinical (i.e. MRI) information only. Results revealed that, clinically, agreement for dissemination over time ($\kappa = 0.69$) exceeded that for space ($\kappa = 0.46$), whereas when it came to MRI analyses, the figures reversed ($\kappa = 0.74$ and $\kappa = 0.25$ for space and time respectively).

Clinically isolated syndromes

Patients with clinically isolated syndromes (CIS) are of particular interest as they are frequently the forerunner of MS. In attempting to describe the natural history of psychiatric and cognitive abnormalities in MS, the study of such patients affords a valuable opportunity to document the earliest evidence of neurological dysfunction before patients progress to the full syndrome. Throughout the book, reference will be made to patients with CIS and a brief description of these conditions is, therefore, given here.

Optic neuritis

Acute unilateral optic neuritis in adults is the presenting feature of MS in 20% of cases. It is characterized by the rapid development of visual loss, usually accompanied by pain, with symptoms progressing for 3–4 weeks and then resolving over 2–3 months, recovery to 6/9 vision occurring in greater than 90% of patients (McDonald, 1983). MRI with contrast enhancement may reveal lesions within the optic nerves (Fig. 1.4). In addition, two thirds of adults presenting with clinically isolated optic neuritis display one or more asymptomatic white matter brain lesions on MRI that appear indistinguishable from those seen in MS (Ormerod *et al.*, 1987).

Brainstem and spinal cord syndromes

Acute brainstem disturbance (e.g. vertigo, diplopia) is the presenting feature of MS in approximately 15% of patients, while twice as many will present with spinal cord

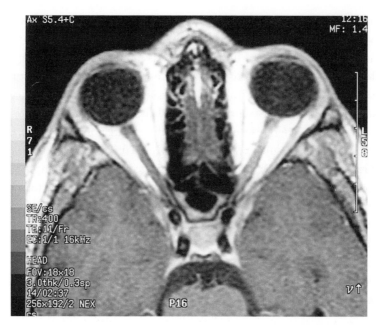

Fig. 1.4.   Magnetic resonance imaging, T_1 weighted, contrast (gadolinium–DPTA)-enhanced, showing pathological changes in the optic nerve in a patient with multiple sclerosis.

symptoms (sensory, motor and sphincter disturbance).[3] The percentage that go on to develop MS is similar to that with optic neuritis (Miller *et al.*, 1992; Brex *et al.*, 2002).

The significance of magnetic resonance abnormalities in patients with clinically isolated syndromes

The presence of brain lesions at index presentation is associated with a high risk of progression to MS. Brex *et al.* (2002), followed a group of 71 patients with CIS for 14 years from symptom onset. Of the 50 patients who had brain lesions to begin with, 44 (88%) had progressed to MS. In addition, a further four (8%) patients with an abnormal index MRI had developed clinically probable MS. Of the remaining two patients, one had new lesions on MRI and the other declined follow-up. Therefore, 49 of 50 patients had clinical and/or radiological evidence at follow-up that was compatible with a diagnosis of MS. This contrasts with the findings from the 21 patients whose initial MRI was normal. Here, only four (19%) patients had gone on to develop MS 14 years later.

Data from patients with CIS can predict not only conversion to MS, but also the level of disability associated with it. For example, an Expanded Disability Status

---

[3] The reader is directed to Polman *et al.* (2005) for a more detailed account of what constitutes MS-related spinal cord pathology.

Score (EDSS) (see below) at 14 years after disease onset correlated reasonably ($r = 0.60$) with lesion volume at the five year follow-up mark and with an increase in lesion volume over the first five years ($r = 0.61$). Collating all the data, the following composite suggested a better long-term prognosis: A CIS presentation of optic neuritis or sensory symptoms, a long period to first relapse, no MRI brain lesions at symptom onset, a small lesion change over the first five years of disease and no disability after five years (Miller *et al.*, 2005).

Of note is that the Poser and McDonald criteria have been compared in a follow-up study of 95 patients with a CIS (Dalton *et al.*, 2002). All subjects underwent a clinical and MRI assessment at baseline and thereafter at three months, one year and three years. The two sets of criteria were applied at each stage to assess the frequency with which MS was diagnosed. The McDonald system gave substantially higher diagnostic yields at every stage. The percentages of patients with MS according to the Poser criteria were 7%, 20% and 38%, respectively, while for the McDonald method the figures were 21%, 48% and 58%, respectively. Given the importance of MRI abnormalities in the McDonald schema, the gist of these findings should not be surprising. It is, however, noteworthy that a diagnosis of MS at one year based on MRI criteria had a high sensitivity (83%) and specificity (83%), and a good predictive value (75%), for clinically definite MS at three years.

Differential diagnosis

The broad array and often subtle nature of neurological signs and symptoms that may herald the onset of MS ensures a formidable list of conditions that make up a differential diagnosis (Rolak, 1996). These include somatization disorder (hysteria), postviral demyelination (acute disseminated encephalomyelitis), vasculitis affecting the CNS (either primary or secondary conditions such as lupus erythematosus), retroviral infections such as acquired immunodeficiency syndrome (AIDS), cerebrovascular accidents (stroke), metachromatic leukodystrophy and tumors (metastases, lymphoma).

To the neuropsychiatrist, dealing primarily with the behavioral sequelae of MS, the somatising patient masquerading with MS-like symptoms can present a considerable therapeutic challenge (Aring, 1965). A follow-up of 400 patients referred to neurologists, and subsequently found not to have MS, revealed 14 with primarily psychiatric problems (Murray and Murray, 1984). These patients were more likely to be female, hospital employees or have a friend with MS and to suffer from anxiety, depression and somatization disorder, the latter formerly called hysteria. Conversely, there are patients with MS who may be incorrectly dismissed as "hysterical." In a defined population of 112 000 Skegg *et al.* (1988) were able to identify 91 patients with MS (a point prevalence of 0.08%) of whom 16% had been referred to a psychiatrist between the onset of neurological symptoms and the diagnosis of MS. Although neurological symptoms were present at the time in the majority of patients, these had been overlooked by the psychiatrist in all but two patients. Instead, patients were given diagnoses such as hysterical personality disorder or conversion disorder.

The clinical course and severity of multiple sclerosis

Clear definitions of disease course are essential for a number of reasons. They are now needed by clinicians before they can assign treatment to patients. From a research perspective they help to frame and interpret all clinical and laboratory data. Historically, the problems encountered in defining terms that describe the course and severity of MS (Whitaker *et al.*, 1995) have stemmed from a reliance on verbal descriptors as opposed to biological markers. This recognition led to an international survey of MS researchers with the aim of assessing agreement pertaining to the various descriptive terms currently in use (Lublin and Reingold, 1996). The survey supplied definitions of the following disease courses and types: relapsing–remitting (RR), relapsing–progressive (RP), primary progressive (PP), secondary progressive (SP), benign and malignant. Definitions of each of these terms were included in the survey, but space was also made available for researchers to provide their own definitions if they disagreed with those enclosed. Of the 215 surveys mailed out, 125 (58%) responded. The results led to the National Multiple Sclerosis Society (USA) providing a set of consensus definitions, which are given below.

Clinical course definitions
Relapsing–remitting (RR)

The consensus definition of RR refers to clearly defined disease relapses with full recovery or with sequelae and residual deficit upon recovery; the periods between disease relapses are characterized by a lack of disease progression. The defining characteriztic of this course is the acute episodes of neurological deterioration with variable recovery but a stable course between attacks (Fig. 1.5).

Primary progressive (PP)

The consensus definition of PP refers to disease progression from symptom onset with occasional plateaus and temporary minor improvements allowed. The cardinal feature here is a gradual, nearly continuous worsening of neurological function from the first presentation, with some minor fluctuations but no discrete relapses (Fig. 1.6).

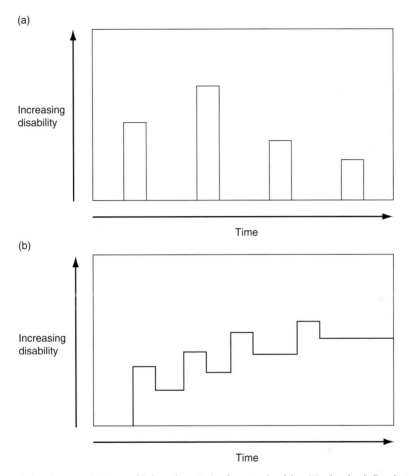

Fig. 1.5.   Relapsing–remitting multiple sclerosis is characterized by (a) clearly defined attacks with complete recovery and (b) sequelae and residual deficit upon recovery. (From Lublin and Reingold [1996] by permission of the American Academy of Neurology.)

Secondary progressive (SP)

The course of SP is defined as initially RR followed by a progression, with or without occasional relapses, minor remissions and plateaus. SP is viewed as the long-term outcome of patients who initially show a RR course. What characterizes the switch from one to the other is when the baseline between relapses begins to worsen (Fig. 1.7).

Relapsing–progressive (RP)

There was no consensus amongst those surveyed, largely because of the overlap between the RP term and some of the other categories. The recommendation was for the term to be abandoned.

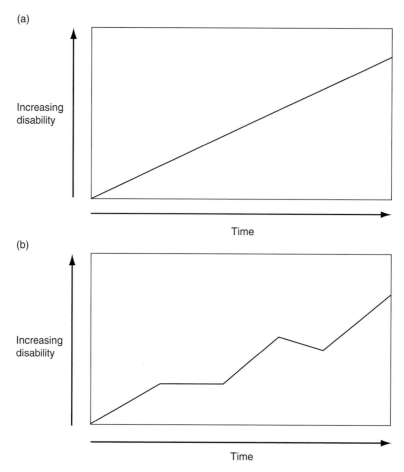

(a)

Increasing
disability

Time

(b)

Increasing
disability

Time

Fig. 1.6.   Primary progressive multiple sclerosis is characterized by disease progression from symptom
onset that is either (a) continual or (b) with some occasional plateaux and temporary minor
improvements but no discrete relapses. (From Lublin and Reingold [1996] by permission of
the American Academy of Neurology.)

Progressive–relapsing (PR)

The generally agreed definition of PR MS was of progressive disease from symptom
onset, with clear, acute relapses, with or without full recovery; the periods between
relapses were marked by continuing disease progression. This was considered an
additional but rare clinical course that warranted a separate definition (Fig. 1.8).

Clinical severity definitions

The merits of defining severity according to two terms, "benign" or "malignant,"
were surveyed and the results indicated a lack of uniformity amongst researchers.
The disagreement was greater for what constituted benign than for malignant

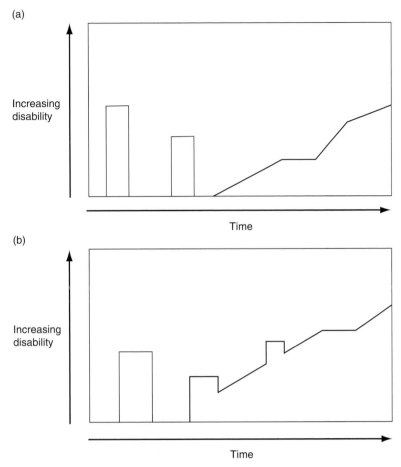

Fig. 1.7.   Secondary progressive multiple sclerosis is initially relapsing–remitting followed by (a) progression of variable rate or (b) progression with occasional relapses, minor remissions and plateaus. (From Lublin and Reingold [1996] by permission of the American Academy of Neurology.)

MS. Many respondents believed that precise definitions were not needed or useful. There was, however, agreement that the terms should not be defined according to scores on the EDSS (Kurtzke, 1983), the most widely used rating scale to assess physical disability in MS, as this would be too restrictive. In the end, definitions were given with the proviso that they be used primarily in a research setting.

Benign multiple sclerosis

The consensus definition of benign MS was of disease in which the patient remains fully functional in all neurological systems for at least 15 years after disease onset.

(a)

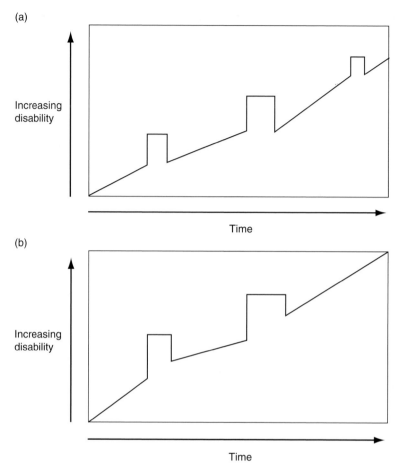

Fig. 1.8.   Progressive–relapsing multiple sclerosis shows progressive disease from symptom onset with clear, acute relapses with (a) or without (b) full recovery. The periods between relapses are marked by continuing disease progression. (From Lublin and Reingold [1996] by permission of the American Academy of Neurology.).

Malignant multiple sclerosis

The consensus definition of malignant MS was of disease with a rapidly progressive course, leading to significant disability in multiple neurological systems or death in a relatively short time after disease onset.

In summarizing their results, Lublin and Reingold (1996) emphasised that their definitions were purely clinically based and descriptive. While acknowledging the usefulness of investigations such as MRI, they concluded that current knowledge was too imprecise to allow for the course of the illness to be defined or influenced by the neuroimaging data.[4]

Rating neurological impairment in multiple sclerosis

The yardstick by which neurological disability is rated in MS patients is the EDSS (Kurtzke, 1983). The scale, routinely used in clinical and research settings, represents a refinement of earlier methods devised to assess physical disability in MS (Kurtzke, 1955, 1970). It consists of eight "functional systems," namely pyramidal, cerebellar, brainstem, sensory, bowel and bladder, visual, cerebral (or mental) and a miscellaneous category termed "other." Each of these functional systems is rated on a 0–5 or 0–6 scale, the score determined by the results of neurological examination. The one exception to this scoring is the miscellaneous system ("other"), which may be given a score of 0 or 1. The complete EDSS is given in Table 1.2.

The results of the functional system ratings are collapsed down to give a total score out of 10, in increments of 0.5; this composite rating is the EDSS. An EDSS score of 0 denotes a normal neurological examination. The only symptom allowed is one of mood change, with the instruction that this should not affect the total EDSS score. An EDSS of 10 signifies death. Between these two extremes, the scale rates the level of disability with a major emphasis on the patient's ability to walk. The EDSS is thus heavily weighted in favor of pyramidal tract and brainstem involvement, with relatively little emphasis on mentation, particularly mood.

This approach is not supported by the neuropsychiatric data. There are some MS patients who are significantly disabled by a mood disorder, be it depression or mania, without a grossly abnormal neurological examination. While it is possible that such cases represent two discrete, unrelated medical disorders, the fact that both major depression and mania occur more frequently in MS patients than chance expectation suggests the possibility of a causal link. These associations are not recognized by the EDSS. As such, sole reliance on this scale as the arbiter of disability may lead to the erroneous impression that all is well with the patient.

The situation is only slightly better with respect to cognitive dysfunction. While the functional system devoted to mentation assigns four grades to cognitive impairment, namely mild (grade 2), moderate (grade 3), marked (grade 4) and demented (grade 5), when it comes to the full EDSS, a patient with profound dementia incapable of independent living will still only score 5.0, which denotes moderate disability. In addition, mild to moderate degrees of cognitive impairment are likely to be frequently missed in the routine neurological examination

---

[4] Insights furnished from MRI have since been used in the revised McDonald criteria to clarify a primary progressive disease course.

Table 1.2. Expanded Disability Status Scale (EDSS)

Scale	Features
0	Normal neurological examination (all grade 0 in FS; grade 1 acceptable)
1.0	No disability, minimal signs in one FS (i.e. grade 1 excluding cerebral grade 1)
1.5	No disability, minimal signs in more than one FS (more than one grade 1 excluding cerebral grade 1)
2.0	Minimal disability in one FS (one FS grade 2, others 0 or 1)
2.5	Minimal disability in two FS (two FS grade 2, others 0 or 1)
3.0	Moderate disability in one FS (one FS grade 3, others 0 or 1) or mild disability in three or four FS (three/four FS grade 2, others 0 or 1) though fully ambulatory
3.5	Fully ambulatory, but with moderate disability in one FS (one grade 3) and one or two FS grade 2, or two FS grade 3, or five FS grade 2 (others 0 or 1)
4.0	Fully ambulatory without aid, self-sufficient, up and about some 12 hours a day despite relatively severe disability consisting of one FS grade 4 (others 0 or 1), or combinations of lesser grades exceeding limits of previous steps; able to walk without aid or rest some 500 meters
4.5	Fully ambulatory without aid, up and about much of the day, able to work a full day but may otherwise have some limitation of full activity or require minimal assistance; characterized by relatively severe disability, usually consisting of one FS grade 4 (others 0 or 1) or combinations of lesser grades exceeding limits of previous steps. Able to walk without aid or rest for some 300 meters
5.0	Ambulatory without aid or rest for about 200 meters; disability severe enough to impair full daily activities (e.g. to work full day without special provisions) (usual FS equivalents are one grade 5 alone, others 0 or 1; or combinations of lesser grades usually exceeding specifications for step 4.0)
5.5	Ambulatory without aid or rest for about 100 meters; disability severe enough to preclude full daily activities (usual FS equivalents are one grade 5 alone, others 0 or 1; or combinations of lesser grades usually exceeding those for step 4.0)
6.0	Intermittent or unilateral constant assistance (cane, crutch or brace) required to walk about 100 meters with or without resting (usual FS equivalents are combinations with more than two FS grade 3+)
6.5	Constant bilateral assistance (canes, crutches or braces) required to walk about 20 meters without resting (usual FS equivalents are combinations with more than two FS grade 3+)
7.0	Unable to walk beyond 5 meters even with aid, essentially restricted to wheelchair; wheels self in standard wheelchair and transfers alone; up and about in wheelchair some 12 hours a day (usual FS equivalents are combinations with more than one FS grade 4+; very rarely, pyramidal grade 5 alone)

Table 1.2. (cont.)

Scale	Features
7.5	Unable to take more than a few steps; restricted to wheelchair; may need aid in transfer; wheels self but cannot carry on in standard wheelchair a full day; may require motorized wheelchair (usual FS equivalents are combinations with more than one FS grade 4+)
8.0	Essentially restricted to bed or chair or perambulated in wheelchair, but may be out of bed itself much of the day; retains many self-care functions; generally has effective use of arms (usual FS equivalents are combinations, generally grade 4+ in several systems)
8.5	Essentially restricted to bed much of the day; has some effective use of arm(s); retains some self-care functions (usual FS equivalents are combinations, generally 4+ in several systems)
9.0	Helpless bed patient; can communicate and eat (usual FS equivalents are combinations, mostly grade 4+)
9.5	Totally helpless bed patient; unable to communicate effectively or eat/swallow (usual FS equivalents are combinations, almost all grade 4+)
10	Death from MS

FS, Functional system.
Source: From Kurtzke, 1983.

(Peyser *et al.*, 1980) and only come to light on more detailed neuropsychological testing. With the emphasis of the EDSS so firmly rooted on ambulation, it is not surprising that correlations with indices of cognitive dysfunction are generally weak to modest, at best (Ch. 6). To be fair to the EDSS, however, its development predates studies that demonstrated a high prevalence of mood disorders (Minden and Schiffer, 1990) and cognitive impairment (McIntosh-Michaelis *et al.*, 1991; Rao *et al.*, 1991) in MS patients.

While the passage of time has revealed the deficiencies in the EDSS, providing solutions has proved more complex. A task force of 16 MS researchers and clinicians from five countries met to address this challenge. The result was the development of a three item scale, the Multiple Sclerosis Functional Composite (MSFC), which better reflects the broad range of disabilities associated with the disease (Rudick *et al.*, 1997). The functions measured are as follows: timed 25-foot walk; nine hole peg test (average of right and left arms); paced auditory serial addition test-3 second version. Scores from the tests can be combined into a single composite score by combining the individual standardized components (Z scores) into an overall score. The committee urged all investigators to include the MSFC measure in their future prospective clinical trials.

A number of studies have used the MSFC and reported encouraging results. Hobart *et al.* (2004) noted that it outperformed the EDSS when it came to differentiating patients of varying disease severity. Furthermore, Fischer *et al.* (1999) reported that the three dimensions of the scale were relatively independent, that the full scale was sensitive to longitudinal change over a one to two year period and that it could predict both current and future EDSS scores. The MSFC has not replaced the EDSS, something it was never meant to do so. Rather, it should be seen as a useful addendum in the assessment of disability secondary to multiple sclerosis.

Summary

- The revised McDonald criteria are used to diagnose MS. Clinical data ("lesions scattered in place and time") are supplemented, when necessary, with paraclinical evidence (MRI, CSF analysis and visual evoked potentials) in making the diagnosis.
- Clinically isolated syndromes affecting the optic nerves, brainstem and spine are frequently the harbingers of MS.
- Definitions are given for relapsing–remitting, primary progressive, secondary progressive, and progressive–relapsing disease courses.
- The most widely used method for rating physical disability in MS remains the EDSS.
- The EDSS is heavily biased in favor of abnormalities affecting the pyramidal, brainstem and cerebellar systems, while difficulties with mentation receive disproportionately little attention. Consequently, the EDSS is an imperfect instrument for those involved in researching the neurobehavioral aspects of MS.
- The MSFC measure is a broader index of disability than the EDSS, taking into account cognitive function together with indexes of ambulation and fine motor coordination.

References

Allen IV. (1991) Pathology of multiple sclerosis. In *McAlpine's Multiple Sclerosis*, ed. WB Mathews, A Compston, IV Allen, CN Martyn. New York: Churchill Livingstone, Ch. 12, pp. 341–378.

Aring SD. (1965) Observations on multiple sclerosis and conversion hysteria. *Brain*, **88**, 663–74.

Barkhof F, Hommes OR, Scheltens P, Valk J. (1991) Quantitative MRI changes in gadolinium–DTPA enhancement after high dose intravenous methylprednisolone in multiple sclerosis. *Neurology*, **41**, 1219–1222.

Barkhof F, Filippi M, Miller DH, *et al.* (1997) Comparison of MR imaging criteria at first presentation to predict conversion to clinically definite multiple sclerosis. *Brain*, **120**, 2059–2069.

Brex PA, Ciccarelli O, O'Riordan JI, *et al.* (2002) A longitudinal study of abnormalities on MRI and disability from multiple sclerosis. *New England Journal of Medicine*, **346**, 158–164.

Bruck W, Stadelman C. (2005) The spectrum of multiple sclerosis: new lesions from pathology. *Current Opinion in Neurology*, **18**, 221–224.

Bruck W, Bitsch A, Kolenda H, *et al*. (1997) Inflammatory central nervous system demyelination: correlation of magnetic resonance imaging findings with lesion pathology. *Annals of Neurology*, **42**, 783–793.

Carone DA, Benedict RH, Dwyer MG, *et al*. (2006) Semi-automated brain region extraction (SABRE) reveals superior cortical and deep gray matter atrophy in MS. *Neuroiamge*, **29**, 505–514.

Charcot J-M. (1868) Histologie de le sclérose en plaques. *Gazette Hôpital Paris*, **141**, 554–555, 557–558.

Compston DAS. (1990) The dissemination of multiple sclerosis. *Journal of the Royal College of Physicians of London*, **24**, 207–218.

Dalton CM, Brex PA, Miszkiel KA, *et al*. (2002) Application of the new McDonald criteria to patients with clinically isolated syndromes suggestive of multiple sclerosis. *Annals of Neurology*, **52**, 47–53.

Dean G. (1967) Annual incidence, prevalence and mortality of multiple sclerosis in white South Africans born and in white immigrants to South Africa. *British Medical Journal*, **2**, 724–730.

Fangerau T, Schimrigk S, Haupts M, *et al*. (2004) Diagnosis of multiple sclerosis: comparison of the Poser and the new McDonald criteria. *Acta Neurologica Scandinavica*, **109**, 385–389.

Ferguson B, Matyszak MK, Esiri MM, Perry VH. (1997) Axonal damage in acute multiple sclerosis. *Brain*, **120**, 393–399.

ffrench-Constant C. (1994) Pathogenesis of multiple sclerosis. *Lancet*, **343**, 271–274.

Fischer JS, Rudick RA, Cutter GR, Reingold SC. (1999) The Multiple Sclerosis Functional Composite measure (MSFC): an integrated approach to MS clinical outcome assessment. National MS Society Clinical Outcomes Assessment Task Force. *Multiple Sclerosis*, **5**, 244–250.

Gilbert JJ, Sadler M. (1983) Unsuspected multiple sclerosis. *Archives of Neurology*, **40**, 533–536.

Gonzalez-Scarano F, Spielman RS, Nathanson N. (1986) Epidemiology of multiple sclerosis. In *Multiple Sclerosis*, Ed. WI McDonald, DH Silberberg. London: Butterworths, pp. 37–55.

Hobart J, Kalkers N, Barkhof F, *et al*. (2004) Outcome measures for multiple sclerosis clinical trials: relative measurement precision of the Expanded Disability Status Scale and Multiple Sclerosis Functional Composite. *Multiple Sclerosis*, **10**, 41–46.

Kurtzke JF. (1955) A new scale for evaluating disability in multiple sclerosis. *Neurology* (Minneapolis), **5**, 580–583.

Kurtzke JF. (1970) Neurological impairment in multiple sclerosis and the Disability Status Scale. *Acta Neurologica Scandinavica*, **46**, 4493–4512.

Kurtzke JF. (1983) Rating neurologic impairment in multiple sclerosis: an expanded disability status scale. *Neurology* (Cleveland), **33**, 1444–1452.

Kurtzke JF, Hyllested K. (1979) Multiple sclerosis in the Faroe Islands. 1. Clinical and epidemiological features. *Annals of Neurology*, **5**, 6–21.

Kutzelnigg A, Lassmann H. (2005) Cortical lesions and brain atrophy in MS. *Journal of Neurological Sciences*, **233**, 55–59.

Kutzelnigg A, Lucchinetti CF, Stadelman C, *et al*. (2005) Cortical demyelination and diffuse white matter injury in multiple sclerosis. *Brain*, **128**, 2705–2712.

Lassmann H, Brück W, Lucchinetti C. (2001) Heterogeneity of multiple sclerosis pathogenesis: implications for diagnosis and therapy. *Trends in Molecular Medicine*, **7**, 115–121.

Lisak RP. (1986) Immunological abnormalities in multiple sclerosis. In *Multiple Sclerosis*. Ed. WI McDonald, DH Silberberg. London: Butterworths, pp. 74–98.

Lublin FD, Reingold SC. (1996) Defining the clinical course of multiple sclerosis: results of an international survey. *Neurology*, **46**, 907–911.

Lucchinetti C, Brück W, Parisi J, *et al.* (2000) Heterogeneity of multiple sclerosis lesions: implications for the pathogenesis of demyelination. *Annals of Neurology*, **47**, 707–717.

Mackay RF, Hirano A. (1967) Forms of benign multiple sclerosis. *Archives of Neurology*, **17**, 588–600.

McDonald WI. (1983) The significance of optic neuritis. *Transactions of the Ophthalmological Society of the UK*, **103**, 230–246.

McDonald WI, Compston A, Edan G, *et al.* (2001) Recommended diagnostic criteria for multiple sclerosis: guidelines from the International Panel on the Diagnosis of Multiple Sclerosis. *Annals of Neurology*, **50**, 121–127.

McIntosh-Michaelis SA, Wilkinson SM, Diamond ID, *et al.* (1991) The prevalence of cognitive impairment in a community survey of multiple sclerosis. *British Journal of Clinical Psychology*, **30**, 333–348.

Merkler D, Ernsting T, Kerschensteiner M, Bruck W, Stadelmann C. (2006) A new focal EAE model of cortical demyelination: multiple sclerosis-like lesions with rapid resolution of inflammation and extensive remyelination. *Brain*, **129**, 1972–1983.

Miller D, Barkof F, Montalban X, Thompson A, Filipi M. (2005) Clinically isolated syndromes suggestive of multiple sclerosis, part 1: natural history, pathogenesis, diagnosis and prognosis. *Lancet Neurology*, **4**, 281–288.

Miller DH, Rudge P, Johnson G, *et al.* (1988) Serial gadolinium enhanced MRI in multiple sclerosis. *Brain*, **111**, 927–939.

Miller DH, Hammond SR, McLeod JG, Purdie G, Skegg DCG. (1990) Multiple sclerosis in Australia and New Zealand: are the determinants genetic or environmental? *Journal of Neurology, Neurosurgery and Psychiatry*, **53**, 903–905.

Miller DH, Morrissey SP, McDonald WI. (1992) The prognostic significance of brain MRI presentation with a single clinical episode of suspected demyelination. A 5 year follow-up study. *Neurology* **42** (Suppl. 3), 427.

Minden SL, Schiffer RB. (1990) Affective disorders in multiple sclerosis. Review and recommendations for clinical research. *Archives of Neurology*, **47**, 98–104.

Murray J. (2005) *Multiple Sclerosis. A history of a disease.* New York: Demos.

Murray TJ, Murray SJ. (1984) Characteristics of patients found not to have multiple sclerosis. *Canadian Medical Association Journal*, **131**, 336–337.

Noseworthy JH, Lucchinetti C, Rodriguez M, Weinshenker BG. (2000) Multiple sclerosis. *New England Journal of Medicine*, **343**, 938–952.

Ormerod IEC, Miller DH, McDonald WI, *et al.* (1987) The role of NMR imaging in the assessment of multiple sclerosis and isolated neurological lesions. *Brain*, **110**, 1579–1616.

Peyser JM, Edwards KR, Poser CM, Filskov SB. (1980) Cognitive function in patients with multiple sclerosis. *Archives of Neurology*, **37**, 577–9.

Polman CH, Reingold SC, Edan G, *et al.* (2005) Diagnostic criteria for multiple sclerosis: 2005 revisions to the "McDonald Criteria." *Annals of Neurology,* **58**, 840–846.

Poser CM. (1984) Taxonomy and diagnostic parameters in multiple sclerosis. *Annals of the New York Academy of Sciences,* **436**, 233–45,

Poser CM, Paty DW, Scheinberg L, *et al.* (1983) New diagnostic criteria for multiple sclerosis: guidelines for research protocols. *Annals of Neurology,* **13**, 227–231.

Prineas JW, Kwon EE, Goldenberg PZ, *et al.* (1989) Multiple sclerosis: oligodendrocyte proliferation and differentiation in fresh lesions. *Laboratory Investigation,* **61**, 489–503.

Prineas JW, Barnard RO, Kwon EE, Sharer LR, Cho ES. (1993) Multiple sclerosis: remyelination of nascent lesions. *Annals of Neurology,* **33**, 137–151.

Prinster A, Quarantelli M, Orefice G, *et al.* (2006) Grey matter loss in relapsing–remitting multiple sclerosis: a voxel based morphometric study. *NeuroImage,* **29**, 859–867.

Rao SM, Leo GJ, Bernardin L, Unverzagt F. (1991) Cognitive dysfunction in multiple sclerosis. 1. Frequency, patterns and prediction. *Neurology,* **41**, 685–691.

Rolak LA. (1996) Multiple sclerosis. In *Office Practice of Neurology* ed., MA Samuels, S Feske. New York: Churchill Livingstone, pp. 350–353.

Rudick R, Antel J, Confavreux C, *et al.* (1997) Recommendations from the National Multiple Sclerosis Society Clinical Outcomes Assessment Task Force. *Annals of Neurology,* **42**, 379–382.

Sadovnik AD, Armstrong H, Rice GP, *et al.* (1993) A population-based study of twins in multiple sclerosis: update. *Annals of Neurology,* **33**, 281–285.

Schumacher GA, Beebe GW, Kibler RF, *et al.* (1965) Problems of experimental trials of therapy in multiple sclerosis. *Annals of the New York Academy of Sciences,* **122**, 552–568.

Sibley WA. (1990) Diagnosis and course in multiple sclerosis. In *Neurobehavioral Aspects of Multiple Sclerosis* Ed. SM Rao. New York: Oxford University Press, pp. 5–14.

Skegg DCG, Cormin PA, Craven RS, Malloch JA, Pollock M. (1987) Occurrence of multiple sclerosis in the north and south of New Zealand. *Journal of Neurology, Neurosurgery and Psychiatry,* **50**, 134–139.

Skegg K, Corwin PA, Skegg DCG. (1988) How often is multiple sclerosis mistaken for a psychiatric disorder? *Psychological Medicine,* **18**, 733–736.

Tintoré M, Rovira A, Martinez MJ, *et al.* (2000) Isolated demyelinating syndromes: comparison of different MR imaging criteria to predict conversion to clinically definite MS. *American Journal of Neuroradiology,* **21**, 702–706.

Trapp BD, Peterson J, Ranschoff RM, *et al.* (1998) Axonal transection in the lesions of multiple sclerosis. *New England Journal of Medicine,* **338**, 278–285.

Tremlett H, Paty D, Devonshire V. (2006) Disability progression in multiple sclerosis is slower than previously reported. *Neurology,* **66**, 172–177.

Whitaker JN, McFarland HF, Rudge P, Reingold SC. (1995) Outcome assessment in multiple sclerosis clinical trials: a critical analysis. *Multiple Sclerosis,* **1**, 37–47.

Zipoli V, Portaccio E, Siracusa G, *et al.* (2003) Interobserver agreement on Poser's and the new McDonald diagnostic criteria for multiple sclerosis. *Multiple Sclerosis* **9**, 481–485.

2

Depression: prevalence, symptoms, diagnosis and clinical correlates

The observation that depression is part of the clinical picture of MS can be traced back to the case reports of Charcot (1877). Of all the mental state changes associated with MS, depression in various forms is by far the most common. Consequently, it is important that the clinician has a good understanding of how the syndrome may present, what factors may underlie causation and how best to approach treatment. Depression is associated with a considerable morbidity, with evidence suggesting it may be the single biggest factor influencing quality of life for MS patients (Lobentanz *et al.*, 2004; Benedict *et al.*, 2005). Moreover, the link between depression and suicide, so often described in a general psychiatric setting, is equally applicable to the MS clinic. Missing the diagnosis, therefore, does patients a grave disservice. The good news, however, is that depression can often be successfully treated. For all these reasons, a higher profile for this particular aspect of MS is long overdue.

Conceptual issues

The term depression is often loosely applied to describe either a symptom or syndromes of varying severity, with the spectrum including transient changes in mood, adjustment disorders to life events, dysthymia and major depression with or without psychotic features. Common to all is the cardinal feature of low mood.

A decade back the taxonomy underwent a major revision, with the fourth edition of the *Diagnostic and Statistical Manual* (DSM-IV) (American Psychiatric Association, 1994) dropping the term "organic mood disorder" and replacing it with the category "Mood disorder due to a general medical condition;" of which four subtypes are specified (Table 2.1). The criteria for major depression are shown in Table 2.2. Omitting the word organic was a major conceptual leap, implying that most symptoms of mental illness are attributable, in varying degrees, to cerebral pathology. While few would doubt the biological basis to mood change, one cannot always assume that, when depression occurs in the context of a general medical condition, the condition is the primary etiological factor. This point is

Table 2.1. Diagnostic criteria for "mood disorders due to a general medical condition" in the *Diagnostic and Statistical Manual,* 4th edition

Criterion	Features
A	A prominent and persistent disturbance in mood predominates in the clinical picture and is characterized by either (or both) of the following: (i) depressed mood or markedly diminished interest or pleasure in all, or almost all, activities (ii) elevated, expansive, or irritable mood
B	There is evidence from the history, physical examination or laboratory findings that the disturbance is the direct physiological consequences of a general medical condition
C	The disturbance is not better accounted for by another mental disorder (e.g., "adjustment disorder with depressed mood" in response to the stress of having a general medical condition)
D	The disturbance does not occur exclusively during the course of a delirium
E	The symptoms cause clinically significant distress or impairment in social, occupational, or other important areas of functioning *Specify* type: With depressive features: if the predominant mood is depressed, but the full criteria are not met for a major depressive episode With major depressive-like episode: if the full criteria are met (except criterion D) for a major depressive episode With manic features: if the predominant mood is elevated, euphoric or irritable With mixed features: if the symptoms of both mania and depression are present, but neither predominates

Source: With permission from American Psychiatric Association, 1994.

well illustrated by the relationship between depression and MS, where despite significant advances in neuroimaging, the brain–behavior yield from MRI studies lags behind that for cognitive dysfunction. Reasons for this will be discussed in this chapter. First, the review will focus on the following: prevalence, symptom constellations, the concept of subsyndromal depression, anxiety, depression as a presenting feature of MS, the natural history of depressive change and depression in relation to physical disability and disease duration.

Prevalence of depression in multiple sclerosis

The frequency of depressive disorders has varied according to the sample studied and method used. In addition, some studies have looked at point and/or lifetime prevalence rates while others at prevalence figures since the onset of MS.

Table 2.2. Criteria for a "major depressive episode" in the *Diagnostic and Statistical Manual,* 4th edition

Criterion	Features
A	Five (or more) of the following symptoms have been present during the same two-week period and represent a change from previous functioning; at least one of the symptoms is either (i) depressed mood or (ii) loss of interest or pleasure
	(i) Depressed mood most of the day, nearly every day, as indicated by either subjective report (e.g. feels sad or empty) or observation made by others (e.g. appears tearful). **Note**: in children or adolescents, can be irritable mood
	(ii) Markedly diminished interest or pleasure in all, or almost all, activities of the day, nearly every day (as indicated by either subjective account or observation made by others)
	(iii) significant weight loss when not dieting or weight gain (e.g. change of more than 5% of body weight in a month), or decrease or increase in appetite nearly every day. **Note**: in children, consider failure to make expected weight gains
	(iv) Insomnia or hypersomnia nearly every day
	(v) Psychomotor agitation or retardation nearly every day (observable by others, not merely subjective feelings of restlessness or being slowed down)
	(vi) Fatigue or loss of energy nearly every day
	(vii) Feelings of worthlessness or excessive or inappropriate guilt (which may be delusional) nearly every day (not merely self-reproach or guilt about being sick)
	(viii) Diminished ability to think or concentrate, or indecisiveness, nearly every day (either by subjective account or observed by others)
	(ix) Recurrent thoughts of death (not just fear of dying), recurrent suicidal ideation without specific plan, or a suicide attempt or a specific plan for committing suicide
B	The symptoms do not meet the criteria for a mixed episode
C	The symptoms cause clinically significant distress or impairment in social. occupational, or other important areas of functioning
D	The symptoms are not due to the direct physiological effects of a substance (e.g., a drug of abuse, a medication) or a general medical condition (e.g., hypothyroidism)
E	The symptoms are not better accounted for by bereavement, i.e. after the loss of a loved one; the symptoms persist for longer than 2 months or are characterized by marked functional impairment, morbid preoccupation with worthlessness, suicidal ideation, psychotic symptoms or psychomotor retardation

Source: With permission from American Psychiatric Association, 1994.

Conflicting evidence exists on whether there is an increase in depression prior to the onset of neurological symptoms in MS. While Whitlock and Siskind (1980) and Joffe *et al.* (1987) are of the opinion there is, this has not been noted by Ron and Logsdail (1989) nor Minden *et al.* (1987), the latter finding that rates did not differ from those in a healthy community sample matched for age. Subsequently, Sullivan *et al.* (1995) examined 45 patients with MS within two months of receiving the diagnosis. Even at that early stage, 40% of the sample met DSM-IV criteria for major depression, with a further 22% suffering from an adjustment disorder. Past psychiatric history was elicited from all patients and the results compared with a demographically matched group of patients suffering from chronic low back pain: 51% of the MS patients reported a prior episode of depression, significantly higher than the 17% figure in the sufferers of back pain. Furthermore, MS patients with a past history of depression were likely to report significantly more symptoms of MS, in particular muscle weakness and fatigue. The subjective nature of these two complaints illustrates one of the limitations of the study, namely that of retrospective bias. Given the distorted prism through which depressed patients evaluate their health both past and present, it is possible that details of premorbid psychological distress may have been inadvertently amplified. Notwithstanding this cautionary note, the data demonstrated that depression bedevils the lives of many MS patients.

If uncertainty hovers over the premorbid data, there is little doubt that following a diagnosis of MS, the rates of depression are significantly elevated. Minden *et al.* (1987) noted a 54% lifetime prevalence while Schiffer *et al.* (1983), in a sample of 30 patients, found a 37% prevalence of major depression since the onset of the MS. In a study of 100 consecutive attenders at an outpatient clinic, Joffe *et al.* (1987) found a 47% lifetime prevalence of major depression and a 14% prevalence of current depression, with a further 13% of the sample experiencing lesser degrees of depressive illness over their lifetime. Subsequently, Sadovnik *et al.* (1996) reported a lifetime prevalence of DSM-111-R major depression in 50% of MS patients.

Of note is that the above data were derived from MS patients attending hospital-based clinics and may, therefore, have an in-built bias leading to inflated estimates. This potential confounder has been addressed as part of the Canadian Community Health Survey (CCHS) of 115 071 subjects (Patten *et al.*, 2003). Using a self-reported diagnosis of MS and a brief interview for major depression the 12 month prevalence was estimated for subjects with and without MS in addition to those with and without other long-term medical illnesses. The result essentially confirmed the gist of the findings from the clinic-based samples, namely that the 12 month prevalence of depression in MS patients was high and exceeded that in subjects without MS (the adjusted odds ratio taking account of age and sex was 2.3). Furthermore, the prevalence was also higher than in subjects with other long-term medical illness. In those aged 18–45 years, the 12 month figure in the MS group was 25.7%, considerably higher than an earlier estimation from the same research group (Patten *et al.*, 2000). Rates of depression fell as the MS patient aged (Patten *et al.*, 2003), but whether this represented a true fall off in low mood or rather a decrease in emotional responsiveness, as suggested by others (Kneebone *et al.*, 2003) was unclear.

These data are matched by prevalence rates obtained from patient question-naires, of which the Beck Depression Inventory has been the most frequently used (Joffe *et al.*, 1987; Minden *et al.*, 1987; Beatty *et al.*, 1988, 1989; Ron and Logsdail, 1989). It should be noted, however, that this approach is not geared towards establishing a diagnosis.

When compared with other neurological disorders, rates of depression remain high. Using a computer search of medical and psychiatric records in Monroe county, New York, Schiffer and Babigian (1984) found a significantly higher rate of depression in patients with MS compared with those with temporal lobe epilepsy and amyotrophic lateral sclerosis. The data with regard to the latter is particularly compelling given the poor prognosis associated with the condition and tends to suggest that depression in MS cannot be construed simply as a reaction to physical disability. These data supported the conclusions of Whitlock and Siskind (1980), who noted that MS patients experienced more depressive episodes than patients with other neurological disorders, such as muscular dys-trophy, motor neurone disease and dystrophica myotonia. While an earlier study by Surridge (1969) comparing patients with MS and those with muscular dys-trophy had failed to find differences in the prevalence of depression, the study was flawed owing to the absence of standardized assessment procedures and a failure to control for levels of disability.

In summary, pooling figures from published reports, the lifetime prevalence for major depression owing to MS varies from 25 to 50% in clinic attendees (Minden and Schiffer, 1990) with a comparably high rate in community-based patients too (Patten *et al.*, 2003). This is almost three times the lifetime prevalence reported in the general population by the national co-morbidity study (Kessler *et al.*, 1994), a ratio that increases even more if only those symptoms associated with occupational and social dysfunction are counted (Narrow *et al.*, 2002). Finally, rates of depression are also elevated relative to other neurological disorders (Schubert and Foliart, 1993).

The symptoms of depression

Mood change associated with MS may present in a number of ways. While the *syndrome* of major depression has been shown to have a 12 month prevalence rate of 34%, individual symptoms making up the syndrome, such as sadness (64%), anger (64%) and discouragement (42%), are more frequently reported (Minden *et al.*, 1987). There is also evidence that a major depressive-like disorder owing to MS differs from uncomplicated major depression. The typical picture commonly found in the latter (i.e. withdrawn and apathetic, with feelings of guilt and worthlessness) is unusual in MS patients. Rather, symptoms such as irritability, worry and discouragement predominate (Minden *et al.*, 1987). A high frequency of irritability has also been confirmed by others (Ron and Logsdail, 1989), with a point prevalence approaching 50% (Feinstein and Feinstein, 2001).

Here another cautionary note must be sounded. The heterogeneous nature of the syndrome and the potential for confusing certain somatic complaints of MS, such as fatigue and sleeplessness, with symptoms of depression may lead to falsely elevated prevalence rates. This raises the question of whether it is advisable when assessing depression in MS to focus primarily on low mood and to consider abnormalities in "vegetative features" of lesser significance. Nyenhuis *et al.* (1995) believed that including non-mood symptoms leads to artificially high estimates of depression in MS patients. Others worry that in paring down the symptoms the baby may be thrown out with the bathwater (Randolph *et al.*, 2000). In their detailed phenomenological inquiry, disinterest in sex emerged as the only unique vegetative symptom of depression in the MS patient. The difficulty in disentangling somatic complaints is best illustrated by how to interpret fatigue. This was one of the symptoms most frequently endorsed by MS patients on the Clinical Interview Schedule, thereby raising the question whether it is a psychological or a physical symptom, or a combination of the two (Ron and Logsdail, 1989). Krupp *et al.* (1988) considered it to be a distinct entity unrelated to neurological impairment or affective disorder and qualitatively different from fatigue experienced by healthy individuals. Whether or not this is a valid assumption, this ubiquitous symptom is unlikely to exist in isolation and may influence other aspects of the mental state such as concentration, memory, irritability and sleep patterns, and, in turn, be aggravated by low mood.

In a study that compared the frequency of eight somatically loaded depressive symptoms from the Beck Depression Inventory in patients with MS, diabetes mellitus, chronic pain or major depression, plus healthy controls, the only significant between-group difference was that MS patients endorsed more work-related disability (Aikens *et al.*, 1999). Overall, the weight of evidence suggested that even if care is taken before attributing symptoms such as "loss of enjoyment of activities" to depression, as opposed to the underlying neurological disorder, depression in all its guises occurs significantly more often in MS than in many other neurological disorders or in healthy control subjects (Minden *et al.*, 1987).

Here it is germane to introduce the concept of subsyndromal or subthreshold depression, which refers to a mental state defined by up to three symptoms of major depression (Sherbourne *et al.*, 1994). The significance of this clinical entity lies in the fact that it may prove the harbinger of major depression and is a risk factor for relapse if present in patients recovering from major depression. It is frequently encountered in MS patients and causes considerable distress to them and their families (Feinstein and Feinstein, 2001).

Anxiety

In the neuropsychiatric literature, anxiety is depression's poor cousin, often overlooked and neglected. The MS literature is not exempt from this critique. Yet preliminary data suggest a quarter of clinic attenders will endorse significant symptoms of anxiety, with females disproportionately represented (Feinstein *et al.*, 1999). Overall, the frequency with which symptoms are endorsed exceeds that for depression (Feinstein *et al.*, 1999; Zorzon *et al.*, 2001), with this difference most marked soon after the diagnosis of MS is given to patients (Janssens *et al.*, 2003). Anxiety comorbid with depression, rather than anxiety or depression alone, was associated with increased thoughts of self-harm, more somatic complaints and greater social dysfunction. Furthermore, anxiety, but not depression, emerged as one of the most powerful, independent predictors of excessive alcohol consumption in MS patients (Quesnel and Feinstein, 2004).

A study that used a structured interview to diagnose specific DSM-IV anxiety disorders reported the following lifetime prevalence data (with general population estimates in parentheses): generalized anxiety disorder, 18.6% (5.1%); panic disorder, 10.0% (3.5%); obsessive–compulsive disorder, 8.6% (2.5%); social phobia, 7.8% (13.3%) (Korostil and Feinstein, 2007).[1]

Rating scales for depression in MS

There are three useful roles for self-report ratings of mood in MS patients. First, given the frequency with which depression occurs in MS patients, valid screening instruments can prove valuable adjuncts to clinical practice. Second, they have become integral to studies of cognition because of the potential for mood to confound results from neuropsychological testing (Ch. 7). Third, they form the mainstay of clinical trials, providing an index of symptom change over time. Confronted by a plethora of self-report scales, clinician–researchers may be stymied by choice. Some basic principles may, therefore, prove helpful.

The potential for symptoms overlap between MS and depression led Mohr *et al.* (1997) to recommend omitting three questions (fatigue, work problems, concerns

---

[1] Anxiety related to the injection of disease-modifying drugs is discussed in Ch. 11.

over health) from the 21 item Beck Depression Inventory. Given that scales like the Beck were not developed with a medically ill population in mind, an alternative approach has been to devise more specialized scales taking into account the phenomenology particular to this group. The Chicago Multiscale Depression Inventory (CMDI; Nyenhuis et al., 1998) consists of 42 self-report questions that may be subdivided into three sections measuring mood (e.g. sadness), vegetative symptoms (fatigue, cognitive difficulties) and evaluative beliefs (eg, depressive beliefs such as feeling useless). The Hospital Anxiety and Depression Scale (Zigmond and Snaith, 1983) is another frequently used example, containing 14 alternating anxiety and depression questions with thresholds specified for each condition. A weakness of the scale, however, is the presence of one depressive question ("I feel as if I am slowed down") that is frequently endorsed by fatigued MS patients who have little if any depression. A newer scale from Aaron Beck's expanding menu of instruments that quantify contemporary society's emotional ill-health avoids this pitfall. The Beck Fast Screen for Medically Ill Patients (B-FS; Beck et al., 2000) is a seven item scale that has been validated for MS patients (Benedict et al., 2003). Cut-off scores help to stratify the severity of depression (0–3, minimal; 4–6, mild; 7–9, moderate; 10–21, severe).

The busy psychiatrist, neurologist or clinic nurse looking for a quick and valid assessment of mood would find the B-FS patient friendly and informative. The even busier neurologist and psychiatrist should not, however, be tempted by the Yale Single Question screen for depression (Lachs et al., 1990). Comparisons between this minimalist construct and the 21 item Beck Depression Inventory revealed that the single question approach missed approximately 35% of depressed MS patients (Avasarala et al., 2003).

Notwithstanding the criticizms levelled at the full Beck Depression Inventory, the scale endures in the MS literature. Revised 35 years after first publication (Beck et al., 1996), it remains the most widely used screening instrument for depression in MS patients and was consequently endorsed in a series of consensus guidelines for the treatment of depression associated with MS (Goldman Consensus Group, 2005). This recommendation was, however, made before the publication of the B-FS validation study in MS.

Depression as a presentation of multiple sclerosis

Although some instances of MS presenting with psychiatric symptoms (including depression) have been reported (Young et al., 1976; Mathews, 1979; Whitlock and Siskind, 1980), the evidence from epidemiological studies suggests it is uncommon and may be a chance finding. A comparison of rates of psychiatric illness in large samples of patients with MS and temporal lobe epilepsy (Schiffer and Babigian,

1984) revealed that, although 17% of the MS group *initially* presented to a psychiatrist, this was significantly less than the 29% reported for temporal lobe epilepsy. This figure is similar to the 19% prevalence reported by Stenager and Jensen (1988) in their MS sample; these authors found the onset of demyelination coincided with psychotic disorders and transient situational disturbances, but not with depressive or anxiety disorders. While both these studies make the point that psychiatric illness may predate the onset of neurological symptoms, often by years, no unequivocal conclusions can be drawn concerning a shared pathogenesis as it is possible the two disorders may have co-existed purely by chance, given that both are common. In addition, it can be notoriously difficult to accurately document retrospectively the first, often subtle neurological symptoms heralding the onset of MS, which makes the interpretation of data such as these difficult.

Despite these disclaimers, some informative data can still be extracted from a study by Skegg *et al.* (1988), who, in a well-defined regional population, were able to identify 91 patients with MS (a point prevalence of 0.08%). Of these, 15 (16%) had been referred to a psychiatrist between the onset of their symptoms and the diagnosis of MS. Although neurological symptoms were present at the time in the majority of patients, these generally had been overlooked by the psychiatrists. Instead, patients were given diagnoses such as hysteria more often than depression.

Suicide in multiple sclerosis

While the presence of a major depressive illness significantly increases the morbidity associated with MS, it may also add to the mortality. Kahana *et al.* (1971) reported that 9 (3%) of 295 patients committed suicide over a six year period, but it is unclear how representative the sample was or how many subjects were suffering from a depressive illness. More recent data tend to confirm these observations. A study of suicide in patients with a wide range of neurological disorders (Stenager and Stenager, 1992) concluded that the rate was increased in disorders such as MS and certain subgroups of epilepsy. In addition, a Scandinavian epidemiological investigation of 5525 MS patients (Stenager *et al.*, 1992) reported a significantly elevated suicide rate, with males and those diagnosed with MS before the age of 30 years most at risk. Once again, no precise estimates of depression were obtained. Confirmatory epidemiological evidence comes from Sadovnik *et al.* (1991) in a study of 3126 MS patients followed over 16 years. Suicide accounted for 15% of all ascertained deaths, which was 7.5 times that for the age-matched, but not sex-matched, general population.

Indirect evidence linking depression and suicide may be traced to low nocturnal melatonin secretion in MS patients with suicidal behavior or intent (Sandyk and Awerbach, 1993). Serotonin is a precursor to melatonin and a reduction in serotonergic activity has been reported in MS (Johansson and Roos, 1974) and in non-MS subjects who were depressed and committed suicide (Shaw *et al.*, 1967).

These findings are supported by a finding that 28.6% of MS patients harbor suicidal intent over the course of their illness (Feinstein, 2002). This is considerably higher than the rate in the general population, where figures have varied according to geographical location as the following percentages illustrate: USA (13.5%), Australia (5%), Beirut (2.1%), New Zealand (18.5%) (Weissman *et al.*, 1999). While suicidal intent is a predisposing factor for a suicidal attempt, only a minority of MS patients will attempt self-harm. Even here, however, the lifetime figure of 6.4% for MS patients in a Canadian tertiary clinic population is almost double that for the comparable general population. A further salient observation from the Canadian data is that over a third of patients with suicidal intent had received no psychological help (either medication or psychotherapy) while six of nine patients with a major depression, all of whom were harboring suicidal intent, were not on antidepressant treatment (Feinstein, 2002). Of the nine patients in this study who had attempted suicide, all of whom met criteria for major depression, four had never received antidepressant medication. Clues that should alert the clinician to this problem are not difficult to elicit, namely the presence of major depression, the severity of the depression, social isolation and alcohol abuse (Feinstein, 2002). While missed diagnoses and failure to pick up clues of suicidal thinking are not unique to clinicians working with MS patients, it is one area where an increased awareness of the data and a heightened sensitivity to managing the emotional well being of patients can reduce not only the morbidity but also the mortality associated with the disease (Feinstein, 1997).

The natural history of mood change in multiple sclerosis

Data suggesting an absence of major depression and a low overall psychiatric morbidity early in the disease process (Logsdail *et al.*, 1988; Feinstein *et al.*, 1992a) have come from studies of patients with clinically isolated syndromes (CIS) (optic neuritis, brainstem and spinal cord presentations), frequently the harbinger of MS. Prevalence rates for emotional distress in this group did not exceed those reported from healthy community samples (Andrews *et al.*, 1977) or those from general practice attenders (Goldberg and Blackwell, 1970). A study of patients with optic neuritis and MS of less than two years' duration reached similar conclusions (Lyon-Caen *et al.*, 1986). These findings have been challenged by Sullivan *et al.* (1995), who reported that high rates of depression within two months of diagnosis were associated with elevated levels of depression premorbidly.

A follow-up study of patients with CIS offered Feinstein *et al.* (1992b) the opportunity to chart the evolution of mood change as demyelination progressed.

After a period of five years (range, 42–67 months) 54% of patients had developed clinically definite MS, 34% with a relapsing–remitting and 20% with a chronic–progressive course. Overall, psychiatric morbidity had increased with time but was confined to patients who had developed MS. In those whose condition had remained unchanged (i.e. CIS at follow-up), mood generally remained euthymic. The chronic–progressive subgroup were more physically disabled and had more extensive brain plaques. Their depression scores were three times those of the CIS and relapsing–remitting MS groups, with low mood correlating with social not brain MRI variables.

While this study demonstrated that patients become significantly more depressed when their disease progresses from CIS to definite MS status, it did not address the question of possible fluctuations in depressed mood, over time, in patients with established MS. Of interest was the relationship between depression on the one hand and alterations in clinical state and brain lesion load on the other. The interaction between these variables is complex because changes in brain MRI are not always mirrored by changes in neurological status and associated physical disability (Thompson et al., 1992). The possibility exists, therefore, that changes in mood and cognition were more sensitive markers of alterations in brain lesion scores than physical signs. A longitudinal study of 10 patients with relapsing–remitting MS individually matched with 10 healthy control subjects provided evidence to support this (Feinstein et al., 1993). Over a six month period, MS patients underwent MRI at intervals of either two (five patients) or four (five patients) weeks depending on whether they were in an active or remitted disease state. At each radiological assessment, patients were assessed neurologically and completed a mood questionnaire. Two of the five patients in an active phase of the disease had increasing lesion scores. There was also an increase in the number and size of lesions that enhanced with gadolinium–diethylenetriaminepentaacetic acid (gadolinium–DTPA), indicating disease activity. Despite the deteriorating MRI picture, there was no concomitant decline in physical disability according to scores on the Expanded Disability Status Scale (EDSS). Both patients had, however, become increasingly depressed and their worsening mood scores were significantly correlated with their MRI changes. The remaining patients demonstrated little disease activity on serial MRI and their EDSS and depression scores remained stable over time.

Arnett and Randolph (2003) have taken a different approach to monitoring longitudinal change. They broke down depression into three symptom clusters, namely mood (e.g. sadness) vegetative (e.g. sleep and appetite) and evaluative (e.g. guilt and worthlessness), and reported that, over a three year period, feelings of sadness and irritability were significantly more likely to improve or worsen than symptoms derived from the other two categories. To what extent these changes were integral to fluctuations in the MS was, however, difficult to tease out. The authors subsequently confirmed these findings while noting that increased use of active coping strategies could mitigate depressed mood over a three year follow-up period (Arnett and Randolph, 2006).

The effect of physical disability and the duration and course of multiple sclerosis on depression

Considerations of whether disease duration and physical disability influence mood have produced discrepant results. While some studies have reported that depression is associated with physical disability (Whitlock and Siskind, 1980; McIvor *et al.*, 1984; Patten *et al.*, 2005) and disease course (Zabad *et al.*, 2005), others have found no relationship between depression and emotional dysfunction, on the one hand, and disease duration, severity or course on the other (Rabins *et al.*, 1986; Minden *et al.*, 1987; Ron and Logsdail, 1989).

The reason for the lack of a clear relationship may be traced to the diversity in the course of MS. Thus, an illness with the same duration may either involve a few, mild relapses or follow a more malignant, rapidly progressive course. It may also encompass patients with either quiescent lesions or a rapidly deteriorating lesion load. In addition, the degree of physical disability may be determined by a combination of cerebral and spinal cord involvement, each having a different influence on mood. The complexities of these various interactions explain the findings from a community-based study of MS-related depression undertaken in King County, Washington. The severity of MS was assessed in 739 MS patients with a self-report version of the EDSS. Depression was documented with the Center for Epidemiologic Studies Depression Scale. While low mood was linked to greater self-reported neurological disability (i.e. high EDSS scores) it was also associated with shorter disease duration (Chwastiak *et al.*, 2002).

Depression and exacerbations of multiple sclerosis

Dalos *et al.* (1983) undertook a longitudinal study over the course of one year, assessing MS patients at monthly intervals with a self-report measure of psychological distress, namely the General Health Questionnaire (GHQ). The instrument contains four subscales measuring depression, anxiety, somatic complaints and social dysfunction. Patients with spinal cord injuries were used as controls. Higher GHQ scores with regard to social dysfunction and somatic complaints were noted in the MS sample, particularly those experiencing disease exacerbations. However, no firm conclusions could be drawn from this study for a couple reasons, namely the weakness of the GHQ in probing the phenomenology of depression in MS and the possibility that elevated GHQ scores following disease exacerbation may simply reflect a non-specific psychological reaction to a deteriorating neurological status rather than a major pertubation in mood.

A second study of 166 patients exploring the association between depression and disease exacerbation arrived at a different conclusion (Kroencke *et al.*, 2001). The pivotal variable in the pathogenesis of lowered mood was the patients' uncertainties over their illness. According to the authors' theory, disease exacerbations leading to greater doubt and apprehension evoked emotion-centered forms of coping such as passive-avoidance and escape-avoidance behaviors. These maladaptive reactions were contrasted with more mood-protective strategies such as problem-focussed coping, cognitive reframing, active constructive coping and planful problem solving. The true significance of disease exacerbations may, therefore, lie in the kinds of coping mechanisms that they generate. It is also important to note that, while these data suggest exacerbations are linked to symptoms of depression in some patients, no study has yet confirmed an association with the syndromal diagnosis of major depression. Transient sadness may presage sustained low mood, but in the absence of empirical data further clarification is needed.

The diverse mental state changes associated with MS, ranging from isolated symptoms of depression through subsyndromal depression to major depression with or without significant anxiety symptoms, are illustrated by the following clinical vignettes.

Vignette 1

A 37-year-old mother of two children aged ten and eight years, working part time as a secretary, was referred to my neuropsychiatry clinic because of low mood. The patient had had MS for four years, was in a relapsing–remitting course, had an EDSS of 3.5 and had recently experienced an exacerbation from which she had made a full recovery. There was no premorbid nor family history of psychiatric illness. Although the patient complained of feeling depressed, closer questioning revealed her main difficulties were fatigue and having to look after her two young children while holding down a job. Her marriage was described as good, but her husband was frequently away from home on business trips and the running of the household was left to her. There was no history of sleep or appetite disturbance, no suicidal thought, but some mild anhedonia, linked specifically to periods of fatigue. Significantly, the patient reported that when her parents took the grandchildren for a weekend she felt "restored" and better able to enjoy a good book or a visit with a friend. Her problem was assessed as primarily situational rather than a mood disorder, and psychosocial intervention, while only partially alleviating her fatigue, rapidly restored her mood.

Vignette 2

A 25-year-old woman, unmarried, working as a receptionist and with a two year history of relapsing–remitting MS and an EDSS of 4.0 presented to my clinic with complaints of tiredness, low mood and loss of emotional control. She had been sleeping poorly for approximately one month and was slowly withdrawing from social contacts as she preferred being alone. There was no premorbid or family history of psychiatric difficulties and she was known to be an outgoing and gregarious person by nature. There had been a couple of incidents at work in which she reported "snapping" at customers over the telephone, and her company had received one complaint about this. The behavior was most uncharacteriztic of her and she found it upsetting. Her boyfriend of three years reported similar, unprovoked outbursts. Despite taking a few weeks off work "to sort herself out," the irritability, sleep difficulties and social withdrawal had not improved and she had begun questioning whether life was indeed worth living. A diagnosis of mood disorder due to MS (major depressive subtype) was made and the appropriate pharmacotherapy instituted.

Summary

- Data from neurological clinics and community-based samples show that rates of major depression in MS patients are high, with a lifetime prevalence rate that approaches 50%.
- Major depression in MS patients is frequently associated with irritability and a sense of frustration, as opposed to symptoms of guilt and worthlessness that are more typically found in major depression without MS.
- Care should be taken in ensuring that somatic complaints associated with MS, like fatigue and insomnia are not incorrectly attributed to depression.
- MS patients do not appear to have a premorbid risk for affective disorder.
- The Beck Depression Inventory-Fast Screen for Medically Ill Patients (B-FS) has been validated for use in MS patients and provides a valid and quick way of screening depressive symptoms.
- MS patients have a significantly increased rate of suicide compared with the general population and patients with other neurological disorders. Suicidal thoughts have been linked to the presence of depression, the severity of the depression, social isolation and heavy alcohol consumption.
- Anxiety may occur with or without depression in at least a quarter of MS patients and leads to an increase in physical complaints, suicidal thinking and alcohol consumption. Generalized anxiety disorder, obsessive–compulsive disorder and panic disorder are particularly common in MS patients.

References

Aikens JE, Reinecke MA, Pliskin NH, *et al.* (1999) Assessing depressive symptoms in multiple sclerosis: is it necessary to omit items from the original Beck Depression Inventory? *Journal of Behavioral Medicine*, **22**, 127–142.

American Psychiatric Association (1994) *Diagnostic and Statistical Manual*, 4th edn. Washington, DC: American Psychiatric Press.

Andrews G, Schonell M, Tennent C. (1977) The relationship between physical, psychological and social morbidity in a suburban community. *American Journal of Epidemiology*, **105**, 324–329.

Arnett PA, Randolph JJ. (2003) Longitudinal course of depression symptoms in multiple sclerosis. *Archives of Clinical Neuropsychology*, **18**, 733.

Arnett PA, Randolph JJ. (2006) Longitudinal course of depression symptoms in multiple sclerosis. *Journal of Neurology, Neurosurgery and Psychiatry*, **77**, 606–610.

Avasarala JR, Cross AH, Trinkaus K. (2003) Comparative assessment of the Yale Single Question and Beck Depression Inventory Scale in screening for depression in multiple sclerosis. *Multiple Sclerosis*, **9**, 307–310.

Beatty WW, Goodkin DE, Monson N, Beatty PA, Hertsgaard D. (1988) Anterograde and retrograde amnesia in patients with chronic–progressive multiple sclerosis. *Archives of Neurology*, **45**, 611–619.

Beatty WW, Goodkin DE, Monson N, Beatty PA. (1989) Cognitive disturbance in patients with relapsing–remitting multiple sclerosis. *Archives of Neurology*, **46**, 1113–1119.

Beck AT, Steer RA, Brown GK. (1996) *Beck Depression Inventory (BDI)-II Manual*. San Antonio, TX: The Psychological Corporation.

Beck AT, Steer RA, Brown GK. (2000) *BDI-Fast Screen for Medical Patients Manual*. San Antonio, TX: The Psychological Corporation.

Benedict RH, Fishman I, McClellan MM, Bakshi R, Weinstock-Guttman B. (2003) Validity of the Beck Depression Inventory-Fast Screen in multiple sclerosis. *Multiple Sclerosis*, **9**, 393–396.

Benedict RHB, Wahlig E, Bakshi R, *et al.* (2005) Predicting quality of life in multiple sclerosis: accounting for physical disability, fatigue, cognition, mood disorder, personality and behavior. *Journal of the Neurological Sciences*, **231**, 29–34.

Charcot JM (1877) *Lectures on the Diseases of the Nervous System delivered at La Salpetriere*. London: New Sydenham Society, pp. 194–195.

Chwastiak L, Ehde DM, Gibbons LE, *et al.* (2002) Depressive symptoms and severity of illness in multiple sclerosis: epidemiologic study of a large community sample. *American Journal of Psychiatry*, **159**, 1862–1868.

Dalos NP, Rabins PV, Brooks BR, O'Donnell P. (1983) Disease activity and emotional state in multiple sclerosis. *Annals of Neurology*, **13**, 573–577.

Feinstein A. (1997) Multiple sclerosis, depression and suicide. *British Medical Journal*, **315**, 691–692.

Feinstein A. (2002) An examination of suicidal intent in patients with multiple sclerosis. *Neurology*, **59**, 674–678.

Feinstein A, Feinstein KJ. (2001) Depression associated with multiple sclerosis. Looking beyond diagnosis to symptom expression. *Journal of Affective Disorders*, **66**, 193–198.

Feinstein A, Youl B, Ron MA. (1992a) Acute optic neuritis: a cognitive and magnetic resonance imaging study. *Brain*, **115**, 1403–1415.

Feinstein A., Kartsounis L, Miller B, Youl B, Ron MA. (1992b) Clinically isolated lesions of the type seen in multiple sclerosis: a cognitive, psychiatric and MRI follow-up study. *Journal of Neurology, Neurosurgery and Psychiatry*, **55**, 869–876.

Feinstein A, Ron MA, Thompson A. (1993) A serial study of psychometric and magnetic resonance imaging changes in multiple sclerosis. *Brain*, **116**, 569–602.

Feinstein A, O'Connor P, Gray T, Feinstein K. (1999) The effects of anxiety on psychiatric morbidity in patients with multiple sclerosis. *Multiple Sclerosis*, **5**, 323–326.

Goldberg DP, Blackwell BB. (1970) Psychiatric illness in general practice. A detailed study using a new method of case identification. *British Medical Journal*, **ii**, 439–443.

Goldman Consensus Group. (2005) The Goldman consensus statement on depression in multiple sclerosis. *Multiple Sclerosis*, **11**, 328–337.

Janssens ACJW, van Doorn PA, de Boer JB, *et al*. (2003) Impact of recently diagnosed multiple sclerosis on quality of life, anxiety, depression and distress of patients and partners. *Acta Neurologica Scandinavica*, **108**, 389–395.

Joffe RT, Lippert GP, Gray TA, Sawa G, Horvath Z. (1987) Mood disorder and multiple sclerosis. *Archives of Neurology*, **44**, 376–378.

Johansson B, Roos B-E. (1974) 5-Hydroxyindoleacetic acid and homovanillic acid in cerebrospinal fluid of patients with neurological disease. *European Neurology*, **11**, 37–45.

Kahana E, Leibowitz U, Alter M. (1971) Cerebral multiple sclerosis. *Neurology*, **21**, 1179–1185.

Kessler RC, McGonagle KA, Shanyang Z, *et al*. (1994) Lifetime and 12 month prevalence of DSM-111-R psychiatric disorders in the United States, Results from the National Co-morbidity Survey. *Archives of General Psychiatry*, **51**, 8–19.

Kneebone II, Dunmore EC, Evans E. (2003) Symptoms of depression in older adults with multiple sclerosis (MS): comparison with a matched sample of younger adults. *Aging and Mental Health*, **7**, 183–185.

Korostil M, Feinstein A. (2007) Anxiety disorders and their clinical correlates in multiple sclerosis patients. *Multiple Sclerosis*, **13**, 67–72.

Kroencke DC, Denney DR, Lynch SG. (2001) Depression during exacerbations in multiple sclerosis: the importance of uncertainty. *Multiple Sclerosis*, **7**, 237–242.

Krupp LB, Alvarez LA, LaRocca NG, Scheinberg LC. (1988) Fatigue in multiple sclerosis. *Archives of Neurology*, **45**, 435–437.

Lachs MS, Feinstein AR, Cooney LM, *et al*. (1990) A simple procedure for general screening for functional disability in elderly patients. *Annals of Internal Medicine*, **113**, 557–558.

Lobentanz IS, Asenbaum S, Vass K, *et al*. (2004) Factors influencing quality of life in multiple sclerosis patients: disability, depressive mood, fatigue and sleep quality. *Acta Neurologica Scandinavica*, **110**, 6–13.

Logsdail SJ, Callanan MM, Ron MA. (1988) Psychiatric morbidity in patients with clinically isolated lesions of the type seen in multiple sclerosis. *Psychological Medicine*, **18**, 355–364.

Lyon-Caen O, Jouvent R, Hauser S, *et al*. (1986) Cognitive function in recent onset demyelinating disease. *Archives of Neurology*, **43**, 1138–1141.

Mathews WB. (1979) Multiple sclerosis presenting with acute remitting psychiatric symptoms. *Journal of Neurology, Neurosurgery and Psychiatry*, **42**, 859–863.

McIvor GP, Riklan M, Reznikoff M. (1984) Depression in multiple sclerosis as a function of length and severity of illness, age, remissions and perceived social support. *Journal of Clinical Psychology*, **40**, 1028–1033.

Minden SL, Schiffer RB. (1990) Affective disorders in multiple sclerosis. Review and recommendations for clinical research. *Archives of Neurology*, **47**, 98–104.

Minden SL, Orav J, Reich P. (1987) Depression in multiple sclerosis. *General Hospital Psychiatry*, **9**, 426–434.

Mohr DC, Goodkin DE, Likosky W, *et al.* (1997) Identification of Beck Depression Inventory items related to multiple sclerosis. *Journal of Behavioral Medicine*, **20**, 407–414.

Narrow WE, Rae DS, Robins LN, Regier DA. (2002) Revised prevalence estimates of mental disorders in the United States. *Archives of General Psychiatry*, **59**, 115–123.

Nyenhuis DL, Rao SM, Zajecka JM, *et al.* (1995) Mood disturbance versus other symptoms of depression in multiple sclerosis. *Journal of the International Neuropsychological Society*, **1**, 291–296.

Nyenhuis DL, Luchetta T, Yamamoto C, *et al.* (1998) The development, standardization, and initial validation of the Chicago Multiscale Depression Inventory. *Journal of Personality Assessment*, **70**, 386–401.

Patten SB, Metz LM, Reimer MA. (2000) Biopsychosocial correlates of lifetime major depression in a multiple sclerosis population. *Multiple Sclerosis*, **6**, 115–120.

Patten SB, Beck CA, Williams JVA, Barbui C, Metz LM. (2003) Major depression in multiple sclerosis. A population-based perspective. *Neurology*, **61**, 1524–1527.

Patten SB, Lavorato DH, Metz LM. (2005) Clinical correlates of CES-D depressive symptom ratings in an MS population. *General Hospital Psychiatry*, **27**, 439–445.

Quesnel S, Feinstein A. (2004) Multiple sclerosis and alcohol: a study of problem drinking. *Multiple Sclerosis*, **10**, 197–201.

Rabins PV, Brooks BR, O'Donnell P, *et al.* (1986) Structural brain correlates of emotional disorder in multiple sclerosis. *Brain*, **109**, 585–597.

Randolph JJ, Arnett PA, Higginson CI, Voss WD. (2000) Neurovegetative symptoms in multiple sclerosis: relationship to depressed mood, fatigue and physical disability. *Archives of Clinical Neuropsychology*, **15**, 387–398.

Ron MA, Logsdail SJ. (1989) Psychiatric morbidity in multiple sclerosis: a clinical and MRI study. *Psychological Medicine*, **19**, 887–895.

Sadovnik AD, Eisen RN, Ebers GC, Paty DW. (1991) Cause of death in patients attending multiple sclerosis clinics. *Neurology*, **41**, 1193–1196.

Sadovnik AD, Remick RA, Allen J, *et al.* (1996) Depression and multiple sclerosis. *Neurology*, **46**, 628–632.

Sandyk R, Awerbuch G. (1993) Nocturnal melatonin secretion in suicidal patients with multiple sclerosis. *International Journal of Neuroscience*, **71**, 173–182.

Schiffer RB, Babigian HM. (1984) Behavioral disturbance in multiple sclerosis, temporal lobe epilepsy and amyotrophic lateral sclerosis; an epidemiologic study. *Archives of Neurology*, **41**, 1067–1069.

Schiffer RB, Caine ED, Bamford KA, Levy S. (1983) Depressive episodes in patients with multiple sclerosis. *American Journal of Psychiatry*, **140**, 1498–1500.

Schubert DSP, Foliart RH. (1993) Increased depression in multiple sclerosis. A meta-analysis. *Psychosomatics*, **34**, 124–130.

Shaw DM, Camps FE, Eccleston EG. (1967) 5-Hydroxytryptamine in the hindbrain of depressive suicides. *British Journal of Psychiatry*, **113**, 1407–1411.

Sherbourne CD, Wells KB, Hays RD, *et al.* (1994) Subthreshold depression and depressive disorder: clinical characteristics of general medical and mental health speciality outpatients. *American Journal of Psychiatry*, **151**, 1777–1784.

Skegg K, Corwin PA, Skegg DCG. (1988) How often is multiple sclerosis mistaken for a psychiatric disorder? *Psychological Medicine*, **18**, 733–736.

Stenager E, Jensen K. (1988) Multiple sclerosis: correlation of psychiatric admissions to onset of initial symptoms. *Acta Neurologica Scandinavica*, **77**, 414–417.

Stenager EN, Stenager E. (1992) Suicide and patients with neurologic diseases. Methodologic problems. *Archives of Neurology*, **49**, 1296–1303.

Stenager EN, Stenager E, Koch-Henrikson N, *et al.* (1992) Suicide and multiple sclerosis: an epidemiological investigation. *Journal of Neurology, Neurosurgery and Psychiatry*, **55**, 542–545.

Sullivan MJL, Weinshenker B, Mikail S, Edgley K. (1995) Depression before and after diagnosis of multiple sclerosis. *Multiple Sclerosis*, **1**, 104–108.

Surridge D. (1969) An investigation into some aspects of multiple sclerosis. *British Journal of Psychiatry*, **115**, 749–764.

Thompson AJ, Miller D, Youl B, *et al.* (1992) Serial gadolinium-enhanced MRI in relapsing/remitting multiple sclerosis of varying disease duration. *Neurology*, **42**, 60–63.

Weissman MM, Bland RC, Canino GJ, *et al.* (1999) Prevalence of suicide ideation and attempts in nine countries. *Psychological Medicine*, **29**, 9–17.

Whitlock FA, Siskind MM. (1980) Depression as a major symptom of multiple sclerosis. *Journal of Neurology, Neurosurgery and Psychiatry*, **43**, 861–865.

Young AC, Saunders J, Ponsford JR. (1976) Mental change as an early feature of multiple sclerosis. *Journal of Neurology, Neurosurgery and Psychiatry*, **39**, 1008–1013.

Zabad RK, Patten SB, Metz LM. (2005) The association of depression wuth disease course in multiple sclerosis. *Neurology*, **64**, 359–360.

Zigmond AS, Snaith RP. (1983) The Hospital and Anxiety Depression Scale. *Acta Psychiatrica Scandinavica*, **67**, 361–370.

Zorzon M, de Masi R, Nasuelli D, *et al.* (2001) Depression and anxiety in multiple sclerosis. A clinical and MRI study in 95 subjects. *Journal of Neurology*, **248**, 416–421.

3

Depression: etiology and treatment

In Ch. 2, data were presented defining the phenomenology of depression associated with MS. This is an essential precursor to studies that have explored the etiology of mood change. Indeed, some of the difficulties in determining which symptoms most accurately reflect mood change in MS patients may account, in part, for the inconsistencies in the neuroimaging data. It is, therefore, no coincidence that as symptom clarification proceeds in tandem with advances in neuroimaging brain–behavior correlations have become more robust.

This chapter will explore, first, putative etiological factors in relation to depression, namely genetics, brain imaging changes, endocrine dysfunction, immune system abnormalities and diverse psychosocial theories. Thereafter, a review of treatment modalities for depressed MS patients will be presented.

Etiology of depression in multiple sclerosis

The pathogenesis of the major depressive-like disorders frequently experienced by MS patients is unclear. Research has been undertaken to examine mood and MS using genetics, structural and functional neuroimaging, endocrine and immune system markers and social variables, and a mixed picture has emerged. The reasons for these partial successes and failures are reviewed and future research options suggested.

Genetics and depression

Evidence suggesting a genetic link between MS and unipolar depression is mixed. Based on the family history method, Joffe *et al.* (1987) did not find an excess of affective illness in the first-degree relatives of patients with MS, a finding in agreement with others (Minden *et al.*, 1987; Schiffer *et al.*, 1988). Patten *et al.* (2000) reported otherwise, with their findings more in keeping with the familial linkage noted in patients with primary major depression (Gershon *et al.*, 1982).

Comparisons between patients with multiple sclerosis and those with spinal cord injuries

Rabins *et al.* (1986) noted higher scores on the 28 item General Health Questionnaire (GHQ) in MS patients with brain involvement on CT scan when compared with a control group with spinal cord injuries. Similarly, Schiffer *et al.* (1983) compared two groups of 15 MS patients with either brain or spinal cord involvement based on clinical assessment and CT scan findings. Despite being matched for age, duration of illness and degree of physical disability, the former had significantly more major depressive episodes.

Neuroimaging

Magnetic resonance imaging

A number of early MRI studies reported equivocal results in their quest for an association between brain involvement and depression. Negative findings (Huber *et al.*, 1987; Logsdail *et al.*, 1988; Ron and Logsdail, 1989; Anzola *et al.*, 1990; Feinstein *et al.*, 1992a,b) outweighed the positive (Honer *et al.*, 1987; Reischies *et al.*, 1988; George *et al.*, 1994), but methodological problems meant that these results have to be interpreted with caution. Limitations pertain to three areas, namely the method of psychiatric assessment (which omitted structured interviews), scanners with weak field strengths, and MRI data analysis that focussed exclusively on T_2 weighted lesion area.

More recent studies that avoided these pitfalls have yielded more promising brain–behavior correlates. Pujol *et al.* (1997) looked at 45 MS patients carefully screened to exclude those on steroid treatment, or with dementia and comorbid medical conditions. Mood assessment was limited to the Beck Depression Inventory, with seven patients meeting criteria for moderately severe depression defined as scores greater than 17. A consistent pattern emerged in their MRI analysis irrespective of whether the brain was viewed in the axial or coronal plains, namely that higher scores were associated with more lesions in the left (dominant) arcuate fasciculus. Of note was that high depression scores also occurred in the absence of lesions in this region and, as a result, the MRI data could account for only 17% of the depression score variance. While this study benefited from detailed computerized MRI lesion analysis, it did not escape some of the criticizms spelled out above.

In a subsequent analysis of the same data, a factor analysis was applied to the Beck questionnaire, breaking it down into four components: affective symptoms, somatic complaints, performance difficulties and cognitive distortions (Pujol *et al.*, 2000). Reexamining brain correlates revealed that lesions in the left arcuate fasciculus could now account for 26% of the variance in the first two categories. The authors concluded that brain lesions were implicated in core depressive features only.

Different anatomical regions emerged from a study that included a structured psychiatric clinical interview, a brief cognitive battery and a series of self-report questionnaires including the Beck Depression Inventory (Berg *et al.*, 2000). Of 78 patients, 31(39.7%) received a DSM-IV diagnosis of mood disorder attributed to MS and of this group, 12 suffered from severe affective symptoms. Depressed patients were found to have a significantly higher T_2 weighted lesion load in the right temporal lobe with trends emerging for the right parietal lobe, cerebellum and total lesion load. Even when controlling for total lesion load, the right temporal lobe lesion score still significantly differentiated depressed from non-depressed subjects.

Bakshi *et al.* (2000) were the first to look beyond hyperintense lesions, incorporating indices of cerebral atrophy and hypointense (T_1 weighted) lesion volume in their analyses. Their study was notable for a failure to detect any association between depression as assessed by self-report measures and T_2 weighted hyperintense lesions. Rather, depressed patients were more likely to have T_1 weighted hypointense lesions in superior frontal and superior parietal brain regions. In addition, the *severity* of depression correlated with these MRI indices plus hypointense temporal lobe lesions and atrophy affecting the frontal lobes and the third and lateral ventricles. No laterality data were reported. The conclusion from this study was that depression was closely linked to "hard" evidence of brain pathology given that T_1 weighted lesions are generally synonymous with more chronic, destructive and thereby irreversible brain damage. While informative, a major weakness of this study was a reliance on visual rating scales to detect all aspects of brain pathology, a methodology considered less sensitive than sophisticated computer driven techniques (Rao *et al.*, 1989). While this could account for the absence of T_2 weighted lesions in the etiological mix, the findings were important in that they highlighted the connection between more ominous markers of brain pathology and depression. These findings should also be seen in the context of functional imaging abnormalities elicited in MS patients (p. 50).

Subsequently, Feinstein *et al.* (2004) demonstrated that hyperintense and hypointense lesions plus atrophy are all integral to the development of depression. In their study, 21 MS patients meeting DSM-IV criteria for major depression and 19 non-depressed MS patients were matched for age, gender, disease course, duration and exacerbations, cognitive function based on the Brief Repeatable Neuropsychological Battery (Rao *et al.*, 1991) and social stress. Subjects taking steroids and disease-modifying drugs were excluded, given the propensity for these treatments to affect MRI lesion load. Regional brain analysis was based on the Talairach proportional grid system, which served as the foundation for the automatic parcellation of each brain into 13 regional volumes of interest per hemisphere. The regional boundaries were delineated using a combination of predefined co-ordinate positions: the three orthogonal plains of the Talairach system, the edges of the brain, and four user defined points on each brain (i.e. central sulcus, sylvian fissure, occipital and parietal sulci). The use of the

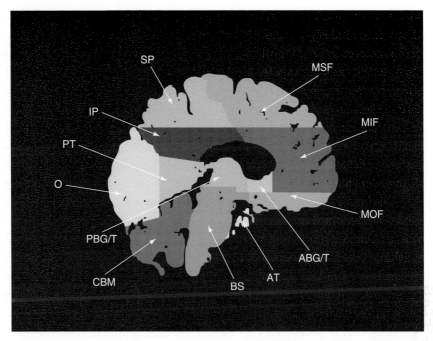

Fig. 3.1.   MRI sagittal (medial) view demonstrating semi-automated brain region extraction (SABRE)-generated brain areas. MIF, medial inferior frontal; MOF, medial orbital frontal; MSF, medial superior frontal; SP, superior parietal; IP, inferior parietal; AT, anterior temporal; PT, posterior temporal; ABG/T, anterior basal ganglia/thalamus; PBG/T, posterior basal ganglia/thalamus; O, occipital; BS, brainstem; CBM, cerebellum. For color image please see plate 1.

proportional grid system to obtain regional volumes reduced the impact of head size variability. Thus, segmentation results for each region were normalized by expressing them as a proportion of the regional volume. Atrophy was defined based on the percentage of CSF in each region. The brain regions demarcated were medial and lateral superior frontal, medial and lateral inferior frontal, medial and lateral orbito frontal, anterior and posterior temporal, anterior and posterior basal ganglia, superior and inferior parietal, and occipital. The cerebellum and brainstem were analyzed separately. For each brain region, volumes were obtained for hyperintense and hypointense lesions, CSF, white and gray matter (Fig. 3.1; see plate section for this figure in color).

The results showed that depressed MS patients had more extensive lesions (hyper and hypointense) in the left medial inferior frontal regions and less gray matter volume and greater CSF volume in the left anterior temporal region. Depressed patients did not have greater total lesion load, nor did they show greater total white matter and gray matter volume loss. The degree to which the brain abnormalities contributed to the development of major depression was explored using a logistic regression analysis and two left-sided brain areas were found to be significant independent predictors of major depression, namely medial inferior hyperintense lesion load and anterior temporal CSF volume (an index of regional cerebral atrophy). These two variables accounted for 42% of the variance when it came to explaining the presence of major depression.

By demonstrating that almost half the variance in the diagnosis of depression was directly attributable to brain pathology, the data extended findings from previous MS studies and provided the most compelling evidence yet of a direct brain–mood relationship in MS patients. These results, with the exception of the laterality data, replicated the findings of Zorzon *et al.* (2001), who also found that frontal lesion load and temporal lobe atrophy differentiated depressed from non-depressed MS patients.

Neuroimaging findings in depressed MS patients overlap with those found in other neurological disorders. Thus, in stroke patients an association between post-stroke depression and lesions situated in the anterior aspect of the left (dominant) frontal lobe has been noted (Robinson *et al.*, 1983; Starkstein and Robinson, 1989), replicated (Eastwood *et al.*, 1989) and disputed (Singh *et al.*, 1998; Carson *et al.*, 2000). It is postulated that depression ensues after lesions disrupt the neural circuits linking the prefrontal cortex to the striatum, in the process interfering with biogenic amine pathways.

Promising as the more recent MRI data are, it nevertheless remains sobering to reflect that more than half the variance in a diagnosis of depression in MS cannot be explained by brain abnormalities. One possible reason for this is the relative insensitivity of conventional MRI techniques in detecting cerebral pathology. Other MR modalities such as diffusion tensor imaging and magnetization transfer ratios that can detect pathological changes embedded within normal-appearing brain tissue offer a useful avenue for further research.

Functional imaging

Although global and regional cerebral hypometabolism have been demonstrated in MS patients (Bakshi *et al.*, 1998), there has been only one study looking specifically at functional brain correlates of depression (Sabatini *et al.*, 1996). Ten depressed and a similar number of non-depressed MS patients underwent cognitive testing and brain imaging with MRI and single photon emission computed tomography (SPECT). Type II error and a rating scale approach to lesion assessment can explain the absence of between-group MRI differences. The most informative data were those from the SPECT imaging where a significant asymmetry in limbic perfusion was noted. Regional cerebral blood flow was higher in the left limbic cortex in depressed patients whereas in non-depressed subjects higher values were noted on the right side. No such findings were found in six other brain regions. The authors' explanation that depression may be associated with a relative increase in dominant limbic cortex metabolism or a relative decrease in the non-dominant side could not be matched with their MRI data.

These findings mesh once more with those from other subcortical disorders. Depressed as opposed to non-depressed patients with Parkinson's disease had lower metabolism in the caudate nuclei and orbital frontal cortex on positron emission tomographic (PET) imaging (Mayberg et al., 1990). Similarly, depressed patients with Huntington's disease had reduced caudate, putamen and cingulate metabolism in addition to orbital frontal and inferior prefrontal hypoperfusion (Mayberg et al., 1992). Similarly, the emergence on MRI of anterior lobe atrophy as a significant independent predictor of depression in MS fits with findings from a PET study comparing depressed and non-depressed patients who had had a stroke and who had single lesions of the basal ganglia restricted to the caudate nucleus. In the former, hypometabolism was found in a number of limbic areas, most prominently the anterior temporal cortex (Mayberg, 1993). In general, there is a consistent theme to the neuroimaging data in patients with depression secondary to heterogeneous neurological disease: neural circuits coursing between the prefrontal cortex and subcortical areas, which include the basal ganglia and medial and anterior aspects of the temporal lobes, are pivotal in regulating mood (Mayberg, 1994).

It remains likely, however, that depression in all its complexity will always defy a neat reductionist approach that posits quantifiable brain pathology as the sole etiological factor. It should, therefore, come as no surprise that an emerging literature incorporating social and temperamental factors now stands alongside the imaging data, making a persuasive argument.

Psychosocial factors

A large literature has explored the relationship between depression and a range of psychosocial variables. Before reviewing these findings, it is important to remember that association does not necessarily imply causality. Unlike the structural imaging data where it is more plausible to suggest that regional lesion burden and atrophy trigger depression, rather than the reverse, with psychosocial variables the direction of attribution becomes less certain. This does not minimize the importance of these factors. Nor should it suggest that biological and psychological theories are competing for the same territory.

The importance of uncertainty (Lynch et al., 2001), inadequate coping strategies (Aikens et al., 1997; Jean et al., 1997; Mohr et al., 1997; Pakenham et al., 1997; Pakenham, 1999; Lynch et al., 2001), helplessness (Shnek et al., 1997; Patten and Metz, 2002; van der Werf et al., 2003), social relationships (Maybury and Brewin, 1984), loss of recreational activities (Voss et al., 2002), high levels of stress (Patten et al., 2000) and fatigue (Lobentanz et al., 2004) have all been emphasised when it comes to accounting for depression. There is a broad consensus that patients who utilize emotion-focussed rather than problem-focussed coping strategies are at increased risk of becoming depressed. In addition, there is evidence that MS patients who are cognitively impaired will, in turn, demonstrate higher levels of depression because they are more likely to utilize high levels of avoidance or low levels of active coping when it comes to managing their disability (Arnett *et al.*, 2002). When the relative contributions of these factors are weighed, some independent predictors of depression emerge, namely uncertainty, hope, disability and emotion-centered coping. These account for 40% of the variance in patients' self-reported depression (Lynch *et al.*, 2001), a figure that approximates the one reported in the MS MRI–depression literature (Feinstein *et al.*, 2004). It is, therefore, tempting, albeit potentially misleading, to conclude that by combining these two strands of inquiry, nearly all the variance in the depression scores can be accounted for. At best, these numbers should be seen as coarse approximations, likely to change in time as newer and improved methodologies in both research domains are developed and applied.

Other causes

Abnormalities in the hypothalamic–pituitary–adrenal axis of patients with MS have been documented (Michelson *et al.*, 1994; Wei and Lightman, 1997), including failure to suppress cortisol in depressed and non-depressed patients after dexamethasone administration (Reder *et al.*, 1987). Whether these changes are etiologically implicated in depression is unclear, although a study that correlated depression with hypothalamic–pituitary–adrenal axis abnormalities and contrast-enhanced brain lesions on MRI suggested that they are (Fassbender *et al.*, 1998).

Similarly, although an association between depression and dysregulation of the immune system has been reported in MS patients (Foley *et al.*, 1992), what is cause and effect is still being teased out. Some intriguing findings have appeared suggesting that successfully treating depression in MS may have the added benefit of also improving the MS (Mohr *et al.*, 2001a). Fourteen patients with relapsing–remitting MS and comorbid major depression were randomly assigned to one of three treatment modalities, namely antidepressant medication, cognitive–behavior therapy (CBT) or group therapy. A control group of eight healthy non-depressed subjects were also studied. Prior to the depressed patients receiving treatment levels of OKT3 stimulated interferon gamma (IFN-γ) were measured. This important pro-inflammatory cytokine is considered central to the pathogenesis of demyelination. Increased production of IFN-γ is associated with disease exacerbations, an accelerated disease course and the development of new lesions on brain MRI. Levels of IFN-γ at baseline were correlated with severity of depression as measured by the Beck Depression Inventory. As scores decreased with treatment, so did the levels of IFN-γ. No such longitudinal variations in IFN-γ levels were found in the healthy control subjects. Given that the mechanism for these interactions are not clearly understood, the authors shied away from concluding that the depression–immune dysregulation relationship was unidirectional, preferring to see it as dynamic and reciprocal.

A better understanding of the complex relationship between mood and immunological status has assumed added clinical importance since the introduction of interferons beta-1a and beta-1b as a treatment for relapsing–remitting MS. Reports of the drugs' effectiveness have been colored by concerns over depression as a side effect (Ch. 11).

Summarizing etiology

Much has been learnt over the past few years about the pathogenesis of depression in MS. The neuroimaging data now appear more compelling. Equally persuasive are the findings emerging from an eloquent set of psychosocial investigations. Here the importance of uncertainty needs repeating because, in an illness frequently characterized by relapses and remissions, this is something most MS patients must confront. The mean age of disease onset in MS is considerably earlier than in stroke, Parkinson's disease and Huntington's disease and the difficulties faced by young patients contemplating lifelong disability, often with little hope of cure, are formidable. In bringing together disparate etiological theories, explanations such as "multifactorial" cannot be avoided. Unsatisfactory as it may seem, particularly in relation to the literature on secondary depression in other neurological disorders, it currently represents the most accurate explanation why so many patients with MS become depressed (Feinstein, 1995).

Treatment

Treatment of MS-related depression need not be the preserve of the psychiatrist (Schiffer, 1987). Rather than leave a depressed patient in limbo awaiting an appointment with a psychiatrist, a more timely intervention with medication and some supportive psychotherapy is the consensus recommendation of the National Multiple Sclerosis Society (USA) (Goldman Consensus Group, 2005). An easy to follow treatment algorithm guides primary care physicians, neurologists and psychiatrists through what is considered the optimal approach. The necessity of having clear guidelines widely distributed is supported by data showing that two thirds of MS patients with major depression within neurological clinics received no antidepressant treatment, while only one quarter were given medication at the correct dose (Mohr *et al.*, 2006).

Missed therapeutic opportunities are not, however, unique to MS. The evolution of the neuropsychiatry of MS provides a historical paradigm for other neurological disorders, with a set sequence of events unfolding over the course of a century or more. First, a clinically astute neurologist, who posterity will treat kindly, described the neurological (and occasionally, psychological) signs and symptoms that come to define the disorder. The new disease entity may bear his name. (In the case of MS this would have created taxonomical confusion given Charcot's multiple, seminal observations in a host of disorders.) Over succeeding decades, the diagnostic criteria are refined with further observation supplemented by data from newly developed technologies. Mental state changes either pass with little notice or are missed. A couple of generations later comes a belated recognition of prominent abnormalities in mentation. Neuropsychiatry redux. A flurry of research defines the prevalence of cognitive dysfunction and the phenomenology of emotional change. Invariably the data reveal major psychiatric problems integral to the disease. And then, with few exceptions, clinical research stops. Few are the double-blind, placebo-controlled treatment trials in neuropsychiatry that provide an evidence-based approach to treating the newly discerned behavioral abnormalities. Not content with anecdotal evidence, the clinician is left with little choice but an uncomfortable retreat back into general psychiatry and the application of principles and regimens that may not be the most effective (Feinstein, 2004).

Medication

Only one double-blind placebo-controlled drug trial in depressed MS patients has been reported (Schiffer and Wineman, 1990). In a sample of 28 patients, 14 were randomly assigned to a five week trial of desipramine and individual psychotherapy and 14 to placebo and psychotherapy. All subjects met the criteria for major depression. The mean daily dose of desipramine was 123.2 ± 60.8 mg and seven patients in the drug treatment group were unable to reach the desired serum level because of untoward side effects. These included postural hypotension, dry mouth and constipation, which were more common in the drug group but also occurred in the placebo-treated patients. Patients taking desipramine showed a statistically significant improvement in mood compared with the placebo group according to scores on the Hamilton Rating Scale. The attainment of the therapeutic window was not of crucial significance in that patients taking the drug still improved at subthreshold levels. The authors concluded that desipramine was of modest benefit to depressed patients with MS, but side effects remained a problem, limiting the dose and thereby the response.

In an open trial, 11 MS patients were treated with 100 mg sertraline, a selective serotonin reuptake inhibitor (SSRI). All 10 patients who remained on treatment for at least three months improved and none reported side effects (Scott et al.,

1995). A retrospective review of 51 depressed MS patients receiving various SSRIs and tricyclic antidepressants confirmed the efficacy of medication in general; depression returned in over 50% of patients if treatment was stopped prematurely (Scott *et al.*, 1996). Data from a different drug class reveal an equally promising picture: 9 of 10 patients reached full remission in their depression when taking 150–400 mg daily of the reversible monoamine oxidase A inhibitor moclobemide (Barak *et al.*, 1999). As with the sertraline study, the small sample size and the open label nature of the trial impose limitations in data interpretation.

The remaining reports of response to psychotropic medication have been anecdotal but also illustrate that other SSRI drugs are likely to be equally effective. Shafey (1992) documented a patient with depression who did not respond to 225 mg/day of a tricyclic antidepressant (doxepin) but returned to an euthymic state when given 40 mg/day fluoxetine. Flax *et al.* (1991) also noted good responses to fluoxetine in 20 patients with MS, who all tolerated the drug well. The one discordant note came from Browning (1990), who reported an exacerbation in neurological symptoms in a single patient just started on fluoxetine. The significance of this one case report is difficult to assess in the absence of controlled treatment trials, but it is likely that the exacerbation was either a chance occurrence or a rare adverse drug reaction.

Until such time as double-blind placebo-controlled trials are undertaken, it would, therefore, seem prudent to use an SSRI or selective noradrenaline reuptake inhibitor as first choice, switching to another drug in the same class if treatment response is unsatisfactory. These drugs are, in theory, better tolerated than the tricyclic antidepressants, but they too are not without side effects in MS patients. Nausea, sexual dysfunction, insomnia, palpitations, tremor and anorexia in varying combinations were reported in one in six patients treated (Scott *et al.*, 1996). There is no evidence in MS patients that any one SSRI is better than another, but the preference for fluoxetine may reflect the perception amongst clinicians that the drug is helpful with some neurological symptoms as well, particularly fatigue. Once again, this evidence is anecdotal. A practical point to follow when starting treatment is not to discontinue the drug in response to complaints such as constipation or dry mouth, but rather to reduce the dosage. Clinical experience dictates that certain patients respond better, with less side effects, to 10 mg fluoxetine daily as opposed to the more frequently prescribed 20 mg. The use of buproprion, the only norepinephrine and dopamine reuptake inhibitor has not been evaluated in MS-related depression, although it has been used as an adjunct in treating SSRI-induced sexual dysfunction.

An impediment to successful maintenance treatment with an SSRI is sexual dysfunction. In itself, MS impairs sexual function in more than 50% of patients (Hussain and Fowler, 2000). An SSRI may successfully treat low mood, but at the

> **Vignette 1**
>
> A 32-year-old married accountant with a five year history of MS and an EDSS of 3.5 presented to his family doctor with a six week history of low mood, irritability, some vegetative features and thoughts of suicide. Desipramine had been started and the dose gradually titrated upwards, with some improvement in mood and partial resolution of insomnia. However, at doses greater than 100 mg/day, the patient reported excessive drowsiness and a very unpleasant dry mouth and requested to come off the treatment. At this point, he was referred to my clinic. The medication was discontinued over the course of a week and 20 mg fluoxetine started as a replacement. A marked improvement in mood was noted within two weeks and the medication was well tolerated apart from erectile dysfunction, not previously reported. Reducing the dosage of fluoxetine to 10 mg daily did not restore sexual function, although mood remained euthymic. The patient elected to remain on the fluoxetine stating he could "live with the (sexual) problem, but not with the depression." However, after six months of normal mood, he changed his mind and asked once again to come off treatment. Given the disabling nature of his depression and the earlier plans for self-harm when depressed I was reluctant to discontinue treatment after only 6 months. The addition of 75 mg buproprion daily, an antidepressant with minimal seretonergic effects, brought about a resolution in the erectile difficulties.

cost of aggravating or inducing sexual difficulties, leaving patients with an uncomfortable choice: a further loss of neurological function versus mood stability (see Vignette 1). Brief drug holidays such as three to four days off treatment before attempting intercourse are not particularly effective. Many young and middle-aged MS patients spontaneously stop treatment because of concerns that relationships will unravel and be lost because of SSRI-induced impotence or low libido. Mirtazepine, a novel antidepressant that selectively blocks the noradrenergic receptor and the serotonergic $5HT_1$, but not the $5HT_2$ or $5HT_3$ receptor, spares sexual function and thus offers one way out of this therapeutic bind. Unfortunately, sedation, which may aggravate fatigue, and weight gain can be troublesome. Nevertheless, mirtazepine in daily doses ranging from 15 to 45 mg theoretically offers some benefits, but as yet there has not been a clinical trial in MS patients.

Cognitive–behavior therapy

Data from a general psychiatric setting suggest CBT is effective in patients with mild to moderate (Rush *et al.*, 1977; Blackburn *et al.*, 1986) and moderate to severe (Derubeis *et al.*, 2005) depression. Furthermore, for those patients unable to tolerate anti-depressant medication, this treatment modality has obvious advantages. Three studies of depressed MS patients confirm its utility, albeit for patients without major cognitive difficulties. The most compelling evidence comes from a treatment trial comparing individual CBT, supportive expressive psychotherapy and the SSRI sertraline. Dosing started at 50 mg daily and where necessary was increased by 50 mg increments up to 200 mg daily, according to clinical response. The results revealed that CBT and medication emerged as equally effective, both surpassing the supportive expressive psychotherapeutic approach (Mohr *et al.*, 2001b). The treatment trial lasted for 16 weeks, but a subsequent analysis at 6 months revealed that the findings held. Although success was judged by fewer diagnoses of major depression and lower scores on the full Beck Depression Inventory and a modified 18 item version, this was not matched by results from the semi-structured Hamilton Rating Scale for depression. No satisfactory explanation was given for this. Notwithstanding this anomaly, the study remains important and a major addition to a small literature short on facts. It shows that CBT offers an alternative, effective treatment for all depressed MS patients, not just those troubled by medication side effects. Patients may not, however, be given a choice of treatments: CBT requires a skilled therapist and the realities of health-care provision are such that it is more likely for a MS patient to receive a prescription than a 16 week course of CBT.

One way of overcoming some of the logistical difficulties in securing access to a cognitive behavior therapist is for the treatment modality to be administered via telephone. In an innovative approach, Mohr *et al.* (2000) showed that eight weeks of telephone-administered CBT significantly improved symptoms of depression in 16 patients compared with the same number who continued to receive the usual care offered to them (in two patients this involved antidepressant medication and in one patient psychotherapy).

These two studies built on Larcombe and Wilson's (1984) earlier conclusions that CBT was more effective than no treatment in alleviating symptoms of depression in MS patients. Sample size in their study was small, with nine patients receiving CBT and 10 put on a waiting list without intervention. CBT took place in groups over a six week period with weekly sessions of 90 minutes each. All subjects had been carefully screened to ensure they met diagnostic criteria for depression without evidence of cognitive dysfunction, the presence of which may have compromised effective therapy. At the end of the trial, the patients receiving CBT showed a significant improvement in mood based on four separate assessment procedures, namely a self-report scale, a clinician rating scale, a rating made by a significant other (close friend, family member) and a measure of daily mood.

A variant of CBT – stress inoculation training (SIT) – is a short-term, CBT approach that targets maladaptive psychological responses to stress, thereby enhancing coping mechanisms. Such a technique, in combination with progressive deep muscle relaxation, has been applied effectively to MS patients in a case–control study (Foley *et al.*, 1987).

Psychotherapy

Individual psychotherapy

An approach to psychotherapy for patients with MS has been eloquently summarized by Minden (1992). She stresses a practical, common sense attitude to therapy, decrying the notion that only supportive therapy is required and debunking the myth that patients have to be "psychologically minded" before they can begin treatment. Varying degrees of psychological distress will be present at different times in the disease course because of the dynamic nature of a disease process characterized by relapses and remissions and the difficulty in predicting what the future holds. The therapist must be flexible in order to deal with the fluctuating feelings of despair, fear and hopelessness alternating with optimism, hope and relative well being. During periods of disease exacerbation and psychological distress, supportive therapy intermingled with practical advice to the patient seems more appropriate than attempts at dealing with unresolved, hidden conflicts, which may be well defended. Conversely, during remissions in the disease, which is often accompanied by greater emotional equanimity, more detailed insight-oriented psychoanalytic therapy may prove beneficial. The use of pharmacotherapy as an adjunct is not ruled out. This flexible approach extends to deciding the duration of treatment, which may vary from a single session to treatment over years, depending on the needs of the patient. Although there are no empirical data to support the efficacy of Minden's approach, the overriding emphasis on humaneness and the intuitive appeal to common sense have much to recommend it.

Group therapy

A number of early reports suggested that group therapy with MS patients was advantageous in relieving psychological distress. The approaches have been varied: psychoanalytic (Day *et al.*, 1953; Barnes *et al.*, 1954), supportive–analytical (Bolding, 1960), supportive (Spielberg, 1980) and educational (Pavlou *et al.*, 1979). What the reports all had in common was their largely anecdotal nature with an absence of control groups and a failure to employ pre- and post-treatment assessment measures.

Crawford and McIvor (1985) corrected many of these shortcomings in their study of 41 MS patients who were divided into three groups: insight-oriented psychotherapy, current events discussion and non-treatment. Patients were assessed over a six month period. Although the groups were equally depressed at entry to the study, only patients receiving the insight-oriented psychotherapy showed a significantly mood improvement. The result has not been replicated.

A meta-analysis of treatment options available to depressed MS – which was based on just five publications meeting criteria for inclusion – concluded that medication and problem-oriented psychotherapy are equally effective (Mohr and Goodkin, 1999). An important caveat is that this conclusion applies to patients with mild to moderately severe depression. Further evidence relating to severe depression and the acutely suicidal patient is still awaited. The meta-analysis also stressed that failure to treat invariably leads to a worsening in the depression. A consensus panel of MS experts has concluded that while treatment should be individualized for each person the "gold standard" for patients with moderate to severe depression should involve the combination of medication and a form of psychotherapy, be it supportive, CBT or interpersonal (Goldman Consensus Group, 2005).

An intriguing observation that requires further investigation is the possibility that response to treatment, be it medication or CBT, may be determined by brain lesion volume, lesion location and cognitive function (Mohr et al., 2003). Higher lesion volume in the temporal lobes was associated with a reduction in treatment efficacy in patients who received either 16 weeks of sertraline 50 mg daily or CBT. Furthermore, neuropsychological functioning emerged as an important mediator between depression and lesion volume (see Ch. 7 for a discussion on the relationship between depression and cognitive function).

Electroconvulsive therapy

The use of electroconvulsive therapy has been reported in a small number of MS patients and found to be effective (Gallineck and Kalinowsky, 1958; Krystal and Coffey, 1997), although treatment has been associated with an exacerbation in MS symptoms in approximately 20% of patients. The presence of contrast-enhancing lesions on MRI prior to therapy has been identified as a possible risk factor for neurological deterioration (Mattingley et al., 1992). Electroconvulsive therapy should be used only if the patient has not first responded to pharmacotherapy or as emergency treatment in the severely depressed, actively suicidal patient. A contrast-enhanced MRI as part of the work-up may also guide the treatment decision.

Herbal remedies

It is not uncommon for MS patients to self-medicate and a host of preparations, available without prescription, have been tried ranging from the legal (e.g. evening oil of primrose) to the outlawed (e.g. cannabis). Depressed MS patients have resorted to St. John's wort (*Hypericum perforatum*) and there is evidence from a meta-analysis that this has some merit. Linde et al. (1996) reviewed the data from 23 randomized clinical trials (none confined to MS patients) and concluded that the herb was more effective than placebo in mild to moderately severe depression. Its use cannot, however, be given an unqualified endorsement, for efficacy in comparison with SSRI or tricyclic antidepressants, or in treating more severe forms of depression, has yet to be established. Furthermore, the pharmacological effects of St. John's wort means that the medication should not be combined with more conventional antidepressant medication because of the risk of a serotonergic syndrome.

Summary

- There is a clear link between major depression and fronto-temporal brain pathology (hyperintense and hypointense lesions and atrophy). Nevertheless, brain changes can explain, at best, less than 50% of the depression variance.
- A limited functional brain imaging literature supports the importance of limbic areas, in particular the temporal lobes, in maintaining euthymic mood in MS patients.
- Psychosocial factors, namely emotion-based coping styles, helplessness, uncertainty and social stressors (relationship difficulties, reduced recreational opportunities) have also been casually implicated in depression.
- There is a suggestion that immune abnormalities in association with dysfunction of the hypothalamic–pituitary–adrenal axis may be the mechanism underlying the high lifetime risk for major depression.
- There is one double-blind, placebo-controlled trail of antidepressant medication in depressed MS patients and this demonstrated the clinical efficacy of the tricyclic antidepressant desipramine. Anecdotal evidence, however, points towards newer antidepressants such as the selective serotonin reuptake inhibitor drugs as the treatment of choice because of their less troublesome side effects.
- Sixteen weeks of cognitive–behavior therapy has been found to be as effective as sertraline (50 mg) in treating MS patients with moderately severe depression.
- Psychotherapy, either individual or group, is also helpful, particularly for less severe depression. In more severe cases, it may prove a useful addition to antidepressant medication.
- In patients who do not respond to antidepressant medication, lithium augmentation of the antidepressant drug may prove effective.
- Electroconvulsive therapy may be used in severe cases of drug refractory depression, although there appears to be a 20% risk of triggering a MS relapse. The presence of active brain lesions on MRI pretherapy is a potential risk factor for neurological relapse following treatment.
- It needs to be emphasised that depression represents a considerable source of morbidity and mortality in MS and missing the diagnosis does the patient a great disservice, more so as the disorder can, in many patients, be successfully treated.

References

Aikens JE, Fischer JS, Namey M, Rudick RA. (1997) A replicated prospective investigation of life stress, coping and depressive symptoms in multiple sclerosis. *Journal of Behavioral Medicine*, **20**, 433–445.

Anzola GP, Bevilacqua L, Cappa SF, *et al.* (1990) Neuropsychological assessment in patients with relapsing–remitting multiple sclerosis and mild functional impairment: correlation with magnetic resonance imaging. *Journal of Neurology, Neurosurgery and Psychiatry*, **53**, 142–145.

Arnett PA, Higginson CI, Voss WD, Randolph JJ, Grandey AA. (2002) Relationship between coping, cognitive dysfunction, and depression in multiple sclerosis. *The Clinical Neuropsychologist*, **16**, 341–355.

Bakshi R, Miletich RS, Kinkel PR, Emmet ML, Kinkel WR. (1998) High-resolution fluorode-oxyglucose positron emission tomography shows both global and regional cerebral hypo-metabolism in multiple sclerosis. *Journal of Neuroimaging*, **8**, 228–234.

Bakshi R, Czarnecki D, Shaikh ZA, *et al.* (2000) Brain MRI lesions and atrophy are related to depression in multiple sclerosis. *NeuroReport*, **11**, 1153–1158.

Barak Y, Ur E, Achiron A. (1999) Moclobemide treatment in multiple sclerosis patients with co-morbid depression: an open label safety trial. *Journal of Neuropsychiatry and Clinical Neuroscience*, **11**, 271–273.

Barnes RH, Busse EW, Dinken H. (1954) Alleviation of emotional problems in multiple sclerosis by group psychotherapy. *Group Psychotherapy*, **6**, 193–201.

Berg D, Supprian T, Thomae J, *et al.* (2000) Lesion pattern in patients with multiple sclerosis and depression. *Multiple Sclerosis*, **6**, 156–162.

Blackburn I. M., Eunson K. M., Bishop, S. (1986) A two-year naturalistic follow-up of depressed patients treated with cognitive therapy, pharmacotherapy and a combination of both. *Journal of Affective Disorders*, **10**, 67–75.

Bolding, H. (1960) Psychotherapeutic aspects in management of patients with multiple sclerosis. *Diseases of the Nervous System*, **21**, 24–26.

Browning WN. (1990) Exacerbation of symptoms of multiple sclerosis in a patient taking fluoxetine. *American Journal of Psychiatry*, **147**, 1089.

Carson AJ, MacHale S, Allen K, *et al.* (2000) Depression after stroke and lesion location: a systematic review. *Lancet*, **356**, 122–126.

Crawford JD, McIvor GP. (1985) Group psychotherapy: benefits in multiple sclerosis. *Archives of Physical Medical Rehabilitation*, **66**, 810–813.

Day M, Day E, Herrmann R. (1953) Group therapy of patients with multiple sclerosis. *Archives of Neurology and Psychiatry*, **69**, 193–196.

Derubeis RJ, Hollon SD, Amsterdam JD, *et al.* (2005) Cognitive therapy vs medications in the treatment of moderate to severe depression. *Archives of General Psychiatry*, **62**, 409–416.

Eastwood MR, Rifat SL, Nobbs H, Ruderman J. (1989) Mood disorder following CVA. *British Journal of Psychiatry*, **154**, 195–200.

Fassbender K, Schmidt R, Mößner R, *et al.* (1998) Mood disorders and dysfunction of the hypothalamic–pituitary–adrenal axis in multiple sclerosis. *Archives of Neurology*, **55**, 66–72.

Feinstein A. (1995) Multiple sclerosis and depression: an etiological conundrum. *Canadian Journal of Psychiatry*, **40**, 573–576.

Feinstein A. (2004). The neuropsychiatry of multiple sclerosis. *Canadian Journal of Psychiatry*, **49**, 157–163.

Feinstein A, Youl B, Ron MA. (1992a) Acute optic neuritis: a cognitive and magnetic resonance imaging study. *Brain*, **115**, 1403–1415.

Feinstein A, Kartsounis L, Miller B, Youl B, Ron MA. (1992b) Clinically isolated lesions of the type seen in multiple sclerosis: a cognitive, psychiatric and MRI follow-up study. *Journal of Neurology, Neurosurgery and Psychiatry*, **55**, 869–876.

Feinstein A, Roy P, Lobaugh N, Feinstein KJ, O'Connor P. (2004) Structural brain abnormalities in multiple sclerosis patients with major depression. *Neurology*, **62**, 586–590.

Flax JW, Gray J, Herbert J. (1991) Effects of fluoxetine on patients with multiple sclerosis. *American Journal of Psychiatry*, **148**, 1603.

Foley FW, Bedell JR, LaRocca NG, Scheinberg LC, Reznikoff M. (1987) Efficacy of stress-inoculation training in coping with multiple sclerosis. *Journal of Consulting and Clinical Psychology*, **55**, 919–922.

Foley FW, Traugott U, LaRocca NG, *et al.* (1992) A prospective study of depression and immune dysregulation in multiple sclerosis. *Archives of Neurology*, **49**, 238–244.

Gallineck A, Kalinowsky LB. (1958) Psychiatric aspects of multiple sclerosis. *Diseases of the Nervous System*, **19**, 77–80.

George MS, Kellner CH, Bernstein H, Goust JM. (1994) A magnetic resonance imaging investigation into mood disorders in multiple sclerosis. *Journal of Nervous and Mental Disease*, **182**, 410–412.

Gershon ES, Hamovit J, Guroff JJ, *et al.* (1982) A family study of schizoaffective, bipolar 1, bipolar 11, unipolar, and normal control probands. *Archives of General Psychiatry*, **39**, 1157–1167.

Goldman Consensus Group. (2005). The Goldman Consensus statement on depression in multiple sclerosis. *Multiple Sclerosis*, **11**, 328–337.

Honer WG, Hurwitz T, Li DKB, Palmer M, Paty DW. (1987) Temporal lobe involvement in multiple sclerosis patients with psychiatric disorders. *Archives of Neurology*, **44**, 187–190.

Huber SJ, Paulsen GW, Shuttleworth EC, *et al.* (1987) Magnetic resonance imaging correlates of dementia in multiple sclerosis. *Archives of Neurology*, **44**, 732–736.

Hussain IF, Fowler CJ. (2000) The cause and management of bladder, sexual and bowel symptoms. In *The Principles and Treatment of Multiple Sclerosis*, Ed. CP Hawkins, JS Wolinsky. Oxford: Butterworth Heinemann, pp. 258–281.

Jean VM, Beatty WW, Paul RH, Mullins L. (1997) Coping with general and disease related stressors by patients with multiple sclerosis: relationships to psychological distress. *Multiple Sclerosis*, **3**, 191–196.

Joffe RT, Lippert GP, Gray TA, Sawa G, Horvath Z. (1987) Personal and family history of affective disorder, *Journal of Affective Disorders*, **12**, 63–65.

Krystal AD, Coffey CE. (1997) Neuropsychiatric considerations in the use of electroconvulsive therapy. *Journal of Neuropsychiatry and Clinical Neurosciences*, **9**, 283–292.

Larcombe NA, Wilson PH. (1984) An evaluation of cognitive–behaviour therapy for depression in patients with multiple sclerosis. *British Journal of Psychiatry*, **145**, 366–371.

Linde K, Ramirez G, Mulrow CD, *et al.* (1996) St. John's wort for depression: an overview and meta-analysis of randomised clinical trials. *British Medical Journal*, **313**, 253–258.

Lobentanz IS, Asenbaum S, Vass K, *et al.* (2004) Factors influencing quality of life in multiple sclerosis patients: disability, depressive mood, fatigue and sleep quality. *Acta Neurologica Scandinavica*, **110**, 6–13.

Logsdail SJ, Callanan MM, Ron MA. (1988) Psychiatric morbidity in patients with clinically isolated lesions of the type seen in multiple sclerosis. *Psychological Medicine*, **18**, 355–364.

Lynch SG. Kroencke DC, Denney DR. (2001) The relationship between disability and depression in multiple sclerosis: the role of uncertainty, coping and hope. *Multiple Sclerosis*, **7**, 411–416.

Mattingley G, Baker K, Zorumski CF, Figiel GS. (1992) Multiple sclerosis and ECT: possible value of gadolinium enhanced magnetic resonance scans for identifying high risk patients. *Journal of Neuropsychiatry and Clinical Neurosciences*, **4**, 145–151.

Mayberg HS. (1993) Neuroimaging studies of depression in neurological disease. In *Depression in Neurological Disease*, ed. SE Starkstein, RG Robinson, pp. 186–216. Baltimore, MD: Johns Hopkins University Press.

Mayberg HS (1994) Frontal lobe dysfunction in secondary depression. *Journal of Neuropsychiatry and Clinical Neurosciences*, **6**, 428–442.

Mayberg HS, Starkstein SE, Sadzot B, *et al.* (1990) Selective hypometabolism in the inferior frontal lobe in depressed patients with Parkinson's disease. *Annals of Neurology*, **28**, 57–64.

Mayberg HS, Starkstein SE, Peyser CE, *et al.* (1992) Paralimbic frontal lobe hypometabolism in depression associated with Huntington's disease. *Neurology*, **42**, 1791–1797.

Maybury CP, Brewin CR. (1984) Social relationships, knowledge and adjustment to multiple sclerosis. *Journal of Neurology, Neurosurgery and Psychiatry*, **47**, 372–376.

Michelson D, Stone L, Galliven E, *et al.* (1994) Multiple sclerosis is associated with alterations in hypothalamic–pituitary–adrenal axis function. *Journal of Clinical Endocrinology and Metabolism*, **79**, 848–853.

Minden SL. (1992) Psychotherapy for people with multiple sclerosis. *Journal of Neuropsychiatry and Clinical Neurosciences*, **4**, 198–213.

Minden SL, Orav J, Reich P. (1987) Depression in multiple sclerosis. *General Hospital Psychiatry*, **9**, 426–434.

Mohr DC, Goodkin D. (1999) Treatment of depression in multiple sclerosis. Review and meta-analysis. *Clinical Psychology: Science and Practice*, **6**, 1–9.

Mohr DC, Goodkin DE, Gatto N, van der Wende J. (1997) Depression, coping and level of neurological impairment in multiple sclerosis. *Multiple Sclerosis*, **3**, 254–258.

Mohr DC, Likosky W, Bertagnolli A, *et al.* (2000) Telephone-administered cognitive–behavioral therapy for the treatment of depressive symptoms in multiple sclerosis. *Consulting and Clinical Psychology*, **68**, 356–361.

Mohr DC, Goodkin DE, Islar J, Hauser SL, Genain CP. (2001a) Treatment of depression is associated with suppression of nonspecific and antigen specific T_H1 response in multiple sclerosis. *Archives of Neurology*, **58**, 1081–1086.

Mohr DC, Boudewyn AC, Goodkin D, Bostrom A, Epstein L. (2001b) Comparative outcomes for individual cognitive–behavior therapy, supportive–expressive group therapy, and sertraline for the treatment of depression in multiple sclerosis. *Journal of Consulting and Clinical Psychology*, **69**, 942–949.

Mohr DC, Epstein L, Luks TL, *et al.* (2003) Brain lesion volume and neuropsychological function predict efficacy of treatment for depression in multiple sclerosis. *Journal of Consulting and Clinical Psychology*, **71**, 1017–1024.

Mohr DC, Hart SL, Fonareva I, Tasch ES. (2006) Treatment of depression for patients with multiple sclerosis in neurology clinics. *Multiple Sclerosis*, **12**, 204–208.

Pakenham KI. (1999) Adjustment to multiple sclerosis: application of a stress coping model. *Health Psychology*, **18**, 383–392.

Pakenham KI, Stewart CA, Rogers A. (1997) The role of coping in adjustment to multiple sclerosis: related adaptive demands. *Psychology, Health and Medicine*, **2**, 197–211.

Patten SB, Metz LM. (2002) Hopelessness ratings in relapsing–remitting and secondary progressive multiple sclerosis. *International Journal of Psychiatry in Medicine*, **32**, 155–165.

Patten SB, Metz LM, Reimer MA. (2000) Biopsychosocial correlates of lifetime major depression in a multiple sclerosis population. *Multiple Sclerosis*, **6**, 115–120.

Pavlou M, Johnson P, Davis FA, Lefebre K. (1979) Program of psychologic service delivery in multiple sclerosis centre. *Professional Psychology*, **10**, 503–510.

Pujol J, Bello J, Deus J, Marti-Vilalta JL, Capdevila A. (1997) Lesions in the left arcuate fasciculus region and depressive symptoms in multiple sclerosis. *Neurology*, **49**, 1105–1110.

Pujol J, Bello J, Deus J, *et al.* (2000) Beck Depression Inventory factors related to demyelinating lesions of the left arcuate fasciculus region. *Psychiatry Research: Neuroimaging*, **99**, 151–159.

Rabins PV, Brooks BR, O'Donnell P, *et al.* (1986) Structural brain correlates of emotional disorder in multiple sclerosis. *Brain*, **109**, 585–597.

Rao SM, Leo GJ, Haughton VM, St. Aubin-Faubert P, Bernardin L. (1989) Correlation of magnetic resonance imaging with neuropsychological testing in multiple sclerosis. *Neurology*, **39**, 161–166.

Rao SM, Leo HJ, Bernardin L, Unverzagt F. (1991) Cognitive dysfunction in multiple sclerosis. *Neurology*, **41**, 685–691.

Reder AT, Lowy MT, Meltzer HY, Antel JP. (1987) Dexamethasone suppression test abnormalities in multiple sclerosis: relation to ACTH therapy. *Neurology*, **37**, 849–853.

Reischies FM, Baum K, Brau H, Hedde JP, Schwindt G. (1988) Cerebral magnetic resonance imaging findings in multiple sclerosis. Relation to disturbance of affect, drive and cognition. *Archives of Neurology*, **45**, 1114–1116.

Robinson RG, Kubos KL, Starr LB, Rao K, Price TR. (1983) Mood disorders in stroke patients: relationship to lesion location. *Comprehensive Psychiatry*, **24**, 555–556.

Ron MA, Logsdail SJ. (1989) Psychiatric morbidity in multiple sclerosis: a clinical and MRI study. *Psychological Medicine*, **19**, 887–895.

Rush AJ, Beck A, Kovacs M, Hollon SD. (1977) Comparative efficacy of cognitive therapy and pharmacotherapy in the treatment of depressed out-patients. *Cognitive Therapy and Research*, **1**, 17–37.

Sabatini U, Pozzilli C, Pantano P, *et al.* (1996) Involvement of the limbic system in multiple sclerosis patients with depressive disorders. *Biological Psychiatry*, **39**, 970–975.

Schiffer RB. (1987) The spectrum of depression in multiple sclerosis. An approach for clinical management. *Archives of Neurology*, **44**, 596–599.

Schiffer RB, Wineman NM. (1990) Antidepressant pharmacotherapy of depression associated with multiple sclerosis. *American Journal of Psychiatry*, **147**, 1493–1497.

Schiffer RB, Caine ED, Bamford KA, Levy S. (1983) Depressive episodes in patients with multiple sclerosis. *American Journal of Psychiatry*, **140**, 1498–1500.

Schiffer RB, Weitkamp LR, Wineman NM, Guttormsen S. (1988) Multiple sclerosis and affective disorder: family history, sex and HLA-DR antigens. *Archives of Neurology*, **45**, 1345–1348.

Scott TF, Nussbaum P, McConnell H, Brill P. (1995) Measurement of treatment response to sertraline in depressed multiple sclerosis patients using the Carroll scale. *Neurological Research*, **17**, 421–422.

Scott TF, Allen D, Price TRP, McConnell H, Lang D. (1996) Characterization of major depression symptoms in multiple sclerosis. *Journal of Neuropsychiatry and Clinical Neurosciences*, **8**, 318–323.

Shafey H. (1992) The effect of fluoxetine in depression associated with multiple sclerosis. *Canadian Journal of Psychiatry*, **37**, 147–148.

Shnek ZM, Foley FW, LaRocca NG, *et al.* (1997) Helplessness, self-efficacy, cognitive distortions, and depression in multiple sclerosis and spinal cord injury. *Annals of Behavioral Medicine*, **19**, 287–94.

Singh A, Herrmann N, Black SE. (1998) The importance of lesion location in poststroke depression: a critical review. *Canadian Journal of Psychiatry*, **43**, 921–927.

Spielberg N. (1980) Support group improves quality of life. *Rehabilitation, Nurses Journal*, **5**, 9–11.

Starkstein SE, Robinson RG. (1989) Affective disorders and cerebral vascular disease. *British Journal of Psychiatry*, **154**, 170–182.

van der Werf SP, Evers A, Jongen PJH, Bleijenberg G. (2003) The role of helplessness as mediator between neurological disability, emotional instability, experienced fatigue and depression in patients with multiple sclerosis. *Multiple Sclerosis*, **3**, 89–94.

Voss WD, Arnett PA, Higginson CI, *et al.* (2002) Contributing factors to depressed mood in multiple sclerosis. *Archives of Clinical Neuropsychology*, **17**, 103–115.

Wei T, Lightman SL. (1997) The neuroendocrine axis in patients with multiple sclerosis. *Brain*, **120**, 1067–1076.

Zorzon M, de Masi R, Nasuelli D, *et al.* (2001) Depression and anxiety in multiple sclerosis. A clinical and MRI study in 95 subjects. *Journal of Neurology*, **248**, 416–421.

4

Multiple sclerosis, bipolar affective disorder and euphoria

Occasionally, it has been my experience to encounter an MS patient with mania, who apart from the abnormal mental state examination is neurologically quite well. Furthermore, I have treated patients with manic episodes heralding the onset of MS and have also come across bipolar patients who subsequently went on to develop MS often years later. Managing the floridly manic MS patient can present a considerable challenge given the potential that neuroleptic and mood-stabilizing medications have in further compromising neurological function. Early detection of the patient going "high" makes management easier, but as a first step to early detection, increased awareness amongst clinicians of the increased rate of co-morbidity is needed. Criteria for diagnosing mania are clearly set out and, as with clinically significant depression, diagnosis and treatment, particularly of patients with mildly elevated mood, does not have to await the arrival of the neuropsychiatrist.

Conceptual and semantic issues

Mania may occur as part of many physical conditions or as a reaction to drug therapy. When this occurs, the mania has been termed "secondary," differentiating it from the more usual occurrence as a primary psychiatric syndrome. The correct DSM-IV (American Psychiatric Association, 1994) terminology for the syndrome is a "mood disorder due to a general medical condition" (MDGMC) (Table 4.1), with the type of mood change specified as "with manic features" (Table 4.2) or "with hypomanic features" (Table 4.3). If the symptoms of mania are present together with depression and neither predominates, the type of mood change is specified as "mixed." The DSM-IV nomenclature has done away with the primary–secondary dichotomy, although the fundamental idea of the mood disorder arising as a result of the medical condition remains unchanged.

This terminology may be somewhat misleading and MS patients presenting with mania or hypomania are more often than not given the diagnosis of bipolar affective disorder, type 1, denoting mania, and type 11, denoting hypomania. This

Table 4.1. Diagnostic criteria for "mood disorder (mania) due to a general medical condition" in DSM-IV[a]

Criterion	Features
A	A prominent and persistent disturbance in mood predominates in the clinical picture and is characterized by an elevated, expansive or irritable mood
B	There is evidence from the history, physical examination or laboratory findings that the disturbance is the direct physiological consequence of the medical condition
C	The disturbance is not better accounted for by another mental disorder (e.g. a bipolar disorder that predates the medical condition by many years)
D	The disturbance does not occur exclusively during the course of a delirium
E	The symptoms cause clinically significant distress or impairment in social, occupational or other important areas of functioning
	The *types* are then specified as either manic or mixed.
	The general medical condition should be mentioned on axis 1 and should also be coded on axis 3

[a] The DSM-IV makes the point that although the clinical presentation of the mood disorder may resemble a manic or hypomanic episode, the full criteria for one of these episodes need not be met (see Table 4.2 and 4.3 for the full criteria for a manic or hypomanic episode).
Source: With permission from the American Psychiatric Association, 1994.

was called manic–depressive disorder in the earlier World Health Organization classifications of mental illness. Confusion is understandable as the signs and symptoms of bipolar affective disorder are indistinguishable from the MDGMC manic subtype. Therefore, the situation with respect to terminology bears many similarities to that found in depression (Ch. 2) and psychosis (Ch. 6). For the purposes of this chapter, mania in the context of MS will be referred to as bipolar affective disorder, even though this is not strictly correct by the criteria of the DSM-IV. The decision is nevertheless a practical one, because the literature makes scant reference to the verbally cumbersome MDGMC subtype.

This chapter will review briefly the literature pertaining to bipolar affective disorder and medical conditions in general before the focus shifts to MS. The epidemiology, etiology and treatment of mania in the context of MS will be discussed and a section is devoted to differential diagnosis, in particular the mental state change of euphoria.

Literature review of mania and medical illness

In a wide-ranging review, Krauthammer and Klerman (1978) found cases of mania occurring in association with infection, neoplasm, epilepsy and metabolic

Table 4.2. Criteria for a manic episode in DSM-IV

Criterion	Features
A	A distinct period of abnormally and persistently elevated, expansive or irritable mood lasting at least one week (or any duration if hospitalization is necessary)
B	During the period of mood disturbance, three or more of the following symptoms have persisted (four if the mood is only irritable) and have been present to a significant degree: (i) inflated self-esteem or grandiosity (ii) decreased need for sleep (e.g. feels rested after only three hours of sleep) (iii) more talkative than usual or pressure to keep talking (iv) flight of ideas or subjective experience that thoughts are racing (v) distractibility (i.e. attention too easily drawn to unimportant or irrelevant external stimuli) (vi) increase in goal-directed activity (either socially, at work or school, or sexually) or psychomotor agitation (vii) excessive involvement in pleasurable activities that have a high potential for painful consequences (e.g. engaging in unrestrained buying sprees, sexual indiscretions, or foolish business investments)
C	The mood disturbance is sufficiently severe to cause marked impairment in occupational functioning or in usual social activities or relationships with others, or to necessitate hospitalization to prevent harm to self or others, or there are psychotic features.

Source: With permission from the American Psychiatric Association, 1994.

disturbances. Drugs implicated included corticosteroids, isoniazid, procarbazine, levodopa and bromide. No cases of MS were reported. Using criteria more restrictive than current DSM-IV guidelines (i.e. manic symptoms had to be present for longer than a week) the authors identified certain characteristics of mania that suggested a link to the associated medical disorder. These included a later age of onset of mania, which in their review was 41 years (as opposed to 25 years in "primary" bipolar illness) and the relative absence of a family history of affective illness. Written during an era when psychiatric disorders were divided into either organic or functional, Krauthammer and Klerman (1978) concluded that secondary mania was organic in origin.

Their observations were replicated in a study comprising 39 manic patients with and without an antecedent medical illness (Cook *et al.*, 1987). Additional differences in the medically ill sample included a predominantly irritable mood, more assaultative behavior, less Schneiderian first rank symptoms and more personality change. Once again, the sample did not contain patients with MS.

Table 4.3. Criteria for a hypomanic episode in DSM-IV

Criterion	Features
A	A distinct period of persistently elevated, expansive or irritable mood lasting throughout at least four days, that is clearly different from the usual non-depressed mood
B	As in the criteria for manic episode
C	The episode is associated with an unequivocal change in functioning that is uncharacteristic of the person when not symptomatic
D	The disturbance in mood and the change in functioning are observable by others
E	The episode is not severe enough to cause marked impairment in social or occupational functioning, or to necessitate hospitalization, and there are no psychotic features

Source: With permission from the American Psychiatric Association, 1994.

Multiple sclerosis and bipolar affective disorder

Prevalence of co-morbidity

Over the years there have been case reports of mania associated with MS (Peselow *et al.*, 1981; Garfield, 1985). In addition, two patients with rapid cycling bipolar disorder and MS have been reported (Kellner *et al.*, 1984). There are also case reports of MS first presenting as mania (Kwentus *et al.*, 1986; Hurley *et al.*, 1999; Ali-Asghar *et al.*, 2004). In all these patients, the neurological examination was either normal or showed minimal signs. Brain MRI and CSF findings gave the clues as to diagnosis. While clinically informative, these case reports have not been able to address the issue of whether the co-occurrence of MS and mania exceeds chance expectation.

One study that purported to show this was by Hutchinson *et al.* (1993), who described a series of seven patients whose bipolar disorder, either presenting as recurrent manic episodes or mania alternating with depression, appeared many years before the onset of their neurological symptoms. The patients were collected over a 10 year period and were part of a database of 550 MS patients, which yielded a prevalence rate of antecedent bipolar disorder in MS of 1.2%. Five of the seven patients had had MRI brain scans during their initial psychiatric assessment and they all revealed white matter changes compatible with a diagnosis of MS, although two also had marked cerebral atrophy. Based on these findings, the authors concluded that mania may, in some patients, be a presenting symptoms of MS. This does not, however, fit with the DSM-IV concept of a temporal association between the medical and psychiatric conditions. In addition, ascertainment bias cannot be ruled out for it is unclear to what extent the 550 patients in the database were representative of MS patients in general.

Firmer evidence of an increased association between the two disorders comes from a study in Monroe County, New York. Schiffer *et al.* (1986) attempted to trace all patients in the county (population 702 238) who had both MS and bipolar affective disorder. Patients were excluded if their manic episode occurred in the context of corticosteroid treatment. Assuming lifetime risks of 0.77% and 100/100 000 for bipolar disorder and MS, respectively, the expected rate of co-morbidity was estimated to be 5.4. However, twice the number of patients were found to have both conditions. In all cases, demyelination preceded the first affective symptom by at least one year. While the absence of a more immediate temporal association between the disorders is once again problematic, the representative nature of the sample studied provides more robust evidence of a link. Indeed, Schiffer *et al.* (1986) acknowledged that their figure may, in fact, be an underestimate of the true co-morbidity because cases of either disorder may not have appeared on the computerized records kept in the county. In addition, MS may have shortened the lifespan of individuals, thereby decreasing the observed prevalence rate of patients with both conditions.

Joffe *et al.* (1987a) supported these conclusions. One hundred consecutive MS clinic attenders were interviewed with the Schedule for Affective Disorders and Schizophrenia-lifetime version that enabled diagnoses compatible with DSM-III criteria to be made. Patients had to have a history of depression and hypomania and to have sought psychiatric help before a diagnosis of bipolar disorder was given. Despite these strict selection criteria, 13% of patients were found to have a lifetime prevalence of bipolar disorder, well in excess of the 1% rate in the general population. Given the small sample size and ascertainment bias (the clinic was part of a tertiary referral process), the figure derived by Joffe *et al.* (1987a) is likely to be an overestimate, but even making allowances for these limitations, the result still points to an increased prevalence of mania associated with MS.

Indirect evidence confirming an increased association comes from a study of 2720 psychiatric inpatients screened for MS. Although only 10 patients with MS were detected, they were more likely to present with manic or hypomanic symptoms than the remainder of the in-patient sample (Pine *et al.*, 1995). In common with the series of Hutchinson *et al.* (1993), almost two thirds of patients had had psychiatric admissions before going on to receive a diagnosis of MS. In a study with a similar methodology, Lyoo *et al.* (1996) evaluated the brain MRI scans of 2783 patients admitted to a private psychiatric facility over a six year period. They found white matter changes suggestive of MS in 23 (0.83%) of their sample. Of these patients, four had been given a bipolar (manic) diagnosis. The comorbid neurological condition did not, however, seem to differentially affect psychiatric outcome. Bipolar patients with white matter lesions on MRI (considered indicative of MS by the authors) and those without lesions did not differ significantly in terms of the number of psychiatric admissions or the length of stay on the psychiatric ward.

Etiology of bipolar disorder in multiple sclerosis

Research on the development of bipolar disorder with MS is limited but has focussed on three areas: a genetic vulnerability, adverse reactions to steroids and regional brain changes demonstrated by MRI.

Genetics

Schiffer *et al.* (1986) in their Monroe County study found that 5 of their 10 patients with bipolar disorder had first- or second-degree relatives with a clinically significant affective disorder while one patient had a family history of schizophrenia. The authors did not comment on what, at first sight, seems to be an increased genetic loading for mental illness. No distinction was made between a family history of unipolar or bipolar depression, and the comparable figures for the MS patients without affective disorders were not given. However, in another study that specifically addressed the question of genetic vulnerability to mood change in MS, Schiffer *et al.* (1988) investigated 56 patients with MS, who were divided into four groups: bipolar (n = 15), unipolar (n = 16), no affective disorder (n = 13) and probably no affective disorder (n = 12). Sufficient data were available in 44 of these patients to allow conclusions to be drawn about a family history of mental illness. Two thirds of the patients with MS and bipolar disorder had a family history of affective disorder whereas only one in the group with a unipolar disorder and two of the group without affective disorders had such a history; the differences between the bipolar and unipolar groups was statistically significant. In addition, 5 of the 44 patients for whom data were available had a family history of MS. Of these, four had bipolar and one a unipolar disorder. While these numbers are small, they reinforced the conclusion that a genetic link was present between MS and affective disorder, predominantly of a bipolar subtype.

Schiffer and colleagues extended their analysis to look at the effects of gender on mood and found that 3 of the 15 bipolar probands and 1 of the 16 unipolar probands were male. Controlling for a known female bias in MS (ratio of 1.5–2 females to 1 male), females with MS were still statistically more likely to have an affective disorder than males. Among the 34 affectively ill relatives of the probands, the proportion of males and females affected was equal; however, when the disorders were split into unipolar or bipolar, female and male predilections for bipolar and unipolar disorders, respectively, were noted. An attempt to validate these findings by looking for associations with various HLA antigen subtypes was inconclusive, the small sample size preventing meaningful statistical analysis.

Although this line of research appeared to offer potentially useful clues as to the familial transmission of affective disorder in MS, in particular bipolar disorder, no further attempts have been made to replicate or extend the findings.

Contradictory results were, however, reported by another study looking at familial risk. Joffe *et al.* (1987b) used the family history method to assess the prevalence of affective disorders in the relatives of MS patients. No excess was found, leading the authors to suggest bipolar mood change in MS was an intrinsic part of the neurological disorder.

Steroid-induced mania

The mood-altering properties of steroids and adrenocorticotropic hormone (ACTH) are well known, and mild to moderate degrees of mania may occur in up to a third of patients (Ling *et al.*, 1981). Minden *et al.* (1988), in a retrospective study, investigated steroid-induced mania in a sample of 50 patients with MS. Although they could not determine dosage, duration of treatment or response to treatment from the case notes, the authors were able to interview informants to ascertain (a) whether the medication was in fact taken, (b) the intervals between starting the medication and the development of psychiatric symptoms, and (c) the duration between stopping the treatment and the cessation of mania. Psychiatric symptomatology and diagnoses were made using the Schedule for Affective Disorders and Schizophrenia-lifetime version, which generated research diagnostic criteria diagnoses. Nine patients developed mania or hypomania (at least one week of elevated or irritable mood and increased activity of various forms) during the course of their treatment. There was a close temporal relationship between symptom onset/resolution and treatment starting and ending. In one patient, the elevated mood persisted and worsened in time, ending in a full-blown manic state with psychotic features that gradually subsided into a depressive disorder on discontinuation of the ACTH.

A search for clinical predictors of mania was limited to the ACTH group as, in the authors' opinion, they were more likely to become manic than the prednisone-treated patients. The most striking finding was that a history of major depression, either before or after the diagnosis of MS, or a family history of unipolar depression or alcoholism, or both, were risk factors for patients becoming manic. There were no differences between the manic and non-manic patients in any demographic or disease-related variables. In addition, manic symptoms did not occur with every drug exposure. Although the study was not without methodological problems, in particular the retrospective nature of the data collected, the evidence suggested that risk factors for mania include ACTH as opposed to prednisone treatment and a premorbid and/or genetic (familial) diathesis for psychopathology, particularly depression or alcoholism.

The prophylactic nature of lithium therapy in corticotropin-induced mania (Falk *et al.*, 1979) means that physicians should not necessarily discontinue treatment if patients become high. Rather, the careful monitoring of the mental state on a reduced dose of ACTH, together with the addition of lithium, may allow treatment to continue.

Cerebral correlates of mania

Before discussing the MRI brain changes reported in manic MS patients, a summary of the MRI findings in bipolar patients without a neurological illness is required. The most replicated findings are those of white matter and periventricular hyperintensities, while the evidence linking bipolar disorders to more regional brain pathology, in particular abnormalities in the limbic structures of the temporal lobes, is more equivocal. Similarly, the support for any definite cerebral laterality effect is inconclusive. The literature has been reviewed by Soares and Mann (1997), who also noted some evidence of a larger third ventricle and perhaps a smaller temporal lobe volume in bipolar patients.

The MRI finding of periventricular white matter lesions has certain similarities with MS and it has been suggested that the two disorders could share an etiology (Young *et al.*, 1997) or that bipolar disorder arises from anomalous myelination (Dupont *et al.*, 1995). Such views, however, lack substance. While there are some imaging similarities in a subset of patients, there are also many more substantial differences. Cerebral white matter changes on MRI are virtually ubiquitous in MS, which is not the case in bipolar disorder. In addition, the pathology of the white matter lesions in patients with bipolar disorders has not been established. At present, a vascular etiology is favored (Soares and Mann, 1997). Consequently, MRI may have good sensitivity in detecting white matter changes, but it lacks the specificity to determine etiology.

No neuroimaging study has addressed the specific question of cerebral changes in MS patients who also have mania. In a MRI study of psychosis in MS, Feinstein *et al.* (1992) noted the presence of increased plaque in the regions surrounding the temporal horns of psychotic as opposed to non-psychotic MS patients. The psychotic sample was equally divided between affective and schizophrenia-like presentations and there were no MRI differences between them. As there is no evidence that the disease process in MS selectively targets these areas, the authors suggested the lesion burden or white matter loss in the temporal lobes may have to exceed a putative critical threshold in patients with a prior diathesis for mood disorders before clinical symptoms are triggered.

There is little in the literature to substantiate or refute this view. Of the five manic patients who underwent MRI of the brain in the series reported by Hutchinson *et al.* (1993), only one had lesions in the temporal lobes. Reischies *et al.* (1988) looked at the relationship between MRI brain changes and individual psychiatric symptoms and reported that periventricular and frontal white matter lesions were closely associated with poor judgement and euphoria. However, their study had a number of shortcomings, in particular a failure to use valid and reliable methods of rating psychiatric symptoms and, consequently, the absence of psychiatric diagnoses. Therefore, it could not be ascertained whether the observed changes in mood and judgement were part of a manic illness. In the study of Lyoo *et al.* (1996) comprising 23 patients admitted to a psychiatric hospital, a fronto-temporal lesion distribution in all patients and generalized atrophy in 15 were the notable MRI findings. Finally, Casanova *et al.* (1996) confirmed at postmortem the presence of marked, diffuse periventricular demyelination in a 81-year-old female with late-onset mania but whose neurological examination had been normal over a 31 year period. Although the case report highlighted the possibility of mania alone being a symptom of MS, a predominantly periventricular lesion distribution in an elderly patient is too non-specific to be regarded as a firm cerebral correlate of mania.

Differential diagnosis

The diagnosis of a hypomanic or manic episode is often straightforward, but two other clinical disorders may have some overlapping features. Hypomania must be differentiated from euphoria, and mania with psychotic features should be distinguished from a non-affective psychosis.

Euphoria

For many years, euphoria was considered virtually pathognomonic of the abnormal mental state in MS. In an influential early paper, Cottrell and Wilson (1926) reported it in over two thirds of their sample and defined four states: mental well being or "euphoria sclerotica" characterized by a persistently cheerful mood; physical well being or "eutonia sclerotica" distinguished by unconcern over physical disability; "pes sclerotica," an incongruous optimizm for the future; and emotional lability. Although the validity of this approach has never been adequately proven, the above criteria, with the exception of emotional lability, are still considered pathognomonic of the disorder. Consequently, as currently defined, euphoria bears some similarity to hypomania with regard to elevated affect, but it lacks the associated motor overactivity and increased energy manifesting as a flurry of new ideas and activities. Euphoria is fixed rather than fluctuating and may best be considered akin to a personality change; this clinical picture is, for the most part, readily discernible from hypomania (Surridge, 1969).[1]

---

[1] An absorbing historical account of disorders of affect in MS has been provided by Finger (1998), who does not, however, make a distinction between euphoria and pseudobulbar affect (Ch. 5). Nevertheless, in the quotes that he includes from such luminaries as Charcot and Gowers amongst others can be discerned the hallmarks of abnormal behavior that would in time come to be called euphoria.

Few studies since Cottrell and Wilson (1926) have reported such high rates. Surridge (1969), comparing his case register of MS patients with a control group with muscular dystrophy found euphoria in 26% of the MS group and in none of the muscular dystrophy group. Poser (1980) reported a 24% rate while Rabins *et al.* (1986), using Cottrell and Wilson's (1926) definition, noted a 48% point prevalence. A reason for this decline in frequency was the recognition that many patients with emotional lability appeared superficially euphoric but, in reality, had subjective evidence of depressed mood. In addition, pseudobulbar affect, which was included in Cottrell and Wilson's rubric of emotional lability came to be considered a distinct entity. Summarizing the various studies up to the late 1980s, Rabins (1990) arrived at a *median* rate of 25%.

Since then, the estimates have fallen further, a fact likely attributable to the introduction of structured interviews coupled with more representative sample selection. Two studies used the Neuropsychiatric Inventory (Cummings *et al.*, 1994) to detect euphoria in MS patients and arrived at similar conclusions. Diaz-Olavarrieta *et al.* (1999) compared the profiles of 44 MS patients and 25 healthy controls. Depressive symptoms were the most common psychiatric disturbances noted, occurring in 79% of patients. Euphoria at 13% came a distant sixth, after agitation (40%), anxiety (37%), irritability (35%) and apathy (20%). However, it was one of two signs and symptoms (the other being hallucinations) that correlated with MRI changes, namely fronto-temporal pathology. In another study using the Neuropsychiatric Inventory, Fishman *et al.* (2004) investigated 75 clinic attendees with MS and compared the results with those from 25 healthy control subjects. Applying a factor analysis to their data, the authors identified euphoria/disinhibition in 9% of the patients. Clinical and social correlates included secondary progressive disease course, poor insight, decreased cognition and higher care-giver stress.

Euphoria is considered a manifestation of advanced MS commensurate with more extensive cerebral damage. Studies have demonstrated an association with greater physical disability and cognitive impairment (Surridge, 1969; Rabins *et al.*, 1986; Fishman *et al.*, 2004), progressive disease course (Rabins *et al.*, 1986; Fishman *et al.*, 2004), enlarged ventricles on CT (Rabins *et al.*, 1986), frontal lesions on MRI (Reischies *et al.*, 1988; Diaz-Olavarrieta *et al.*, 1999) and more widespread lesions on MRI (Ron and Logsdail, 1989).

Before leaving the topic, it is important to note that frontal pathology, although implicated in the pathogenesis of euphoria, may also give rise to other very different behaviors, one being apathy. In a study that utilized the Frontal Systems Behaviour Scale, MS patients were found to have two significant difficulties, apathy and executive dysfunction (Chiaravalloti and DeLuca, 2003). Disorders of self-regulation, like euphoria, were not found. This observation is not, however, at odds with the literature reviewed this far. Rather, it is a good illustration of how behavior reflects the involvement of discreet fronto-subcortical circuits, three of which have been described: a dorso lateral prefrontal circuit subserving executive function, an orbito frontal circuit linked to self-regulation (which includes euphoria) and an anterior cingulate circuit associated with motivation (Cummings, 1993; Ch. 12). Each may be affected individually or in various combinations, hence clinical presentations that can vary considerably, ranging from disinhibition to disinterest.

Non-affective psychosis

Differentiating a psychotic manic patient from a patient with a non-affective psychosis may also present a clinical challenge as the latter may display considerable agitation and emotional arousal, leading to an erroneous impression of mania. It is, however, the prominence and persistence of mood change that suggests an affective diagnosis.

The importance of establishing the correct diagnosis is self-evident, determining both the treatment and prognosis.

Treatment

In the absence of published treatment trials of bipolar affective disorder associated with MS, anecdotal evidence has to suffice (see the vignette on p. 77).

The clinical data in this vignette illustrates the many potential difficulties posed by treating the floridly manic MS patient and highlights the range of drug treatments that may be required. Lesser degrees of mania, without psychosis, are easier to treat and frequently respond well to monotherapy in the form of a mood-stabilizing drug. Here, the clinician is faced with a number of choices, the most widely used medications being lithium carbonate, carbamazepine and sodium valproate. More recently, newer antiseizure drugs such as gabapentin and lamotrigine have also been reported to have mood-stabilizing properties, but their use in MS patients with bipolar disorder awaits clarification.

Of all the drugs available, the most data have accrued with respect to lithium. Although it is generally an effective treatment for mania in patients with neurological disease (Young *et al.*, 1977), the information pertaining to its use in MS patients with bipolar disorder remains limited, contradictory and anecdotal. Kemp *et al.* (1977) and Solomon (1978) found the drug was effective while Kellner *et al.* (1984) and Kwentus *et al.* (1986) did not. As lithium is known to produce a diuresis, MS patients with bladder problems may have difficulty tolerating the drug. Furthermore, Solomon (1978) cautioned against mistaking the development of neurological impairment as a sign of lithium toxicity. Should the manic episode be suggestive of an exacerbation in a patient's MS, Peselow *et al.* (1981) endorsed a combination of prednisone plus lithium. Should the mania be steroid induced, a dose reduction or the addition of litium may prove helpful (Falk *et al.*, 1979; Minden *et al.*, 1988).

Vignette

A 40-year-old married female on long-term disability payments because of a 10 year history of MS (EDSS of 6.0) was brought to the emergency room by her husband one evening. The emergency services had been called to assist him with this. The husband reported his wife had been sleeping poorly, had recently spent a large sum of money on trivial items of no practical use while internet shopping and had assaulted him with her walking stick. The patient appeared irritable and was verbally threatening during questioning. She did not understand why a psychiatrist had been called and demanded an immediate release so that she could pursue a plan that she was convinced would rid the world of AIDS. She spoke grandiosely of writing a book explaining her ideas and was convinced this work would make her famous and rich.

A diagnosis of bipolar affective disorder, manic episode was made; the patient was admitted to hospital and detained under a provision of the Mental Health Act. She refused all medication and had to be declared incapable of consenting to treatment. Her behavior on the ward was dismissive and angry and her cane was confiscated because of assaults on the nursing staff. Without the cane, her balance was precarious, but such was her degree of motor overactivity and manically driven behavior, she refused a wheelchair or any form of assistance and had a number of falls. Sedation was needed and had to be given by the intramuscular route. Lorazepam was injected at a dose of 2 mg four times per day, as required. This sedated the patient but produced further unsteadiness, leaving her at an added risk of falling. A nursing assistant was, therefore, assigned to remain constantly with her. While the lorazepam was effective in slowing the patient down, it did not produce a lessening in her grandiose delusional beliefs. An antipsychotic drug, olanzapine 10 mg/day, was, therefore, given intramuscularly as she still refused to take oral treatment. After 24 hours, the dose was raised to 10 mg twice daily and one week later the patient's irritability and grandiosity gradually began improving.

At this point, she agreed to take medication orally and the olanzapine administration was changed accordingly. Lithium carbonate 300 mg three times a day was introduced, but the patient was unable to tolerate the drug because it exacerbated her urinary incontinence, thereby causing renewed distress. Sodium valproate was substituted and 250 mg given twice daily with food. Soon thereafter, the olanzapine was gradually tapered off over the course of a week while the sodium valproate increased by increments of 250 mg until she was taking a dose of 500 mg twice a day. Lorazepam was no longer required and three weeks after admission the patient's mood was judged to be euthymic and her thought content normal. She was on monotherapy and tolerating the sodium valproate well. She was discharged from hospital and given an outpatient follow-up appointment. Five years later, she remains well on sodium valproate.

An alternative mood stabilizer is sodium valproate, which may be equally effective but better tolerated (Stip and Daoust, 1995). Given that both MS and bipolar disorder may run relapsing–remitting courses, prophylaxis with mood-stabilizing drugs may be required for many years.

Should sedation be required for agitation, the benzodiazepine clonazepam is recommended. If patients with mania become psychotic, antipsychotic treatment will often be required. There are no drug trials on which to base recommendations, but the newer antipsychotic drugs (olanzapine, quetiapine and risperidone) are anecdotally effective and produce fewer extrapyramidal symptoms than the less expensive phenothiazines (e.g. chlorpromazine, perphenazine) and butyrophenones (e.g. haloperidol). They are, therefore, less likely to exacerbate preexisting motor, balance and co-ordination difficulties.[2]

Finally, returning to the theme of mania heralding the onset of MS, Ali-Asghar *et al.* (2004) have described such a patient in whom psychotropic medication was largely ineffective. Instead, monthly intravenous cyclophosphamide and alternate day subcutaneous interferon beta-1b brought about some improvement in her mental state, although not enough to allow her to live independently after discharge from hospital. This bleak outcome is, however, the exception.

Summary

- Bipolar affective disorder (manic episodes) in association with MS occurs more frequently than chance expectation.
- The possibility of a shared genetic diathisis could explain the association, although preliminary results need replication.
- Both MS and bipolar disorder are associated with white matter changes on MRI, but the pathogenesis of these lesions is likely to be different.
- There is MRI evidence suggesting manic patients with psychosis have plaques that are distributed predominantly in bilateral temporal horn areas.
- MS patients who become hypomanic or manic on steroid therapy are more likely to have a family history of affective disorder and/or alcoholism or a premorbid psychiatric history of these disorders. This should not be a contra-indication to treatment with steroids although caution is advised.
- Lithium carbonate is an effective treatment for manic and hypomanic (including steroid-induced) episodes. Sodium valproate is an effective alternative treatment for patients unable to tolerate lithium.
- Should mania be accompanied by psychosis, antipsychotic medication, preferably newer drugs like olanzapine and quetiapine, will be required. Benzodiazepines are useful if sedation is needed.

---

[2] It must not be forgotten that, when encountering a depressed MS patient, the physician should always inquire about a past history of mania. Should there be one, the correct diagnosis is bipolar affective disorder and the treatment plan may need to be modified by including a mood-stabilizing drug in addition to the required antidepressant.

- Euphoria should not be confused with hypomania. It represents a fixed mental state change and is generally associated with more severe disease, greater physical disability, cognitive dysfunction, lack of insight and a significant brain lesion load, often more frontal in distribution.

References

Ali-Asghar AA, Taber KH, Hurley R, Hayman LA. (2004) Pure neuropsychiatric presentation of multiple sclerosis. *American Journal of Psychiatry*, **161**, 226–232.

American Psychiatric Association (1994) *The Diagnostic and Statistical Manual*, 4th edn. Washington, DC: American Psychiatric Press.

Casanova MF, Kruesi M, Mannheim G. (1996) Multiple sclerosis and bipolar disorder: a case report with autopsy findings. *Journal of Neuropsychiatry and Clinical Neurosciences*, **8**, 206–208.

Chiaravalloti ND, DeLuca J. (2003) Assessing the behavioral consequences of multiple sclerosis: an application of the Frontal Systems Behavior Scale (FrSBe). *Cognitive and Behavioral Neurology*, **16**, 54–67.

Cook BL, Shukla S, Hoff AL, Aronson TA. (1987) Mania with associated organic factors *Acta Psychiatrica Scandinavica*, **76**, 674–677.

Cottrell SS, Wilson SAK (1926) The affective symptomatology of disseminated sclerosis. *Journal of Neurological Psychopathology*, **7**, 1–30.

Cummings JL. (1993) Frontal-subcortical circuits and human behavior. *Archives of Neurology*, **50**, 873–880.

Cummings JL, Mega M, Gray K, *et al.* (1994) The Neuropsychiatric Inventory: comprehensive assessment of psychopathology in dementia. *Neurology*, **44**, 2308–2314.

Diaz-Olavarrieta C, Cummings JL, Velasquez J, Garcia de la Cadena C. (1999) Neuropsychiatric manifestations of multiple sclerosis. *Journal of Neuropsychiatry and Clinical Neurosciences*, **11**, 51–57.

Dupont RM, Jernigan TL, Heindel WN, *et al.* (1995) Magnetic resonance imaging and mood disorders: localisation of white matter and other subcortical abnormalities. *Archives of General Psychiatry*, **52**, 747–755.

Falk WE, Mahnke MW, Poskanzer DC. (1979) Lithium prophylaxis of corticotropin-induced psychosis. *Journal of the American Medical Association*, **241**, 1011–1012.

Feinstein A, du Boulay G, Ron MA. (1992) Psychotic illness in multiple sclerosis. A clinical and magnetic resonance imaging study. *British Journal of Psychiatry*, **161**, 680–685.

Finger S. (1998) A happy state of mind: A history of mild elation, denial of disability, optimism and laughing in multiple sclerosis. *Archives of Neurology*, **55**, 241–250.

Fishman I, Benedict RHB, Bakshi R, Priore R, Weinstock-Guttman B. (2004) Construct validity and frequency of euphoria sclerotica in multiple sclerosis. *Journal of Neuropsychiatry and Clinical Neurosciences*, **16**, 350–356.

Garfield DAS. (1985) Multiple sclerosis and affective disorder: 2 cases of mania with psychosis. *Psychotherapy and Psychosomatics*, **44**, 22–33.

Hurley RA, Taber KH, Zhang J, Hayman LA. (1999) Neuropsychiatric presentation of multiple sclerosis. *Journal of Neuropsychiatry and Clinical Neurosciences*, **11**, 5–7.

Hutchinson M, Stack J, Buckley P. (1993) Bipolar affective disorder prior to the onset of multiple sclerosis. *Acta Neurologica Scandinavica*, **88**, 388–393.

Joffe RT, Lippert GP, Gray TA, Sawa G, Horvath Z. (1987a) Mood disorder and multiple sclerosis. *Archives of Neurology*, **44**, 376–378.

Joffe RT, Lippert GP, Gray TA, Sawa G, Horvath Z. (1987b) Personal and family history of affective illness in patients with multiple sclerosis. *Journal of Affective Disorders*, **12**, 63–65.

Kellner CH, Davenport Y, Post RM, Ross RJ. (1984) Rapid cycling bipolar disorder and multiple sclerosis. *American Journal of Psychiatry*, **141**, 112–113.

Kemp K, Lion JR, Magram G. (1977) Lithium in the case of a manic patient with multiple sclerosis: a case report. *Diseases of the Nervous System*, **38**, 210–211.

Krauthammer C, Klerman GL. (1978) Secondary mania. Manic syndromes associated with antecedent physical illness and drugs. *Archives of General Psychiatry*, **35**, 1333–1339.

Kwentus JA, Hart RP, Calabrese V, Hekmati A. (1986) Mania as a symptom of multiple sclerosis. *Psychosomatics*, **27**, 729–731.

Ling MHM, Perry PJ, Tsuang MT. (1981) Side effects of corticosteroid therapy. *Archives of General Psychiatry*, **38**, 471–477.

Lyoo IK, Seol HY, Byun HS, Renshaw PF. (1996) Unsuspected multiple sclerosis in patients with psychiatric disorders. *Journal of Neuropsychiatry and Clinical Neurosciences*, **8**, 54–59.

Minden SL, Orav J, Schildkraut JJ. (1988) Hypomanic reactions to ACTH and prednisone treatment for multiple sclerosis. *Neurology*, **38**, 1631–1634.

Peselow ED, Deutsch SI, Fieve RR, Kaufman M. (1981) Coexistent manic symptoms and multiple sclerosis. *Psychosomatics*, **22**, 824–825.

Pine DS, Douglas CJ, Charles E, Davies M, Kahn D. (1995) Patients with multiple sclerosis presenting to psychiatric hospitals. *Journal of Clinical Psychiatry*, **56**, 297–306.

Poser CM. (1980) Exacerbations, activity and progression in multiple sclerosis. *Archives of Neurology*, **37**, 471–474.

Rabins PV. (1990) Euphoria in multiple sclerosis. In *Neurobehavioral Aspects of Multiple Sclerosis*, ed. SM Rao. New York: Oxford University Press, pp. 180–185.

Rabins PV, Brooks BR, O'Donnell P, *et al.* (1986) Structural brain correlates of emotional disorder in multiple sclerosis. *Brain*, **109**, 585–597.

Reischies FM, Baum K, Bräu H, Hedde JP, Schwindt G. (1988) Cerebral magnetic resonance imaging findings in multiple sclerosis. Relation to disturbance of affect, drive and cognition. *Archives of Neurology*, **45**, 1114–1116.

Ron MA, Logsdail SJ. (1989) Psychiatric morbidity in multiple sclerosis: a clinical and MRI study. *Psychological Medicine*, **19**, 887–895.

Schiffer RB, Wineman M, Weitkamp LR (1986) Association between bipolar affective disorder and multiple sclerosis. *American Journal of Psychiatry*, **143**, 94–95.

Schiffer RB, Weitkamp LR, Wineman M, Guttormsen S. (1988) Multiple sclerosis and affective disorder. Family history, sex and HLA-DR antigens. *Archives of Neurology*, **45**, 1345–1348.

Soares JC, Mann JJ. (1997) The anatomy of mood disorders: review of structural neuroimaging studies. *Biological Psychiatry*, **41**, 86–106.

Solomon JG. (1978) Multiple sclerosis masquerading as lithium toxicity. *Journal of Nervous and Mental Disease*, **166**, 663–665.

Stip E, Daoust L. (1995) Valproate in the treatment of mood disorder due to multiple sclerosis. *Canadian Journal of Psychiatry*, **40**, 219–220.

Surridge D. (1969) an investigation into some psychiatric aspects of multiple sclerosis. *British Journal of Psychiatry*, **115**, 749–764.

Young CR, Weiss EL, Bowers MB, Mazure CM. (1997) The differential diagnosis of multiple sclerosis and bipolar affective disorder. *Journal of Clinical Psychiatry*, **58**, 123.

Young LD, Taylor I, Holmstrom V. (1977) Lithium treatment of patients with affective illness associated with organic brain symptoms. *American Journal of Psychiatry*, **134**, 1405–1407.

5

Multiple sclerosis and pseudobulbar affect

Pseudobulbar affect (PBA) has also been called pathological laughing and crying, emotional incontinence and excessive emotionalism. More recently, the term involuntary emotional expression disorder was coined (Cummings *et al.*, 2006). In this chapter, for the sake of consistency and with an eye of historical verisimilitude, the syndrome will be referred to as PBA. It has been described with diverse neurological disorders, such as Alzheimer's disease (Starkstein *et al.*, 1995), stroke (Morris *et al.*, 1993), cerebral tumors (Monteil and Cohadon, 1996), amyotropic lateral sclerosis (Gallagher, 1989) and multiple sclerosis (Minden and Schiffer, 1990). Most of the research on PBA in MS was completed prior to 1970, and the studies are beset by problems with methodology. Of the five pre-1970 papers, only Cottrell and Wilson's (1926) frequently cited article was devoted exclusively to the topic, the remainder discussing PBA in the context of other mental state abnormalities occurring in MS.

Review of earlier studies

Cottrell and Wilson (1926) studied 100 patients with MS seen in a tertiary referral center. They developed a standardized interview of 44 questions probing the patient's mood, thoughts, somatic complaints and affect. By separating mood from affect, the authors made an important distinction between what patients felt and what they expressed, the two conditions not always being synonymous. The study contained a wealth of descriptive data, including demographic characteristics, the duration of neurological symptoms, and physical disability divided according to predominant system involvement (i.e. cerebellar, spinal, etc.). Abnormalities of affect were split into three categories: "euphoria sclerotica," "eutonia sclerotica" and "pes sclerotica," respectively. The first referred to a mood of serenity and cheerfulness, the second to a sense of somatic well being despite physical disability and the third to an incongruous and misplaced optimizm of eventual full recovery from the MS.

The study's most notable finding was that 63% of patients had euphoria and 10% depression. A further 25% were noted to have increased variability in mood since the onset of MS. Therefore, the overwhelming majority of patients had experienced a disordered mood since the onset of demyelination. With regard to a sense of physical well being ("eutonia sclerotica"), this was endorsed by 84% of patients.

It was however Cottrell and Wilson's comments on affect that are germane to PBA. Ninety five percent of their sample were deemed to have various degrees of pathological affect; 71% smiling and laughing constantly, 19% with mixed smiling and laughing plus crying, 2% displaying rapid shifts from laughing to crying and 3% crying constantly. These signs were noticeable for occurring "in season and out of season, under slight provocation, at the bidding of minimal stimuli and make their appearance when there is certainly no obvious warrant for them." A more conservative reading of the study suggests that in only half the patients was the emotional display inappropriate, something the authors also acknowledged. No association was noted with the degree of physical disability, duration of illness, or grouping of neurological symptoms. Another important observation was the presence of outward displays of happiness unmatched by comparable, subjective feelings. The authors concluded that "emotional facility and overaction form one of the cardinal features of the disease."

The study was important for it was the first to investigate the problem of PBA in MS in considerable detail. However, there were a number of flaws that compromised the validity of the conclusions. Patients were seen at a tertiary referral center and no details were given about how they were selected. Consequently, the sample was unlikely to reflect a representative group of patients with MS. Furthermore, there were no attempts to validate the structured interview or the arbitrarily defined categories. This failure to define exactly what constituted the syndrome of PBA was to bedevil subsequent studies too. It is, however, important to view Cottrell and Wilson's (1926) findings in a historical context. Judged by the more rigorous standards applied to research methodology today, the weaknesses are apparent. But, the study served an important function by focussing attention on mentation in patients with MS and highlighted the fact that disturbances in affect were common.

Langworthy *et al.* (1941), in a study of behavioral abnormalities seen in 199 patients with MS attending an outpatient clinic; noted that in the later stages of the disease some patients presented with uncontrollable laughter and/or crying. They regarded the condition as part of pseudobulbar palsy and postulated a freeing of bulbar mechanisms from cortical control. Thirteen patients displayed the phenomenon, establishing a point prevalence of 6.5%, considerably lower than Cottrell and Wilson's figure. The majority of their patients displayed uncontrollable crying, with some patients alternating rapidly between laughing and crying. The authors stressed that pathological laughing and euphoria were two distinct states, but then equivocated and wondered whether the latter was not perhaps a mild variant of forced laughing. The splitting of affective categories accounts, at least in part, for the substantially different prevalence rates between this study and Cottrell and Wilson's earlier effort. Langworthy and Hesser (1940) also speculated as to the etiology of the syndrome and concluded that bilateral rather than unilateral pathology, primitive reflexes, intellectual enfeeblement and difficulties with swallowing and speech were frequent concomitant findings.

The definition of "emotional dyscontrol" was subsequently loosened by Sugar and Nadell (1943). Their sample consisted of 28 inpatients, all with long-standing MS. Forty three percent displayed constant smiling and laughing, 25% had a mixed picture (smiling, laughing and crying), 4% changed rapidly between the two states and 7% cried constantly. Overall, 79% of their patients were deemed to have exaggerated emotional expression. The study suffered from the same methodological limitations as Cottrell and Wilson's, without the virtue of good sample size.

In a wide-ranging investigation of psychiatric aspects of MS, Pratt (1951) selected 100 outpatients with MS, excluding those with more advanced disease. Once again, the interview formulated by Cottrell and Wilson was used, but the study differed because of the inclusion of a control group of 100 non-MS patients, all but three having "organic disease of the nervous system." The disorders that constituted the control group were not revealed, but patients and controls were matched for age and gender. The patients with MS were found to laugh ($n = 22$) and cry ($n = 29$) more easily, giving a 51% prevalence rate for pathological affect. Although Pratt excluded patients with marked neurological disability, he concluded that impaired control over laughing and crying was more often associated with a more severe degree of physical disability and intellectual impairment.

Finally, Surridge (1969) compared psychiatric abnormalities in 108 MS patients and 39 patients with muscular dystrophy. The latter were chosen as a control group because of the debilitating nature of their disease, despite a sparing of cerebral involvement. By controlling for the effects of disability, attribution of psychopathology could be assigned either to cerebral or reactive causes. Although the principle was a sound one, any advantage was offset by applying arbitrary definitions and severity ratings to mental state changes such as depression, euphoria and intellectual deterioration. In addition, a cut-off age of 40 years was stipulated, in order to avoid the possible complicating factor of menopause. Some patients were also excluded prior to the study onset because of signs of mental illness, as were patients who had had MS for less than two years. Within this tightly selected sample, exaggerated emotional responses were reported in 11 (10%) MS patients and no controls. There was no concomitant subjective emotional distress in 9 of these 11 patients, suggesting a split between what patients felt and what they expressed. A significant association was noted between the emotional dyscontrol and intellectual decline, as in the anecdotal report of Langworthy (1940) and Hesser, but in contrast to Cottrell and Wilson's (1926) observation that such a change was rare. Given this finding, Surridge concluded that emotional dyscontrol was a product of cerebral disease and akin to that seen in pseudobulbar palsy.

In summary, these five studies produced markedly different point prevalence rates, ranging from 6.5% to 95%. Arbitrary and inadequate definitions of "emotional dyscontrol" (used synonymously with PBA or emotional exaggeration), biased sample selection, and the use of non-standardized interviews of unproven validity and reliability explain the inconsistent findings.

Definition of pseudobulbar affect

An attempt to bring some diagnostic rigor to a general definition of PBA, irrespective of the underlying neurological disorder, was supplied by Poeck (1969), who distinguished PBA and a number of other symptom complexes. These included emotional lability, which he regarded as episodes of crying (and less frequently laughing) that were excessive but appropriate to the situation in which it occurred; "witzelsucht" (facetiousness) and euphoria, associated with a fluctuating and congruent affective tone; and laughing or crying secondary to substance abuse, psychosis or as part of histrionic behavior. In contrast, PBA was regarded as a distinct syndrome caused by a release of inhibition of the motor component of facial expression. According to Poeck, the full syndrome had four components: response to non-specific stimuli, absence of an association between affective change and the observed expression, absence of voluntary control of facial expression, and an absence of a corresponding change in mood exceeding the period of laughing or crying. This is the definition that has been adopted in this chapter, although it is acknowledged that such clear subdivisions are not always possible. In practice, a degree of overlap may characterize many presentations begging questions, as yet unresolved, about etiology.

It is useful to conceptualize changes in mood and affect along a continuum. At one end are patients with a clear diagnosis of major depression, who have the subjective complaints of low mood coupled with objective signs of altered affect. At the other end are patients who meet strict criteria for PBA, with loss of affective control but without the subjective complaints of low or elevated mood. Between these two clearly defined syndromes come a large number of patients who display varying degrees of emotional lability, without meeting criteria for either disorder. These patients, to date, have slipped through the diagnostic cracks, their clinical distress caught in a taxonomical limbo where uncertainty over their status runs the risk of obscuring treatment options.

Prevalence and neurobehavioral correlates of pseudobulbar affect

The prevalence and behavioral correlates of PBA were ascertained in a consecutive, outpatient sample of 152 patients with clinically or laboratory definite MS (Feinstein *et al.*, 1997). Subjects were assessed with the Pathological Laughing and Crying Scale (PLACS) (Robinson *et al.*, 1993), which quantifies aspects of laughing and crying including duration, relationship to external events, degree of voluntary control, inappropriateness in relation to emotions and extent of subsequent distress. Furthermore, subjects had to meet Poeck's stringent criteria for PBA before they were deemed to have the syndrome.

A group of control subjects with MS, but without PBA, were used as controls. They were matched to the patients with PBA on relevant demographic and disease-related variables. All study participants underwent a neurological examination on the day of testing and overall disability was assessed with the Expanded Disability Status Score (EDSS). Subscale scores for each of the eight systems were recorded (pyramidal, sensory, brainstem, cerebellar, visual, bladder and bowel, mentation and "other"). The psychometric evaluation included a measure of premorbid intelligence (American National Adult Reading Test [ANART; Nelson, 1982], the Wechsler Adult Intelligence Scale-Revised [WAIS-R; Wechsler, 1981]), from which verbal, performance and full-scale IQ values were obtained, and two self-report questionnaires, namely the Hospital Anxiety and Depression Scale (Zigmond and Snaith, 1983) and the 28 item General Health Questionnaire (GHQ; Goldberg and Hillier 1979), containing four subscales (anxiety, somatic complaints, social dysfunction and depression) scored in a simple Likert way (0-1-2-3).

Results showed that of the 152 subjects screened, 15 had PBA, thereby establishing a point prevalence of 9.9%. Comparisons between them and the remainder of the sample revealed no significant age or gender differences. Eleven of the patients with PBA agreed to participate in further cognitive testing and their results were compared with those from 13 matched control subjects. Six subjects displayed prominent crying, three had difficulties with uncontrollable laughing and two had a mixed picture. The four subjects with PBA who refused participation did not differ significantly from the remainder with regard to demographic or disease characteristics.

The PBA group had had MS for approximately 2.5 years longer than the remainder of the sample, but this difference did not reach statistical significance. They were also more likely to have entered a chronic–progressive disease course. The mean EDSS score for the PBA group was 6.4 (standard deviation [SD], 1.7). There were no differences between patients with PBA and controls on any of the EDSS subscales, including brainstem involvement. Given the reported association between brainstem involvement and displays of pathological affect (Wilson, 1924), the data were further analyzed by dichotomizing the variable "brainstem involvement" into either "present" or "absent" and the patients with PBA were compared with their controls. This too did not produce a significant difference, with 7 of the 11 PBA patients (64%) and 7 of the 13 controls (53.8%) having brainstem signs on neurological examination.

Subjects with PBA were not more likely than their controls to have a premorbid or family history of mental illness. The mean PLACS score for the PBA group was significantly higher than for the control group, but there were no group differences with respect to the Hospital Anxiety and Depression Scale scores. None of the patients who displayed pathological laughing were judged clinically to be euphoric. The most frequently endorsed GHQ items were in the subscale devoted to social dysfunction. There was a significant correlation ($r = 0.3$; $p = 0.001$) between the GHQ social dysfunction score and physical disability (EDSS) for the entire sample ($n = 152$). However, patients with PBA did not have higher social dysfunction scores than their control group.

Premorbid IQ according to the ANART in the PBA group was estimated at 110 (SD = 4.1) and did not differ significantly from the control sample (112.0; SD, 5.8). In both groups, performance IQ on the WAIS-R was more adversely affected than verbal IQ. The PBA patients had substantially lower performance and full scale scores, but not verbal IQ scores. Analyses of the WAIS-R data revealed that the PBA patients were much more impaired on the arithmetic subscale and on two of the performance tasks, namely "digit symbol" and "picture arrangement." A more detailed analysis of the raw "digit span" scores showed that the PBA and control groups did not differ on "digits forwards," but significant differences were apparent on "digits backwards."

Summarizing the findings, 10% of a large, consecutive sample of community-based patients with MS had PBA, with uncontrollable crying proving more common than laughing. The study was careful to exclude patients whose problem was primarily one of emotional lability. However, the group scores on the PLACS demonstrated that such a clear-cut separation was not always possible. The demographic and disease profile to emerge was one without gender predilection, of fairly long-standing disease duration and associated with progressive, significant physical disability, not necessarily of brainstem origin. In conformity with Poeck's 1969 notion of PBA, patients did not experience greater subjective emotional distress. In addition, they were more cognitively impaired.

Etiology

General theories of pseudobulbar affect

The precise etiology of PBA is unclear and theories abound (Davison and Kelman, 1939; Ironside, 1956; Black, 1982; Ross and Stewart, 1987; Shaibani et al., 1994;

Dark *et al.*, 1996;). Embedded within the theory, however, are some well-established facts. Kinnear Wilson (1924) in his classic paper entitled "Pathological laughing and crying" delineated three key anatomical areas central to the pathogenesis: (a) the bulbar nuclei in the brainstem exert functional control over the facial and respiratory muscles; (b) voluntary control of these bulbar nuclei resides in the cortex; (c) connections between the brainstem and cortex run in the corticospinal, corticobulbar and corticopontine tracts. Should the brainstem nuclei become disconnected from the cortex, voluntary control over the expression of emotion may be lost, resulting in uncontrollable laughing or crying divorced from subjective feelings of mirth or sadness. Useful as a starting point in our understanding, this model leaves many questions unanswered. For example, what are the relevant cortical regions involved in PBA? And what explains the presence of PBA in patients whose pathology is primarily subcortical? Clearly, the search for cerebral correlates demands a more elaborate explanation and, moreover, one that casts a wider net than the corticobulbar axis.

Kinnear Wilson's (1924) seminal paper did, however, provide more clues. The distinction between patients with volitional and emotional facial paresis was highlighted. In the former, there is an inability to demonstrate a smile voluntarily, for example smiling before the camera (the "Kodak" smile). Here the lesion is likely to be found in the primary motor cortex. In emotional facial paresis, there is a loss of reflexive facial responses, which manifests as the inability to smile in response to something funny. This problem is linked to lesions in frontal or limbic areas. While the inability to smile at something considered funny is the phenomenological opposite of PBA, what the two conditions share is a breakdown in the control of facial expression, something mediated, in part, by the limbic system. Limbic areas are also considered pivotal in modulating unconscious or visceral emotion. Central to this neural circuit are the amygdala and its reciprocal connections to the orbito frontal cortex (Mega *et al.*, 1997; Arciniegas and Topkoff, 2000). These regions process information from cortical association areas and, in turn, modulate visceral and motor responses to this information through projections to the brainstem, basal ganglia and hypothalamus (Fig. 5.1; see plate section for this figure in color).

The sensory afferents (e.g. smell, taste, etc.) not only exert their visceral responses but also trigger unconscious or involuntary emotions, which may be pleasant or unpleasant depending on the stimulus. Examples here would be the pleasant associations linking the aroma of delicious cooking and the eager anticipation of a meal, or the negative associations of witnessing a gory sight and feeling sick to one's stomach.

The circuit underpinning unconscious emotions is connected, via the infracallosal cingulate, to a different circuit that subserves conscious emotion. Here the

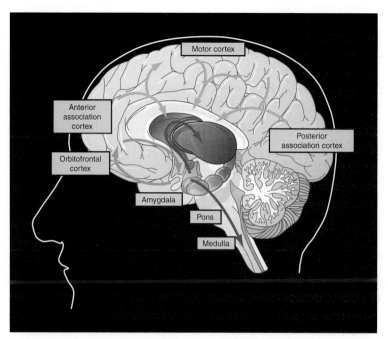

Fig. 5.1.   Neural circuits processing unconscious/visceral emotion. (By permission of the American Geriatric Society and with thanks to Joshua Grill.) For color image please see Plate 2a.

important areas are the hippocampus and cingulate limbic division. These areas process multimodal sensory information and are involved in associative learning and declarative memory. Reciprocal connections run to the dorso lateral prefrontal cortex, a region involved in working memory and considered important in processing information and assigning conscious awareness to it (Fig. 5.2; see plate section for this figure in color).

For example, recalling an anniversary date requires intact declarative memory, but the emotion attached to that date, be it happy in the case of a birthday, or sad when associated with loss and bereavement, challenges the functional integrity of this circuit (Mega *et al.*, 1997; Arciniegas and Topkoff, 2000).

One final anatomical locus needs to be considered in relation to PBA, namely the cerebellum (Fig. 5.3; see plate section for this figure in color). In an elegant case report, Parvisi *et al.* (2001) described a patient who developed the syndrome after a stroke. Detailed MRI analysis revealed five discrete lesions in the brainstem and cerebellum, disrupting cortic-ponto-cerebellar projections, and essentially disconnecting telencephalic structures from the cerebellum.

The significance of this finding lies is the putative role of the cerebellum as a modulator of affect, in essence fine tuning displays of emotion according to

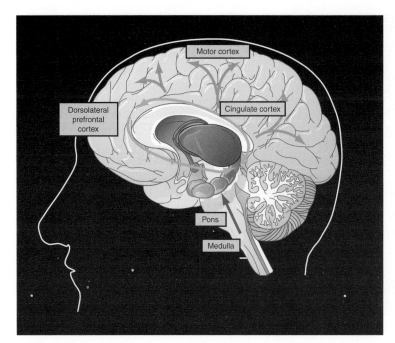

Fig. 5.2.   Neural circuits processing conscious/cognitive emotion. (By permission of the American Geriatric Society and with thanks to Joshua Grill.) For color image please see Plate 2b.

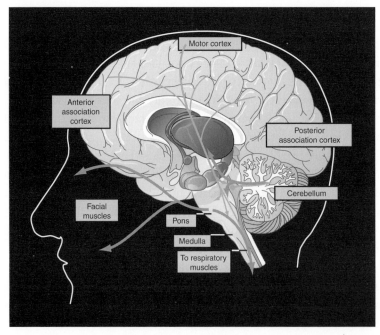

Fig. 5.3.   The cortico-ponto-cerebellar circuit processing emotion. (By permission of the American Geriatric Society and with thanks to Joshua Grill.) For color image please see Plate 3a.

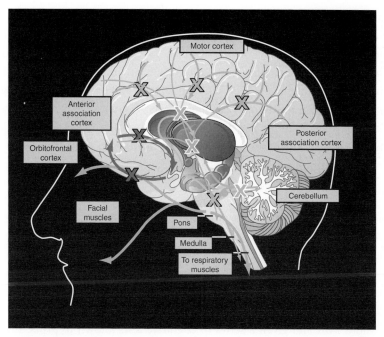

Fig. 5.4.   Pseudobulbar affect associated with lesions at multiple anatomical sites. (By permission of the American Geriatric Society and with thanks to Joshua Grill.) For color image please see Plate 3b.

cognitive and social circumstances. With disruption of this circuit, the patient may receive incomplete information that fails to connect a stimulus to its proper social or cognitive context, thereby promoting laughter or tears that are inappropriate or grossly excessive.

Bringing together these many strands, what emerges is a widely dispersed yet integrated neural network that regulates affect (Fig. 5.4; see plate section for this figure in color).

Encompassing the brainstem, cerebellum, hippocampus, cingulate, amygdala, orbito frontal and dorso lateral prefrontal cortices and sensory association areas, it is evident that disorders such as MS and stroke may disrupt pathways at multiple sites with the same result, namely PBA, What remains unclear, however, is whether bilateral brain involvement is necessary for the syndrome to develop, as postulated by Kinnear Wilson (1926). Here, contrary views have been expressed, with Sackheim *et al.* (1982) reporting an association between pathological affect and specific hemisphere dysfunction. In particular, pathological laughing was linked to mainly right-sided, and pathological crying to predominantly left-sided (dominant) pathology. The associations are by no means clear cut. Destructive unilateral lesions may free the contralateral hemisphere, which then drives the emotional response.

Similarly, unilateral irritative lesions may have the same effect as contralateral destructive ones. An example is gelastic epilepsy, where a left-sided focus produces uncontrollable laughter. Sackheim *et al.* (1982) also concluded, on the basis of three retrospective studies, that pathological laughing was associated significantly more often with males and crying with females and felt that this finding could not be solely attributed to ascertainment bias. Rather, the three-way relationship between affect, gender and laterality suggested that males and females differed in terms of dominant and non-dominant hemisphere function when it came to the expression of positive and negative emotions.

Theories relating to research in patients with multiple sclerosis

Much of the literature devoted to the etiology of pathological affect is either based on retrospectively collected data or confined to theorizing that draws on neuro-anatomical and neuropathological knowledge. However, two MS studies prospectively investigated the role of the prefrontal cortex in the pathogenesis of PBA. Eleven MS subjects with PBA were matched to a control group of 13 MS patient without PBA and given a series of cognitive tests known to probe the functional integrity of the prefrontal cortex (Feinstein *et al.*, 1999). The tests were the Stroop, the Controlled Oral Word Association Test (COWAT) and three indices of the Wisconsin Card Sort Test (WCST) (i.e. number of perseverative responses, total errors and number of categories achieved).

Although the two groups did not differ with respect to age, sex, physical disability, disease course, duration of MS, years of education, premorbid IQ, and depression, the PBA group performed significantly less well on the Stroop Test and the COWAT. They also showed a trend to make more total errors on the WCST, providing evidence from a cognitive perspective that PBA was mediated, at least in part, by dysfunction of the prefrontal cortex. Neurological data from the study, however, failed to demonstrate that patients with PBA were not more likely to have frontal release signs.

There are also some brain MRI data that support the neural networks hypotheses described earlier in this chapter (Ghaffar *et al.*, 2007). Fourteen MS patients with tightly defined PBA according to the criteria of Poeck (1969) were compared with 14 MS patients without PBA (Ghaffar *et al.*, 2007). Both groups were closely matched on demographic and relevant neurological variables and screened for the absence of depression. All subjects underwent brain MRI and regional brain lesions were quantified (see Ch. 3 for a description of the SABRE methodology). The results showed that subjects with PBA had a higher hyperintense total lesion volume ($p < 0.001$) and significantly more hyperintense lesions in the left and right medial inferior frontal regions ($p < 0.004$ and $p < 0.002$, respectively), left medial

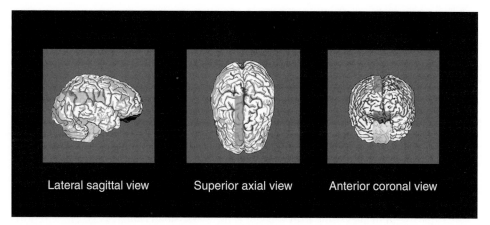

Fig. 5.5.   Brain regions implicated in pseudobulbar affect demarcated by MRI. For color image please see Plate 4.

superior frontal ($p < 0.008$), and left and right inferior parietal lobes ($p < 0.0001$ and $p < 0.001$, respectively). They also had more hypointense lesions in the brainstem ($p < 0.003$) (Fig. 5.5; see the plate section for a color version of this figure).

These data fit well with the networks described earlier (Figs. 5.1–5.4) and highlight the importance of three regions in particular, namely the sensory association areas in the parietal lobes, the prefrontal cortex (in particular medial inferior or orbito frontal regions) and the brainstem, in the pathogenesis of PBA. A logistic regression analysis revealed that lesions (both hyper- and hypointense) in these areas accounted for 75% of the PBA variance. Of note was that while the most destructive lesions (i.e. hypointense) were confined to the brainstem, not every patient with PBA had brainstem pathology discernible on MRI, providing further evidence that PBA was often the product of diaschisis. The imaging findings also differed from those noted in MS patients with major depression, where parietal and brainstem pathology was absent (Feinstein *et al.*, 2004). Some overlap in frontal imaging findings between the depressed and PBA groups may be partly accounted for by a shared symptomatology. Depressed patients show the outward manifestations of sadness, as do patients with PBA. However, a notable difference was the presence of bilateral medial inferior frontal pathology in the PBA but not the major depressive group, where dominant hemisphere lesions only were implicated in the mood change.

Treatment

Pseudobulbar affect can be effectively treated with a number of different drugs at doses that do not cause troublesome side effects. In a double-blind, crossover trial, the efficacy of amitriptyline compared with placebo was clearly demonstrated with two thirds of patients responding significantly to the tricyclic drug (Schiffer *et al.*, 1985). Dosages were without exception small, no patient requiring more than 75 mg daily, well below that generally considered optimal for antidepressant effect. In addition, the improvement in pathological affect occurred rapidly (within 48 hours of starting treatment) and independently of any antidepressant effect, adding support to the theory that PBA entails a dissociation between subjective and objective evidence of disturbed affect. Given the low dosages, side effects (dry mouth, drowsiness) were for the most part mild and well tolerated, although in four patients the dosage had to be reduced.

Evidence suggests that fluoxetine, a selective serotonin reuptake inhibitor (SSRI) is also useful in alleviating PBA (Seliger *et al.*, 1992; Sloan *et al.*, 1992). These reports were based on open trials without control groups, patients having either MS or traumatic brain injury. Sample sizes were small (13 and 6, respectively), but in all cases rapid improvement without unpleasant side effects was noted. Other medications that have proved effective include imipramine after traumatic brain injury (Allman, 1992), citalopram after stroke (Andersen *et al.*, 1993) and traumatic brain injury in a six-year-old boy (Andersen *et al.*, 1999), sertraline following stroke (Burns *et al.*, 1999) and nortriptyline following ischemic brain injury (Robinson *et al.*, 1993). A study that compared the efficacy of paroxetine and citalopram in PBA after traumatic brain injury found the drugs were equally effective, but citalopram was better tolerated and caused less nausea (Müller *et al.*, 1999).

An open label trial of levodopa (0.6–1.5 g/day) and amantadine (100 mg/day) in patients with PBA of vascular origin also furnished positive results (Udaka *et al.*, 1984). Patients responded well within days to treatment, relapsed equally quickly when the medication was stopped and improved once more when treatment was recommenced. Biochemical evidence implicating abnormal dopamine metabolism was demonstrated by patients with PBA having significantly lower CSF concentrations of homovanillic acid, but not 5-hydroxyindoleacetic acid, the former being a major metabolite of dopamine.

More recently, a serendipitous finding has led to a potentially useful drug emerging as the treatment of choice for PBA. AVP-923 is a compound containing dextromethorphan (DM) and quinidine (Q), the latter inhibiting the rapid first pass metabolism of the former. Dextromethorphan was initially envisaged as a neuroprotective agent in amyotrophic lateral sclerosis (ALS) owing to its anti-glutamate properties, but it was subsequently noted to modulate affect. This observation led to a treatment trial of PBA in patients with ALS (Brooks *et al.*, 2004). Subjects were divided into three groups: 30 taking DM, 34 taking Q and 65 taking DM plus Q. The frequency of laughter and crying was charted with the Center for Neurological Study – Lability Scale (CNS-LS), a self-report seven item questionnaire. Quality of life and quality of relationships were rated by questionnaire too and all subjects were assessed at baseline (day 1) and thereafter on days 15 and 29 of treatment. The results revealed that DM/Q (a combination of 30 mg DM and 30 mg quinidine) given twice a day significantly reduced the number of episodes of laughter and crying compared with either of the drugs given alone at the same dosages. This improvement in PBA was accompanied by enhanced quality of life and relationship measurements as well. The drug was generally well tolerated in the ALS group except for nausea, which was largely responsible for the 24% discontinuation rates (versus 6% for DM alone and 8% for Q alone).

A subsequent study investigated the efficacy of DM/Q in 150 patients with MS randomized to drug (DM/Q) ($n = 76$) or placebo ($n = 74$) (Panitch *et al.*, 2006). Once more, symptoms of PBA were recorded using the CNS-LS, which has been validated for MS patients (Smith *et al.*, 2004). Patients on treatment experienced significantly fewer episodes of laughing ($p < 0.008$) and crying ($p < 0.0001$), with a corresponding increase in their quality of life and relationships. Unlike the ALS study, dizziness instead of nausea emerged as the most troubling side effect, occurring in 26.3% of subjects versus 9.5% in the placebo arm. The US Food and Drug Administration has yet to approve DM/Q, but the data from this novel preparation look promising and offer a new direction to future treatment options (Schiffer and Pope, 2005). Advantages over the SSRI drugs are twofold: less sexual side effects, and potentially a greater willingness on the part of PBA patients to take a "neurological" medication as opposed to a "psychiatric" drug, an unfortunate product of the taint still attached to labels such as "antidepressant" and "psychotropic" (Vignette 1).

Summary

- Varying degrees of severity of PBA is found in 10% of MS patients.
- Although PBA may overlap with emotional lability, the two terms are not synonymous. Rather, PBA should be regarded as uncontrollable laughing and/or crying without the associated subjective feelings of happiness or sadness, the syndrome usually occurring without any discernible stressor.
- Generally, PBA is associated with disease of long duration, a chronic–progressive course and moderate to severe physical disability.
- Cognitively impairment is greater in MS patients with PBA than in those without PBA.
- Patients with PBA have difficulty with cognitive tasks that rely on the functional integrity of the prefrontal cortex.
- Lesion data from MRI studies confirm and extend the cognitive observations. Bilateral medial inferior frontal and bilateral inferior parietal hyperintense lesions and brainstem hypointense lesions account for three quarters of the PBA variance.

> **Vignette 1**
>
> A 43-year-old man with a 10 year history of MS and an EDSS of 4.5 was referred after a series of embarrassing events that all pertained to his difficulty controlling outbursts of laughter. The most recent episode of laughter had led to his eviction from a relative's funeral service and the patient felt deeply distressed by what had occurred. He did not, however, present with features of depression or mania, but instead noted that for the past year his ability to control where and when he laughed had steadily lessened. Rather than feel happy while laughing, he reported feeling embarrassed and ashamed. He had noticed that stressful situations, on occasion, brought out the laughter, although more recently it had started occurring in response to minimal provocation. A diagnosis of pseudobulbar affect was made and 25 mg of amitriptyline started, with partial cessation of laughing. The dosage was increased to 50 mg, at which point the uncontrollable laughing ceased.

- The syndrome often responds quickly to small doses of amitriptyline, fluoxetine or levodopa, and complete symptom resolution may be obtained.
- A new treatment for PBA that combines dextromethorphan and quinidine may prove to be the future treatment of choice.

References

Allman P. (1992) Drug treatment of emotionalism following brain damage. *Journal of the Royal Society of Medicine*, **85**, 423–424.

Andersen G, Vestergaard K, Riis J. (1993) Citalopram for post stroke pathological crying. *Lancet*, **342**, 837–839.

Andersen G, Stylsvig M, Sunde N. (1999). Citalopram treatment of traumatic brain damage in a 6 year old boy. *Journal of Neurotrauma*, **16**, 341–344.

Arciniegas DB, Topkoff J. (2000) The neuropsychiatry of pathologic affect: an approach to evaluation and treatment. *Seminars in Clinical Neuropsychiatry*, **5**, 290–306.

Black DW. (1982) Pathological laughter: a review of the literature. *Journal of Nervous and Mental Disease*, **170**, 67–71.

Brooks BR, Thisted RA, Appel SH, *et al.* (2004) Treatment of pseudobulbar affect in ALS patients with dextromethorphan/quinidine. A randomized trial. *Neurology*, **63**, 1364–1370.

Burns A, Russell E, Stratton-Powell H, *et al.* (1999). Sertraline in stroke-associated lability of mood. *International Journal of Geriatric Psychiatry*, **14**, 681–685.

Cottrell SS, Wilson SAK. (1926) The affective symptomatology of disseminated sclerosis. *Journal of Neurology and Psychopathology*, **7**, 1–30.

Cummings JL, Arciniegas DB, Brooks BR, *et al.* (2006) Defining and diagnosing involuntary emotional expression disorder. *CNS Spectrums*, **11** (Suppl. 6), 1–7.

Dark FL, McGrath JJ, Ron MA. (1996) Pseudobulbar affect. *Australian and New Zealand Journal of Psychiatry*, **30**, 472–479.

Davison C, Kelman H. (1939) Pathologic laughing and crying. *Archives of Neurology and Psychiatry*, **42**, 595–643.

Feinstein A, Feinstein KJ, Gray T, O'Connor P. (1997) The prevalence and neurobehavioral correlates of pathological laughter and crying in multiple sclerosis. *Archives of Neurology*, **54**, 1116–1121.

Feinstein A, O'Connor P, Gray T, Feinstein K. (1999) Pathological laughing and crying in multiple sclerosis: a preliminary report suggesting a role for the prefrontal cortex. *Multiple Sclerosis*, **5**, 69–73.

Feinstein A, Roy P, Lobaugh N, Feinstein KJ, O'Connor P. (2004) Structural brain abnormalities in multiple sclerosis patients with major depression. *Neurology*, **62**, 586–590.

Ghaffar O, Chamelian L, Feinstein A. (2007) The neuroanatomy of pseudobulbar affect. *Journal of Neuropsychiatry and Clinical Neurosciences*, in press.

Gallagher JP. (1989) Pathologic laughter and crying in ALS: a search for their origin. *Acta Neurologica Scandinavica*, **80**, 114–117.

Goldberg DP, Hillier VF. (1979) A scaled version of the General Health Questionnaire. *Psychological Medicine*, **9**, 139–145.

Ironside R. (1956) Disorders of laughter due to brain lesions. *Brain*, **79**, 589–609.

Langworthy OR, Hesser FH. (1940) Syndrome of pseudobulbar palsy. An anatomic and physiologic analysis. *Archives of Internal Medicine*, **65**, 106–121.

Langworthy OR, Kolb LC, Androp S. (1941) Disturbances of behavior in patients with disseminated sclerosis. *American Journal of Psychiatry*, **98**, 243–249.

Mega MS, Cummings JL, Salloway S, Malloy P. (1997) The limbic system: an anatomic, phylogenetic and clinical perspective. In *The Neuropsychiatry of Limbic and Subcortical Disorders*, ed. S. Salloway, P Malloy, JL Cummings. Washington DC: American Psychiatric Press, pp. 3–18.

Minden SL, Schiffer RB. (1990) Affective disorders in multiple sclerosis. *Archives of Neurology*, **47**, 98–104.

Monteil P, Cohadon F. (1996) Pathological laughing as a symptom of a tentorial edge tumour. *Journal of Neurology, Neurosurgery and Psychiatry*, **60**, 370.

Morris, PLP, Robinson RG, Raphael B. (1993) Emotional lability after stroke. *Australian and New Zealand Journal of Psychiatry*, **27**, 601–605.

Müller U, Murai T, Bauer-Wittmund T, von Cramont D. (1999) Paroxetine versus citalopram treatment of pathologic crying after brain injury. *Brain Injury*, **13**, 805–811.

Panitch HS, Thisted RA, Smith RA, *et al.* (2006) Randomized controlled trial of dextromethorphan/quinidine for pseudobulbar effect in multiple sclerosis. *Annals of Neurology*, **59**, 780–787.

Parvisi J, Andersen SW, Martin CO, Damasio H, Damasio AR. (2001) Pathological laughter and crying. A link to the cerebellum. *Brain*, **124**, 1708–1719.

Poeck K. (1969) Pathophysiology of emotional disorders associated with brain damage. In *Handbook of Clinical Neurology*, Vol. 3, ed. PJ Vinken, GW Bruyn. Amsterdam: North Holland, pp. 343–367.

Pratt RTC. (1951) An investigation of the psychiatric aspects of disseminated sclerosis. *Journal of Neurology, Neurosurgery and Psychiatry*, **14**, 326–335.

Robinson RG, Parikh RM, Lipsey JR, Starkstein SE, Price TR. (1993) Pseudobulbar affect following stroke: validation of a measurement scale and double-blind treatment study. *American Journal of Psychiatry*, **150**, 286–293.

Ross ED, Stewart RE. (1987) Pathological display of affect in patients with depression and right frontal brain damage. *Journal of Nervous and Mental Disease*, **175**, 165–172.

Sackheim HA, Greenberg MS, Weinman AL, *et al.* (1982) Hemisphere asymmetry in the expression of positive and negative emotions. *Archives of Neurology*, **39**, 210–218.

Schiffer RB, Pope L. (2005) Review of pseudobulbar affect including a novel and potential therapy. *Journal of Neuropsychiatry and Clinical Neurosciences*, **17**, 447–454.

Schiffer RB, Herndon RM, Rudick RA. (1985) Treatment of pathologic laughing and weeping with amitriptyline. *New England Journal of Medicine*, **312**, 1480–1482.

Seliger GM, Hornstein A, Flax J, Herbert J, Schroder K. (1992) Fluoxetine improves emotional incontinence. *Brain Injury*, **6**, 267–270.

Shaibani AT, Sabbagh M, Doody R. (1994) Laughter and crying in neurologic disease. *Neuropsychiatry, Neuropsychology and Behavioral Neurology*, **7**, 243–250.

Sloan R L, Brown KW, Pentland B. (1992) Fluoxetine as a treatment for emotional lability after brain injury. *Brain Injury*, **6**, 315–319.

Smith RA, Berg JE, Pope LE, *et al.* (2004) Validation of the CNS emotional lability scale for pseudobulbar affect (pathological laughing and crying) in multiple sclerosis patients. *Multiple Sclerosis*, **10**, 679–685.

Starkstein SE, Migliorelli R, Teson A, *et al.* (1995) Prevalence and clinical correlates of pathologic affective display in Alzheimer's disease. *Journal of Neurology, Neurosurgery and Psychiatry*, **59**, 55–60.

Sugar C, Nadell R. (1943) Mental symptoms in multiple sclerosis. *Journal of Nervous and Mental Disease*, **98**, 267–280.

Surridge D. (1969) An investigation into some psychiatric aspects of multiple sclerosis. *British Journal of Psychiatry*, **115**, 749–764.

Udaka F, Yamao S, Nagata H, Nakamura S, Kameyama M. (1984) Pathologic laughing and crying treated with levodopa. *Archives of Neurology*, **41**, 1095–1096.

Wechsler D. (1981) *Manual for the Wechsler Adult Intelligence Scale-Revised*. New York: Psychological Corporation.

Wilson SAK. (1924) Some problems in neurology. 11. Pathological laughing and crying. *Journal of Neurology and Psychopathology*, **4**, 1299–1333.

Zigmond AS, Snaith RP. (1983) The Hospital Anxiety and Depression Scale. *Acta Psychiatrica Scandinavica*, **67**, 361–370.

6

Multiple sclerosis and psychosis

Introduction

The association between MS and psychosis has until recently been considered uncommon, which helps to explain the paucity of research devoted to the topic. Nevertheless, the relationship is of interest for a number of reasons. These include the possibility that both demyelination and psychosis have a shared, viral pathogenesis, the role of coarse cerebral pathology in the etiology of psychosis, and problems posed by the treatment of psychosis in the neurologically compromised patient.

The DSM-IV diagnosis for psychosis in the context of multiple sclerosis is "psychosis due to a general medical condition" (PDGMC [American Psychiatric Association 1994]; see Table 6.1 for the criteria). The equivalent *International Classification of Disease* (10th edition; ICD-10; World Health Organization [WHO], 1992) category is one of either "organic hallucinosis," "organic catatonic disorder," or "organic delusional (schizophrenia-like) disorder." This difference in terminology reflects a philosophical divide that separates the taxonomies. Inherent in the DSM approach is the belief that all mental disorders (not just psychotic ones) are "organic" and that the functional–organic dichotomy is needlessly divisive. The ICD-10, mindful of serving a different constituency (i.e. first and third world countries) has retained the word "organic." Irrespective of which classification is subscribed to, references on both sides of the Atlantic abound in descriptive terms such as "schizophrenia-like," "secondary psychosis" and "organic psychosis."

The plethora of terminology also confronts the clinician–researcher with another important dilemma, one that is common to both systems. Is the psychosis caused by the MS or is it a chance occurrence? To make a DSM-IV (or ICD-10) diagnosis, there has to be a high index of suspicion that MS has caused the psychosis, which on an individual basis is often difficult. Given that the lifetime prevalence for a psychotic illness such as schizophrenia is approximately 1% and for MS is 0.1–0.01% (varying according to latitude), the two disorders can be expected to appear together by chance in 0.5–1 per 100 000 cases, which

Table 6.1. Criteria for the diagnostic category "psychosis due to a general medical condition" (PDGMC) in DSM-IV

Criterion	Features
A	Prominent hallucinations or delusions
B	There is evidence from the history, physical examination or laboratory findings that the disturbance is the direct physiological consequence of a general medical condition
C	The disturbance is not better accounted for by another mental disorder
D	The disturbance does not occur exclusively during the course of a delirium

The condition may then be coded according to whether delusions or hallucinations are the most prominent psychotic feature. The general medical condition would also be coded on axis 111

Source: With permission from the American Psychiatric Association.

approaches the lifetime prevalence of a disorder such as amyotrophic lateral sclerosis. Therefore, to make an etiological inference with any degree of certainty, factors supporting face, descriptive, predictive and construct validity should be present. This applies not only to MS, but to all CNS disorders causally implicated in psychosis. This chapter will review the evidence supporting each of these criteria and also provide guidelines on treatment and assessing outcome.

Literature review

Most reports of MS and psychosis are single case studies, with the earliest dating from the nineteenth century. In their comprehensive review of "schizophrenia-like psychoses associated with organic disorders of the central nervous system (CNS)," Davison and Bagley (1969) devoted a section to demyelinating disease. They reviewed every published report (irrespective of language) of MS that occurred concurrently with a psychotic illness that fulfilled the 1957 WHO criteria for schizophrenia. Given their belief that the presence of coarse cerebral pathology would render some psychiatric signs and symptoms invalid, they excluded catatonia, autism and change in personality from the WHO guidelines and were left with the following: the presence of an unequivocal disorder of the CNS; the presence at some stage of shallow, incongruous affect, thought disorder, hallucinations and delusions; and the absence, when psychotic, of features suggesting a delirium, dementia, dysmnesic syndrome and affective psychosis. Applying these criteria to their literature review, they came across 39 reports, a frequency judged not to exceed chance expectation.

This view has been cautiously supported by studies investigating the number of MS patients found in large, inpatient psychiatric populations. The percentages from the Massachusetts State Hospital (0.07%), Manhattan State Hospital (0.05%), and Queensland Mental Hospitals (0.06%) are similar and do not exceed chance probability, but they may be misleadingly low because of a greater community tolerance for mental disturbance in the presence of MS or alternative admissions to hospitals caring for the physically disabled (Davison and Bagley, 1969).

A more recent study has, however, challenged prevailing assumptions. Population-based evidence from Alberta, Canada suggests psychosis in MS patients is more common than previously thought (Patten *et al.*, 2005). As part of universal health-care insurance in Alberta, all subjects seen by physicians are given diagnoses coded by the *International Classification of Diseases*, Ninth Edition Clinical Modification (ICD-9-CM). In 2002, of 2.45 million residents of this Canadian province over 15 years of age, 10 367 were found to have MS, giving an estimated prevalence of 330 per 100 000, in keeping with Alberta's historically high prevalence rate. The authors also looked for the co-occurrence of two ICD-9-CM psychiatric diagnoses in these MS patients. The first was "non-organic/non-affective psychoses" (which included schizophrenia-spectrum disorders, delusional disorders and other non-organic psychoses) and the second category was broadly defined as organic psychotic disorders (drug-induced psychotic disorders, other transient organic psychotic disorders and other organic psychotic disorders). Care was taken to exclude patients with dementia and alcohol-related psychoses.

Results were given separately for each of these two large categories and were stratified according to the following age groups: 15–24, 25–44, 45–64 and 65+ years. Consistent findings emerged across all age groups and in both psychiatric categories, namely that the prevalence of psychosis in MS patients significantly exceeded that reported in patients without MS. The odds ratios (OR) are worth reporting in detail as they tell a compelling story. In the "non-organic" psychotic group, the OR values were 6.6, 2.2, 1.9 and 1.1 in the age groups 15–24, 25–44, 45–64 and 65+ years, respectively. For the "organic" psychotic group the corresponding OR figures were 11.1, 7.4, 5.6 and 1.9, respectively. Sex, unlike age, was not found to modify the observed association.

The main weakness of this study was an offshoot of its greatest strength. The large sample size precluded detailed psychiatric data being collected, so the ICD-9 categories provide only bare bones phenomenology. Nevertheless, under the very broad descriptive rubric of psychosis, an unequivocal picture emerged of elevated rates of psychosis, in the order of 2–3%, occurring in patients with MS. This study provides the most compelling evidence to date that psychosis in MS occurs more frequently than chance dictates, a situation analogous to that found in other neuropsychiatric conditions such as epilepsy and basal ganglia disorders (Dewhurst *et al.*, 1969; Cummings, 1985; Popkin and Tucker, 1994).

Distinguishing characteristics

According to the DSM-IV, to make a diagnosis of PDGMC, the clinician must first establish the presence of the general medical condition and then relate the psychosis to it via a physiological mechanism. It is acknowledged there are no infallible guidelines for doing this, hence the reported diagnostic uncertainty and poor inter-rater reliability, with a kappa score lower than that for other less "organic" disorders. The latter observation goes against a well-established pattern in the classification of mental illness (Lewis, 1994). Despite these limitations, some pointers to a diagnosis of PDGMC are discussed below.

Temporal association

A temporal association between the onset, exacerbation and remission of the medical condition and the psychotic disturbance should be present. While this makes intuitive sense, an examination of the DSM-IV sourcebook reveals inconsistent data. The majority of citations pertain to epilepsy and psychosis where, on average, 14 years have elapsed between the onset of seizures and subsequent psychosis (Slater *et al.*, 1963, Feinstein and Ron, 1990). In a case–control study of 10 psychotic MS patients, the mean duration of neurological symptoms before the onset of psychosis was 8.5 years (range, 0–19). In only one case was the diagnosis of MS made at the time of psychosis onset (Feinstein *et al.*, 1992). In contrast to these results, the MS review of Davison and Bagley (1969) revealed that in 36% of reported cases the neurological and psychiatric symptoms appeared at approximately the same time. In a further 61.5%, the psychosis appeared in either the two years before or the two years after the onset of neurological symptoms. This temporal association in approximately two thirds of patients led the authors to conclude that, although psychosis secondary to MS was rare, when it did occur demyelination was most likely implicated in the pathogenesis.

Clinical features

A unique diagnostic category should have a distinct symptom profile. The DSM-IV alludes to descriptive validity when it notes that the category PDGMC contains symptoms considered atypical for a primary psychosis (e.g. olfactory and visual hallucinations). In a study that specifically addressed this issue, Feinstein *et al.* (1992) examined the case notes of 10 psychotic MS patients treated at a tertiary referral center. All mental states were assessed retrospectively using the symptom

Table 6.2. Commonest symptoms and signs (PSE) in a psychotic group of 10 MS patients

Symptom	Percentage
Lack of insight	100
Persecutory delusions	70
Non-specific evidence of psychosis	60
Irritability	60
Agitation	50
Anxiety	40
Sexual delusions	30
Passivity phenomena	30
Delusions of reference	20
Grandiose delusions	20
Second-person auditory hallucinations	20
Visual hallucinations	20
Thought disorder	20
Third-person auditory hallucinations	10
Thought broadcast	10

Source: From Feinstein *et al.* (1992); reproduced with permission of the Royal College of Psychiatry.

checklist derived from the Present State Examination (Wing *et al.*, 1974). From the symptom checklist, half the subjects were given a diagnosis of schizophrenia and half an affective psychosis. The most common symptoms and signs are shown in Table 6.2 and from this it can be seen that lack of insight characterized all the patients' presentations. Persecutory delusions occurred in over two thirds, whereas non-specific evidence of psychosis (which included heightened or changed perception, "minor" hallucinations, viz. music, noises) was recorded in 60%. Delusions of control (passivity) and delusions with a sexual or fantastic content were present in a third of patients and delusions of reference noted in one in five patients. The symptom profile was notable for the relative infrequency of well-formed hallucinations. Second-person auditory hallucinations were present in 20% of patients, as were visual hallucinations. Third-person auditory hallucinations (two or more voices commenting on the person) were found in only one case. Therefore, delusions in various forms, but particularly with a persecutory content, predominated. The findings lend support to the ICD-10 notion of the psychosis being more akin to an "organic delusional disorder," with perceptual disturbances less noticeable and of secondary import.

Persecutory delusions were also the most common symptom of psychosis found in other neurological disorders (Slater *et al.*, 1963; Davison and Bagley, 1969;

Feinstein and Ron, 1990), with Cummings (1985) noting that relative preservation of cognitive function was necessary for the formation of complex delusional beliefs. Another frequently cited clinical concomitant of PDGMC, namely the preservation of affective responses, also received empirical support (Feinstein *et al.*, 1992). Thus, it would appear that, when patients with MS (or any other CNS disorder) become psychotic, the predominant presentation is one of "positive" psychotic symptoms (delusions, less often hallucinations) with relative preservation of affective responses. The "negative" or "defect" state associated with schizophrenia, (i.e. apathy, impoverished speech and thought), together with blunted affect, is seldom seen. Notwithstanding these well-documented group differences that demarcate the clinical picture of MS psychosis from schizophrenia, it must be emphasised that on an individual level it is often difficult to tell the conditions apart. Consequently, Slater's view that a patient with psychosis associated with epilepsy is indistinguishable from a patient with schizophrenia (Slater *et al.*, 1963) applies equally well to the MS patient who becomes psychotic. Not surprisingly, therefore, in MS patients with no obvious neurological deficits, a diagnosis of schizophrenia is readily made (Schmalzbach, 1954; Parker, 1956). Even in patients with clear neurological symptoms, the mental state may closely mimic schizophrenia.

Age of presentation

The mean age of first presentation of psychosis in patients with schizophrenia is 23 years (Lieberman *et al.*, 1992), which is considerably younger than that reported in two studies of MS patients with psychosis. Davison and Bagley's review (1969) noted a mean age of onset of psychosis a decade older and the average age of onset was 36.6 years in the study of Feinstein *et al.* (1992). A similar picture emerges from studies of other CNS disorders (Slater *et al.*, 1963; Cummings, 1985; Feinstein and Ron, 1990) and is further evidence setting PDGMC apart as a distinct diagnostic entity.

The Alberta population-based study did not specifically address the age of onset of psychosis. However, the prevalence figures stratified by age are nevertheless informative (Patten *et al.*, 2005). For example, the prevalence of "organic" psychosis was found to increase with age, with peak prevalence in the 65 years and over group, but the strongest relative effect (i.e. highest OR) was in the 15–24 year age group. While this observation can be explained by the fact that "organic" psychosis is extremely rare in young patients *without* MS, it cannot negate the conclusion that even young MS patients have a heightened risk of psychosis.

Gender ratio

The gender ratio noted in psychotic MS patients differs from that found in either MS or late-onset schizophrenia. Davison and Bagley reported 21 of 39 cases were male, which is at odds with the 2:1 female to male ratio in MS. Similarly, although the genders are equally represented in schizophrenia (see Lewis, 1992 for a dissenting view), males present earlier than females (Goldstein *et al.*, 1989). If one accepts that the mean age of onset of psychosis in MS patients is approximately a decade older than in schizophrenia, a preponderance of female psychotic MS patients could be anticipated, which is not the case (Davison and Bagley, 1969; Feinstein and Ron 1990; Feinstein *et al.*, 1992). The Alberta study did not discuss this point directly as there were no data regarding age of psychosis onset, but the authors did explore the relationship between gender, age and "organic psychosis" in a logistic regression analysis. The most robust predictor of "organic psychosis" to emerge was the interaction between females and age in the 25–44 year range (Patten *et al.*, 2005). Overall, however, it must be acknowledged that insufficient data precluded any firm conclusions here, other than to suggest that the gender discrepancies between psychotic patients with MS and those with schizophrenia point to a central role for demyelination in the pathogenesis of the psychosis.

Etiology

Genetic links

If the psychosis associated with MS was simply the chance co-occurrence of schizophrenia, then one would expect to find increased evidence of schizophrenia in the relatives of the affected proband. Evidence is scanty on this point but does not support a familial link (Davison and Bagley, 1969). Clinical experience also suggests that premorbid schizoid traits are absent. Once again, it is helpful to look at other CNS disorders for any possible clues to this questions. Feinstein and Ron (1990) found that 4% of their sample of 65 psychotic patients with heterogeneous neurological disorders had a family history of schizophrenia, four times the rate in the general population. This result is, however, difficult to interpret for the data were not age corrected and the family history method used to assess relatives may have underestimated the true psychiatric morbidity (Andreasen *et al.*, 1986). In addition, the heterogeneous nature of the sample meant that some patients with late-onset schizophrenia as opposed to PDGMC may have been included in the sample, thereby increasing the familial yield.

An alternative explanation is that a prevalence rate of 4%, falling between that in the general population and that in families with a schizophrenic proband, still suggests a genetic vulnerability. When coarse brain pathology is superimposed on this genetic diathesis, psychosis can ensue.

Viral hypothesis

Stevens (1988) has postulated that similarities in disease course, age of onset, geographical distribution and immunological response of patients with schizophrenia and those with MS imply some overlap with respect to pathogenesis. In particular, exposure to a virus at a crucial developmental stage (in utero, child-birth, childhood) may be the common thread linking what are clinically two very different conditions. This viewpoint fits well with a theory of schizophrenia as a neurodevelopmental disorder triggered by insult to the fetal brain (Torrey *et al.*, 1994). Support for this comes from the observation that women infected with the influenza virus during the second trimester of pregnancy appear to have an increased risk of producing schizophrenic offspring (O'Callaghan *et al.*, 1991; see Crow and Done, 1992 for a dissenting view). While the developmental hypothesis has its adherents when it comes to schizophrenia (Castle and Murray, 1991; Murray *et al.*, 1992; O'Connell *et al.*, 1997), support weakens considerably when it is applied to MS. Nevertheless, it has been reported that infection with the herpes virus during childhood may leave some patients prone to develop MS in later life (Sanders *et al.*, 1996), while migration studies have shown that for those who emigrate after adolescence, the risk of developing MS does not change from that of their country of origin (Dean, 1967).

While theorizing offers intriguing possibilities, the marked differences in clinical presentations between the two disorders outweigh any similarities, making a shared pathogen unlikely.

Brain changes seen with magnetic resonance imaging

Evidence linking brain changes in MS to psychosis comes from a case–control MRI study of MS patients with (n = 10) and without (n = 10) psychosis, who were matched for age, sex, duration of illness and physical disability (Feinstein *et al.*, 1992). The following Present State Examination (Wing *et al.*, 1974) diagnoses were assigned: schizophrenia (2), schizoaffective psychosis (2), paranoid disorder (1), psychotic depression (1), mania with psychotic features (4).

Subjects and controls underwent contiguous, multislice axial MRI of the brain. All scanning protocols included T_2 weighted images that optimized lesion detection. Patients and controls were scanned over a period of 6 years, during which changes to the MRI scanner and software upgrades ensured better images were obtained. Despite these factors, the imaging protocols and slice thickness were the same in all patient and control groups. It was not, however, possible in one case to match the images for strength of magnetic field. The EDSS and MRI were performed when the patients were psychotic in eight cases. In the remaining two patients, MRI was undertaken one and three years after the psychotic episode, with a normal mental state at the time.

Subjects were compared with controls with respect to site and extent of lesions. The MRI analysis was undertaken by a neuroradiologist blind to psychiatric diagnosis. In assessing the MRI, a system derived by Ormerod *et al.* (1987) was used. The size and presence of lesions were recorded in the following periventricular areas: body of the ventricles; frontal, temporal and occipital horns; trigone; and third and fourth ventricles. These seven areas provided a periventricular score. A further eight areas of brain parenchyma were also examined, namely internal capsule; basal ganglia; frontal, parietal, temporal and occipital lobes; brainstem; and cerebellum. The lobes of the cerebrum were defined as including not only cortex but also underlying white matter. Planes separating lobes were projected from their cortical boundaries to the foramen of Munro or the lateral ventricular trigone, as appropriate. The largest lesion in each particular area was scored using a four point scale according to the greatest diameter measured. A total lesion score was obtained by adding scores from all the areas assessed. The percentage of the total lesion score in each particular area was obtained by dividing the score for each area by the total lesion score and multiplying by 100. This was termed the "percentage score."

Table 6.3 compares the MRI results of psychotic patients and their matched controls. The psychotic patients had a greater total lesion and periventricular lesion score, but this was not statistically significant. Trends emerged for a higher

Table 6.3. Lesion scores in psychotic and control MS patients detected by magnetic resonance imaging[a]

	Mean lesion score (SD)	
	Psychotic patients	Control patients
Total lesion score	32.6(13.6)	27.4(13.8)
Periventricular score	19.3(8.1)	14.0(6.6)
Temporal (bilateral)	8.6(4.3)	6.9(4.4)
Temporal-parietal (bilateral)	12.1(6.2)	9.4(5.6)
Temporal horn R	1.8(0.9)	1.0(0.8)
Temporal horn L	1.7(0.8)	1.0(0.8)
Trigone R	2.2(1.2)	1.7(0.8)
Trigone L	2.3(0.9)	1.5(0.9)
Third ventricle	0.7(0.5)	0.3(0.5)
Temporal lobe R	0.2(0.6)	0.6(0.9)
Temporal lobe L	0.4(0.8)	1.1(1.5)
Temporal horn + trigone R	4.0(2.1)	2.7(1.6)
Temporal horn + trigone L	4.0(1.6)	2.5(1.4)

L, left; R, right; SD, standard deviation.

[a] No differences were found for frontal lobes/horns, occipital lobes/horns, parietal lobes, internal capsule, basal ganglia, Fourth ventricle and cerebellum.

Source: From Feinstein *et al.* (1992); reproduced with permission of the Royal College of Psychiatry.

lesion score in the psychotic group for areas surrounding the temporal horns bilaterally. A similar result was also obtained in the left trigone. Combining the left temporal horn and adjacent left trigone area scores produced a statistically significant difference between the psychotic and control groups.

A clearer picture of the difference in the distribution of lesion scores between the psychotic and control MS patients was demonstrated by observing what percentage of the total lesion score was present in each particular area. In the controls, the total lesion score was distributed equally between periventricular and other brain areas, while in the psychotic patients the periventricular lesion score contributed more than 60% of the total lesion score. This difference was not, however, statistically significant. The most marked differences were present around the temporal horns, where the percentage score in the psychotic patients was almost double that of the control group. Therefore, not only did the psychotic patients have a greater lesion score but lesions were also differentially distributed in periventricular areas and in particular around the temporal horns of the lateral ventricles. A closer look at the individual patient data demonstrated that in all but one case–control pair, the psychotic patient had a greater temporal horn lesion score than their matched control (Fig. 6.1).

The various brain areas were also analyzed to determine whether the presence or absence of lesions, rather than their size, was the crucial factor, but no differences were found between the groups. In the psychotic group, lesion scores between

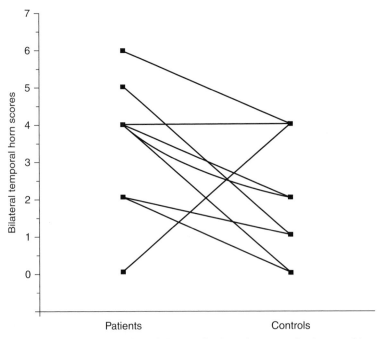

Fig. 6.1.   Temporal horn/scores (bilateral) for psychotic and non-psychotic MS subjects.

right and left hemispheres did not differ significantly. In addition, there were no significant correlations between individual psychotic symptoms and MRI lesions.

The study firmly linked psychosis in MS patients with the presence of increased lesion load in temporal areas and in doing so confirmed the importance of the region in the pathogenesis of psychosis in general. Enlargement of the left temporal horn at postmortem (Crow *et al.*, 1989) and MRI evidence of reduction in temporal lobe (Suddath *et al.*, 1989), and in particular in hippocampal volume (Suddath *et al.*, 1990), in patients with schizophrenia attests to this. An association between temporal lobe pathology and PDGMC has also been reported by some (Slater *et al.*, 1963; Davison and Bagley, 1969), but not others (Feinstein and Ron, 1990), although the heterogeneous composition of the latter's sample could explain the discrepant result.

Although the MRI data are compelling, the study had shortcomings and left questions unanswered. Limitations pertained to small sample size, the possible confounding effects of artefact on MRI quantification, and the scanning of two patients after their psychosis had long resolved. These difficulties were largely offset by a careful case–control design with individual patient–control matching. However, this still left the perplexing question why only certain patients with temporal lobe involvement became psychotic. While the study suggested a "threshold" lesion volume had to be exceeded before psychosis ensued, this did not invariably apply as some patients with a large temporal lesion score did not become delusional. The presence of brain plaques in the temporal lobes is, therefore, unlikely to explain fully the development of psychosis in all cases. Rather, brain lesions superimposed on a premorbid vulnerability (genetic, developmental, premorbid psychiatric history) seems a more plausible explanation.

Treatment

There are no empirically based treatment studies of psychosis associated with MS. Early reports found electroconvulsive treatment (Schmalzbach, 1954) and insulin coma (Parker, 1956) to be ineffective in individual cases. The mainstay of present treatment is antipsychotic medication (Feinstein *et al.*, 1992) and given the often severe nature of the behavioral disturbance, psychiatric hospitalization may be required in the acute stages.

In an analogous situation to that encountered with the floridly manic patient, treatment can present a considerable therapeutic challenge. Experience has taught that MS patients are frequently sensitive to the side effects of neuroleptic medication. Consequently, high-potency drugs such as the butyrophenones (e.g. haloperidol), which are associated with extrapyramidal side effects, may further compromise patients' mobility and balance, resulting in falls that prove distressing to patients, family and nursing staff. A choice of less-potent neuroleptics, such as the phenothiazine groups of compounds, lessens the risk of extrapyramidal symptoms, but anticholinergic difficulties are more prominent, which may aggravate other difficulties such as bladder and bowel control and impaired vision. The associated dry mouth may add to dysarthric problems. All antipsychotic medication, irrespective of class, can produce excessive sedation, which may similarly effect already impaired coordination and balance.

With these difficulties in mind, small doses of antipsychotic medication are recommended. Such an approach is supported by the results of a functional imaging study in schizophrenia, which has shown that 2 mg haloperidol blocks up to three quarters of dopamine D_2 receptors, thereby exerting substantial clinical improvement without troubling side effects (Kapur *et al.*, 1996). The authors have recommended treating psychotic patients with daily doses of haloperidol that do not exceed 2–4 mg although even doses this small may physically compromise the MS patient. The old treatment maxim, "start low and go slow" should not be forgotten here.

Newer antipsychotic drugs offer less-prominent side effects. Furmaga *et al.* (1995) have reported that risperidone was helpful in 10 patients with PDGMC who had not previously responded to a conventional neuroleptic. Clozapine, which has the advantage of few extrapyramidal problems, has a proven efficacy in patients with movement disorders who become psychotic (Chako *et al.*, 1995) and is an alternative to risperidone. Weekly blood checks are required to monitor for the development of agranulocytosis, which affects 1% of patients on treatment. Postural hypotension early in the treatment carries with it the risk of falls in patients who are neurologically impaired, but this difficulty is transient and lessens significantly after a few weeks of treatment. Seizures are another risk factor at higher doses (in excess of 600 mg/day), but such doses are rarely needed. Olanzapine, a thiobenzodiazepine, potentially offers the benefits of clozapine, without the risk of agranulocytosis. It also has the advantage of a convenient once a day dose (recommended daily dose of 10 mg), which can be started immediately. Its efficacy in psychotic MS patients has not yet been ascertained. Similarly, quetiapine fumarate (Seroquel), a psychotropic dibenzothiazepine derivative, potentially offers the same benefits, albeit in a slightly less friendly dosing schedule. Adverse side effects with both olanzapine and quetiapine have been reported in one psychotic MS patient, whereas ziprasidone (a member of the benzothiazolylpiperazine class of antipsychotic drugs) was well tolerated and effective (Davids *et al.*, 2004).

Should behavioral control still be required despite adequate antipsychotic dosage, benzodiazepines may be added. Lorazepam has the advantage of being given via either the oral or the intramuscular route. Oral dosage rarely exceeds 8 mg/day and the clinician should bear in mind that the intramuscular dose is equivalent to 2–2½ times the oral dose, because it avoids the first pass metabolism.

Some of these points are illustrated by the following vignette.

Vignette

A 38-year-old, single, unemployed woman with a seven year history of MS (EDSS of 3.5) was brought to hospital by a friend who had become concerned about her behavior. There was no family history of mental illness and the patient had been well until, at 31 years, a bout of optic neuritis followed soon thereafter by a loss of balance led to a diagnosis of MS. The patient made a good neurological recovery, but six years later, after a second episode of optic neuritis, she began worrying that the CIA had placed her under surveillance. She was convinced her telephone calls were being monitored and that she was being followed by men wearing yellow jackets. She also claimed the secret service had been present at an operation she had undergone a number of years earlier and had planted an electrical device in her uterus.

By the time a psychiatry consult was requested, she had been symptomatic for six months. The presence of persecutory delusions was confirmed. Mood, however, was noted to be normal despite her distress at what she perceived was her unfair treatment at the hands of the CIA agents. A diagnosis of PDGMC (i.e. MS) was made and outpatient treatment began with olanzapine 10 mg/day. Compliance with medication was, however, problematic because the patient soon became concerned with her weight gain on treatment. Furthermore, she failed to see how medication would lead to the CIA "backing off." By the time she returned for her fourth outpatient appointment, she had stopped the treatment and her behavior had turned belligerent. She was no longer talking to her friend and more worryingly was making thinly veiled threats to harm her, accusing her of being in league with the men in yellow jackets. Given the potential for violence, the patient was committed to hospital as an involuntary patient, deemed incapable of consenting to treatment and substitute consent to treat obtained from her next of kin.

The patient's refusal to take oral medication meant that injectable antipsychotic medication had to be used and intramuscular haloperidol 2 mg daily was given. Over the course of 10 days, her hostility lessened together with her fears of persecution, but at the cost of bradykinesia and akathisia. By now, however, her mental state had improved to a point where she no longer refused oral medication. The haloperidol was stopped and risperidone introduced, the dose starting at 0.5 mg twice daily and increased over a week to 1.5 mg twice daily. A short course of benztropine (benzatropine) 2 mg daily dealt with the bradykinesia, while propranolol 10 mg three times a day alleviated the discomfort of her akathisia. On a divided dose of 3 mg of risperidone daily, the patient was no longer delusional and the side effects apparent on haloperidol treatment had dissipated. She was discharged from hospital.

The patient remained well on risperidone for a period of 6 months and then insisted on coming off treatment. The medication was tapered over the course of a month before being stopped. A year later her mental state remained essentially normal and the remission in her MS continued.

Outcome

Earlier literature, much of it predating the appearance of antipsychotic medication in the early 1950s, reported that psychotic MS patients either recovered spontaneously, progressed from psychosis to dementia or ran a relapsing–remitting course with respect to psychosis and MS that ultimately went on to dementia. More recent data demonstrate that antipsychotic medication has substantially altered this outlook. Of 10 psychotic patients followed for approximately six years, the median duration of their first psychotic episode was 5 weeks (range, 1 to 72). Six (60%) of the patients did not experience another psychotic episode, three patients had one further relapse, and a single patient had multiple recurrences. Overall, the psychosis remitted in 90% of patients with a chronic, paranoid psychosis ensuing in a single patient. In general, patients did not require long-term oral or depot neuroleptic use. If a relapse occurred, short-term neuroleptic medication was reintroduced and subsequently discontinued after improvement in the mental state (Feinstein *et al.*, 1992).

The outcome is, therefore, better than in schizophrenia and is similar to other neurological disorders giving rise to psychosis (Slater *et al.*, 1963; Feinstein and Ron, 1990). The outcome data also overlap with that in late-onset schizophrenia (Harris and Jeste, 1988), suggesting age is an important modifier of outcome. Although the duration of follow-up in the study of Feinstein, *et al.* (1992) did not exceed six years, this result may also accurately reflect long-term outcome. Long-term follow-up of patients with schizophrenia has shown that decline is most rapid within the first 5 years after initial presentation, after which the condition tends to plateau (Keith and Mathews, 1994).

Summary

- Although psychosis associated with MS is a rare occurrence, population-based data suggests that the prevalence rates exceed chance expectation.
- A case–control study has demonstrated that psychotic MS patients are more likely to have plaques involving the temporal horn areas bilaterally.
- There are data to suggest that MS-related psychosis is distinct from schizophrenia, based on a later age of presentation, preservation of affective response, quicker resolution of symptoms, fewer psychotic relapses, and a more favorable long-term outcome.
- Antipsychotic drugs such as olanzapine, quetiapine, risperidone and ziprasidone in small doses are the treatment of choice, although reports of their efficacy are anecdotal. Benzodiazepines may be used as an adjunct for sedation.

References

American Psychiatric Association (1994) *Diagnostic and Statistical Manual of the American Psychiatric Association*, 4th edn., Washington DC: American Psychiatric Press.

Andreasen NC, Rice J, Endicott J, Reich T, Coryell W. (1986) The family history approach to diagnosis: how useful is it? *Archives of General Psychiatry*, **43**, 421–429.

Castle D, Murray RM. (1991) The neurodevelopmental basis of sex differences in schizophrenia. *Psychological Medicine*, **21**, 565–575.

Chako RC, Hurley RA, Harper RG, Jankovic J, Cardoso F. (1995) Clozapine for acute and maintenance treatment of psychosis in Parkinson's disease. *Journal of Neuropsychiatry and Clinical Neurosciences*, **7**, 471–475.

Crow TJ, Done DJ. (1992) Prenatal exposure to influenza does not cause schizophrenia. *British Journal of Psychiatry*, **161**, 390–393.

Crow TJ, Ball J, Bloom SR, *et al.* (1989) Schizophrenia as an anomaly of development of cerebral asymmetry: a post mortem study and a proposal concerning the genetic basis of the disease. *Archives of General Psychiatry*, **46**, 1145–1150.

Cummings JL. (1985) Organic delusions: phenomenology, anatomical correlations and review. *British Journal of Psychiatry*, **146**, 184–197.

Davids E, Hartwig U, Gastpar M. (2004) Antipsychotic treatment for psychosis associated with multiple sclerosis. *Progress in Neuropsychopharmacology and Biological Psychiatry*, **28**, 743–744.

Davison K, Bagley CR. (1969) Schizophrenia-like psychoses associated with organic disorders off the central nervous system. A review of the literature. In *Current Problems in Neuropsychiatry*, ed. RN Herrington. Ashford, UK: Hedley, pp. 113–184.

Dean G. (1967) Annual incidence, prevalence and morbidity of multiple sclerosis in white South African-born and in white immigrants to South Africa. *British Medical Journal*, **2**, 724–730.

Dewhurst K, Oliver J, Trick KLK, McKnight AL. (1969) Neuropsychiatric aspects of Huntington's disease. *Confinia Neurological*, **31**, 258.

Feinstein A, Ron MA. (1990) Psychosis associated with demonstrable brain disease. *Psychological Medicine*, **20**, 793–803.

Feinstein A, du Boulay G, Ron MA. (1992) Psychotic illness in multiple sclerosis. A clinical and magnetic resonance imaging study. *British Journal of Psychiatry*, **161**, 680–685.

Furmaga KM, DeLeon O, Sinha S, Jobe T, Gaviria M. (1995) Risperidone response in refractory psychosis due to a general medical condition. *Journal of Neuropsychiatry and Clinical Neurosciences*, **7**, 417.

Goldstein JM , Tsuang MT, Faraone SV. (1989) Gender and schizophrenia: implications for understanding the heterogeneity of the illness. *Psychiatry Research*, **28**, 243–253.

Harris MJ, Jeste D. (1988) Late onset schizophrenia: an overview. *Schizophrenia Bulletin*, **14**, 39–55.

Kapur S, Remington G, Jones C, *et al.* (1996) High levels of dopamine D_2 receptor occupancy with low dose haloperidol treatment: a PET study. *American Journal of Psychiatry*, **153**, 948–950.

Keith SJ, Mathews SM. (1994) The diagnosis of schizophrenia: a review of onset and duration issues. In *DSM-IV Sourcebook*, ed. T Widiger, A Francis, H Pincus, *et al.* Washington, DC: American Psychiatric Press, pp. 393–418.

Lewis S. (1992) Sex and schizophrenia: vive la difference. *British Journal of Psychiatry*, **161**, 445–450.

Lewis SW. (1994) ICD-10: a neuropsychiatric nightmare. *British Journal of Psychiatry*, **164**, 157–158.

Lieberman JA, Alvir A, Woerner M, *et al.* (1992) Prospective study of psychopathology in first episode schizophrenia at Hillside Hospital. *Schizophrenia Bulletin*, **18**, 351–371.

Murray RM, O'Callaghan E, Castle DJ, Lewis SW. (1992) A neurodevelopmental approach to the classification of schizophrenia. *Schizophrenia Bulletin*, **18**, 319–332.

O'Callaghan E, Sham P, Takei N, Glover G, Murray RM. (1991) Schizophrenia after exposure to 1957 A2 influenza epidemic. *Lancet*, **i**, 1248–1250.

O'Connell P, Woodruff PWR, Wright I, Jones P, Murray RM. (1997) Developmental insanity or dementia praecox: was the wrong concept adopted. *Schizophrenia Research*, **23**, 97–106.

Ormerod IEC, Miller DH, McDonald WI, *et al.* (1987) The role of NMR imaging in the assessment of multiple sclerosis and isolated neurological lesions. *Brain*, **110**, 1579–1616.

Parker N. (1956) Disseminated sclerosis presenting as schizophrenia. *Medical Journal of Australia*, **1**, 405–407.

Patten SB, Svenson LW, Metz LM. (2005) Psychotic disorders in MS: population-based evidence of an association. *Neurology*, **65**, 1123–1125.

Popkin MK, Tucker GJ. (1994) Mental disorders due to a general medical condition and substance-induced disorders. Mood, anxiety, psychotic, catatonic and personality disorders. In *DSM-IV Sourcebook*, ed. TA Widiger, AJ Frances, HA Pincus, *et al.* Washington, DC: American Psychiatric Association, Ch. 17, pp. 243–276.

Sanders VJ, Waddell AE, Felisan SL, *et al.* (1996) Herpes simplex virus in postmortem multiple sclerosis brain tissue. *Archives of Neurology* **53**, 125–133.

Schmalzbach O. (1954) Disseminated sclerosis in schizophrenia. *Medical Journal of Australia*, **1**, 451–452.

Slater E, Beard AW, Glithero E. (1963) The schizophrenia-like psychoses of epilepsy. *British Journal of Psychiatry*, **109**, 95–150.

Stevens JR. (1988) Schizophrenia and multiple sclerosis. *Schizophrenia Bulletin*, **14**, 231–241.

Suddath RL, Casanova MF, Goldberg TE, *et al.* (1989) Temporal lobe pathology in schizophrenia: a quantitative magnetic resonance imaging study. *American Journal of Psychiatry*, **146**, 464–472.

Suddath RL, Christison GW, Torrey EF, Casanova MF, Wenberger DR. (1990) Anatomical abnormalities in the brains of monozygotic twins discordant for schizophrenia. *New England Journal of Medicine*, **322**, 789–794.

Torrey EF, Taylor E, Bracha HS, *et al.* (1994) Prenatal origin of schizophrenia in a subgroup discordant monozygotic twins. *Schizophrenia Bulletin*, **20**, 423–432.

Wing JK, Cooper JE, Sartorius N. (1974) The measurement and classification of psychiatric symptoms. *An Instruction Manual for the Present State Examination and CATEGO Programme*. Cambridge, UK: Cambridge University Press.

World Health Organization (1992) *The International Classification of Diseases*, 10th edn. Geneva: World Health Organization.

7

Cognitive impairment in multiple sclerosis

That most perceptive of behavioral neurologists, Charcot (1877), observed that MS patients may show "marked enfeeblement of the memory, conceptions are formed slowly and intellectual and emotional faculties are blunted in their totality." Despite this early recognition of potential cognitive difficulties in MS patients, for the greater part of a century clinicians held to the belief that cognitive difficulties were seldom part of the clinical picture in MS, and if present, generally confined to patients with severe physical disability. Therefore, on the basis of a clinical examination, Kurtzke (1970) estimated that cognitive difficulties affected less than 5% of patients. Even more striking were the conclusions from the influencial study of Cottrell and Wilson (1926) of 100 MS patients seen in a tertiary referral center. Noting intellectual decline in only two patients, the authors considered the problem "minimal and negligible."

With the advent of MRI in the early 1980s, clinicians and researchers were able to visualize the brain's white matter changes with a new found clarity. The ability to detect cerebral lesions in vivo was the impetus for researchers to look for clinical correlates, be they neurological or related to mentation, and MS became attractive to researchers as the prototypical subcortical, white matter dementing process. However, first the prevalence and nature of cognitive changes had to be re-examined, using the more sensitive methods of neuropsychological testing. The result was an outpouring of research data documenting cognitive dysfunction in MS. Within less than 20 years, Kurtzke's figure of less than 5% was shown to be a gross underestimate. When in 1990, the Cognitive Function Study Group of the National Multiple Sclerosis Society published their guidelines for neuropsychological research in MS, they estimated that 54–65% of MS patients were cognitively impaired (Peyser *et al.* 1990).

However, it was also becoming clear that amidst this enthusiastic renaissance, the pendulum may have swung too far in the other direction. MS patients are a heterogeneous group, comprising individuals whose illness differs with respect to duration of symptoms, physical disability, frequency of disease exacerbations, disease course and site of lesions. Furthermore, the studies that had consistently found cognitive impairment in well over half the sample contained an in-built bias for they utilized clinic attenders, a group who were potentially more severely affected by their disease than a community-based sample. New studies were, therefore, needed, using a more representative sample selection and controlling for a host of disease- and demographic-related variables.

Prevalence of cognitive impairment

Two studies followed a more selective approach and their results are comparable. Rao *et al.* (1991) initially approached 730 community-based MS patients via mail. Approximately 10% refused participation, while a number of other factors (uncertainties over diagnosis, previous psychometric assessment, a history of alcohol or drug abuse or a concomitant neurological disorder) reduced the number of subjects to 100. All subjects had a neurological examination and information was obtained on disease course, physical disability, duration of illness from symptom onset and from diagnosis, and current medication use. One hundred healthy control subjects were matched to the MS group with respect to age, gender and number of years of education. Both groups then completed a neuropsychological battery of 31 tests that included the Mini-Mental State Examination (Folstein *et al.*, 1975) and tests of verbal intelligence; immediate, recent and remote memory; abstract reasoning; attention and concentration; language; and visuospatial perception. Cognitive function was rated as impaired if scores fell below the fifth percentile scores of the control subjects.

Compared with healthy controls, the results revealed that MS patients failed significantly more tests: means of 4.64 (standard deviation [SD], 4.9) and 1.13 (SD, 1.8), respectively. If subjects failed on four or more cognitive indices, they were deemed cognitively impaired, which was the case in 48 MS patients and five controls. The false five-positive rate (i.e. five) was subtracted from the true-positive rate, leaving a 43% frequency of cognitive impairment.

This result has been replicated by McIntosh-Michaelis *et al.* (1991), in a community-based sample of 147 patients with MS. A group of 34 patients with rheumatoid arthritis were included for comparison as the authors wanted to control for any possible effects of depression on psychometric performance. The two groups were matched for gender and number of years of schooling, but not age (the patients with rheumatoid arthritis were significantly older). All subjects completed a neuropsychological battery that included the Rivermead Behavioral Memory Test (RBMT), the modified Wisconsin Card Sort Test (WCST), the Controlled Oral Word Association Test (COWAT) and two tests of general intellectual ability, namely the verbal subscale of the Wechsler Adult Intelligence

Scale-Revised (WAIS-R) and the Raven's Standard Progressive Matrices, the last chosen instead of the performance subscale of the WAIS-R to reduce the effects of sensorimotor impairment on performance. Cognitive impairment was defined as deficits on three measures: verbal and performance IQ and any one of the RBMT, COWAT and the modified WCST. The result was that 46% of MS patients and 12% of the patients with rheumatoid arthritis were found to be impaired.

An indication of how important sample selection can prove in determining the prevalence of cognitive dysfunction is shown by van den Burg *et al.* (1987). Although also utilizing a community-based sample drawn from a well-defined epidemiological catchment area in Holland, the authors restricted sample selection to patients with an EDSS not exceeding 4. In addition, the distribution of subjects over the EDSS range of 1 to 4 was kept uniform. Selection was further restricted by excluding patients who had experienced a disease exacerbation within the previous two months. With the emphasis on targeting a less disabled subgroup of patients, and comparing neuropsychological performance with that of an age-, sex- and education-matched group of healthy controls, the number of MS patients found to be cognitively impaired was less than half that reported in the samples analyzed by Rao *et al.* (1991) and McIntosh-Michaelis *et al.* (1991).

A more detailed review of the salient aspects of cognition in MS follows.

General intelligence

As a group, MS patients have IQs within the normal range when examined cross-sectionally and when premorbid IQ is inferred from educational and employment records. However, this broad generalization is misleading. Canter (1951) administered the Army General Classification Test to 23 men who had developed MS after joining the military. The men had all completed the same test prior to enrollment and Canter, therefore, had the unique opportunity of comparing premorbid performance with that post-MS onset. The test–retest duration was up to four years and a significant drop of 13.5 IQ points was noted. This remains the only study that can directly call on a premorbid cognitive examination as a means of comparison. An alternative approach has been to infer premorbid IQ from a reading test such as the American National Adult Reading Test (ANART; Nelson, 1982) and then compare this estimate with a current measure of IQ. Using this method, Ron *et al.* (1991) found a significant decline in MS patients compared with a group of disabled control subjects who had neurological disorders sparing the brain.

Further evidence of decline in IQ comes from a study of 100 MS patients living in the community (Rao *et al.*, 1991). Based on the five verbal subscales of the WAIS-R, 21% of subjects had verbal IQs below the fifth percentile relative to healthy, demographically matched controls. Thirty years earlier, Reitan *et al.* (1971) had also described lower verbal IQs in MS patients compared with healthy controls. However, the ecological validity of this group's findings is questionable, given that the IQ of MS patients remained within the normal range even after decline occurred. One, therefore, has to turn to other psychometric measures to get a better understanding of the deleterious effects of cognitive decline.

Attention and information processing speed

Slowness of thinking, observed Charcot, was one of the hallmarks of mentation in MS patients. A century later, Cummings (1986) reiterated the significance of the symptom and went on to suggest it was one of the defining features of a broad category of dementing illnesses that were primarily subcortical in origin. Speed of information processing has been assessed in MS patients with a number of different tests of which the Symbol–Digit Modality Test (Smith, 1982) is one of the most widely used. The test requires subjects to substitute numbers for symbols and responses are timed. Instead of writing their answers, subjects may respond orally, thereby removing the motor component to testing. Many studies have reported deficits in MS patients (Caine *et al.*, 1986; Franklin *et al.*, 1988; Feinstein *et al.*, 1992a, 1993; Christodoulou *et al.*, 2003; Benedict *et al.*, 2004) and the test is recommended as a sensitive screening procedure for cognitive deficits (Beatty and Goodkin, 1990) and is part of the Brief Repeatable Battery of Neuropsychological tests (Rao *et al.*, 1991) and the Screening Examination for Cognitive Impairment (SEFCI) (Beatty *et al.*, 1995a).

Another measure of cognitive speed is provided by the Paced Auditory Serial Addition Task (PASAT; Gronwall and Wrightson, 1974). Initially devised as a means of assessing cognitive difficulties following traumatic brain injury, it has since been applied to other neurological disorders. In this test, subjects are presented aurally with a series of digits from one to nine and instructed to add each new digit to the one that preceded it. The speed at which the digits are presented can be controlled and has generally varied from 1.2 seconds to 4 seconds. Abnormalities on the PASAT in MS patients have been reported in numerous studies (Litvan *et al.*, 1988a; Feinstein *et al.*, 1992a, 1993; Bobholz and Rao, 2003), with almost a quarter of community-living MS patients performing below the fifth percentile relative to healthy controls (Rao *et al.*, 1991). Generally, impairments are more noticeable when digits are presented at the faster rates (Litvan *et al.*, 1988a). A visual adaptation of the PASAT, whereby the numbers are presented on a computer monitor, has been developed and has replicated the auditory findings (Feinstein *et al.*, 1992a). While the test is regarded as a sensitive marker of cognitive function in MS patients, Fisk and Archibald (2001) have cautioned that a scoring system based on the total number of correct responses may not be the best way of assessing performance. This stems from their observation that some patients may ignore test items and chunk their responses instead. As this negates in part one of the central constructs of the PASAT, they suggest an alternative scoring system, one that sums the number of dyads (i.e. consecutive correct responses).

An indirect measure of assessing information processing speed is via the use of simple and choice reaction time tests. In the former, subjects only have to respond to a stimulus – the appearance of a symbol on a computer monitor – by pressing a button. The responses are timed and the test is thus a measure of basic psycho-motor speed. Studies have reported slowed reaction times in MS patients (Elsass and Zeeberg, 1983; Jennekens-Schinkel *et al.*, 1988a). In the choice reaction time test, subjects are presented with a choice of responses, only one of which is correct. An element of problem solving is, therefore, introduced. Surprisingly, Jennekens-Schinkel *et al.* (1988b) reported that this did not lead to further slowing in the responses of MS patients. The problems with this approach, however, are that it lacks the sensitivity of tests such as the PASAT, while the long duration of the task leaves performances vulnerable to the effects of fatigue. This symptom is endorsed by over 80% of MS patients (Krupp *et al.*, 1988) and may adversely affect "vigilance," defined as the ability to attend to a stimulus over time. Evidence of this comes from a study by Kujala *et al.* (1995). The performances of three groups, mildly cognitively impaired MS patients, cognitively intact MS patients and healthy controls, were compared on various measures of attention, vigilance and information processing speed. The findings illustrated a two-way split, in that cognitively intact MS patients demonstrated signs of motor and fatigue-related slowness, whereas the mildly cognitively impaired group showed more prominent features of cognitive slowness. This result is supported by a study that controlled for the effects of fatigue and depression and still revealed slowed information processing speed in MS subjects (Denney *et al.*, 2004).

Kujala *et al.* (1994) also investigated information processing speed by dividing it into three separate stages. The first division referred to automatic processing of information and did not require conscious effort. An example is the recognition of numbers presented in the center of the visual field. The second stage was one of controlled processing and demands not only attention that but also working memory. An example is conscious decision making, which can be tested with choice reaction time tasks. The third component was motor programming, which refers to the time a subject needs to prepare a motor program before executing a task. This too is assumed to be automatic. The authors investigated these three aspects in two matched MS samples, one deemed cognitively intact and the other mildly impaired. Not surprisingly, the latter performed more poorly at every stage of processing information, but of additional note was that MS subjects thought to be cognitively preserved also showed mild slowing in automatic processing. This may be a result, in part, of the slowness of the visual input system (i.e. delayed conduction in the optic nerves) in the absence of discernible cerebral involvement.

In summary, problems with delayed information processing speed are common in MS and may be regarded as a core, defining feature of cognitive dysfunction in MS. Adding to their significance is the observation that these difficulties may also impact on other aspects of cognition. Deficits cannot be explained on the basis of fatigue or depression alone. Furthermore, a meta-analysis of neuropsychological dysfunction in MS has shown that tests which challenge the rapidity of processing speed are *the* most sensitive in eliciting abnormalities in MS patients (Wishart and Sharpe, 1997).

Executive functions

The executive system is a theoretical construct: a putative cognitive system that controls other aspects of cognition. A helpful analogy is to think of an orchestra, made up of different sections, strings, woodwinds, brass, percussion, all controlled by the conductor. In cognitive neuroscience, the conductor is the executive and because of its pivotal role it has also been termed the central or "higher" executive. Executive function involves planning, abstract thinking, goal setting, problem solving, initiating appropriate behavior and inhibiting incorrect or self-defeating actions. To fulfill these broad, behavior-defining functions, the executive system interacts closely with neural networks subserving attention and is an integral part of working memory.

Prompted by an observation of Canter (1951) that in MS "the most striking psychological loss is [an] inability to analyze and synthesize abstract problems," researchers have set about providing further empirical proof. The earliest attempt was by Parsons *et al.* (1957), who used the Grassi Block Substitution Test (GBST), which requires the subject to shift construct several times at both a simple and complex level during a series of duplications of block designs. Contrasting the performance of 17 MS patients (with the unusual gender distribution of 14 males and 3 females; the study took place in a Veteran's hospital) with 14 males and 3 female patients without CNS involvement recruited from the general medical wards, all subjects initially completed the verbal subscale of the Wechsler–Bellevue Intelligence Scale and four of the performance subscales, excluding the "block design test." Following this, all subjects were given the GBST in which they had to copy five designs of varying difficulty by utilizing four colored blocks. Cognisant of potential motor difficulties in the MS group, subjects were allowed five as opposed to the usual three minutes to complete each step. The results revealed significant deficits in the MS group, although taking into account the broad SD values, there was a degree of overlap in performance between the two groups. These differences could not be ascribed to IQ deficits in the MS patients as the two groups were evenly matched for verbal scores. Although the MS patients had lower perform-ance IQs, the authors controlled for this by taking a subgroup of nine MS patients whose performance IQs matched those of the controls. Once again the MS patients demonstrated significantly more deficits. In keeping with results from other cognitive paradigms, there was a subgroup of MS patients whose performances showed no impairment.

Since then, a number of studies have replicated this finding using a different task of abstracting ability, namely the WCST, with Berg's (1948) original test giving way to a revised and expanded methodology (Heaton, 1981). Given the frequency with which this test has been used in MS research, a description of the method-ology appears warranted. A subject is given a pack of 128 cards that contain four symbols (star, cross, triangle and circle) in four colors (red, blue, green, yellow). Four stimulus cards are placed before the subject in the following left to right order: one red triangle, two green stars, three yellow crosses, four blue circles. The subject is then instructed to match each consecutive card from the deck with one of the four stimulus cards, in whichever way he or she thinks they match. Subjects are only told whether they are right or wrong and the correct sorting principle is never divulged. Once a certain number of correct responses have been made, the sorting principle is changed (e.g. from color to form). This occurs without warning and subjects have only the examiner's responses to alert them to the change. The test proceeds in similar fashion through a number of shifts in set, namely form, color and number. Scores are provided for indices such as the number of categories completed, the total number of errors made and the number of perseverative errors made – to name three of the most sensitive markers of deficits in conceptual reasoning.

The WCST has proved effective in differentiating MS patients from healthy controls (Heaton *et al.*, 1985, Beatty *et al.*, 1989a; Rao *et al.*, 1991; Mendozzi *et al.*, 1993) and disabled patients without brain involvement (Rao *et al.*, 1987; Ron *et al.*, 1991). There is confirmatory evidence from other similar neuropsychological tests that MS patients have difficulty problem solving, with a tendency to perseverate in their responses. This has been demonstrated with the Raven's Progressive Matrices (Rao *et al.*, 1991) and the Category Test (Peyser *et al.*, 1980; Heaton *et al.*, 1985; Rao *et al.*, 1991). All these tests are, however, measures of non-verbal abstracting ability, prompting Beatty *et al.* (1995b) to investigate whether MS patients con-front similar difficulties with verbal abstraction. Their tests included two non-verbal measures (i.e. the WCST and a shortened version of the California Card Sort Test [CCST]) and one verbal measure of abstracting ability (i.e. the Shipley Institute of Living Scale [SILS]). The SILS measures both concept formation and abstracting ability, while taking into account overall verbal (vocabulary) performance. In relation to healthy controls, MS patients were impaired across all three measures. Their deficits on the SILS went beyond problems with vocabulary and illustrated that MS patients solve verbal abstraction problems more slowly and less accurately than controls.

Beatty and Monson (1996) have also commented on a potential short-coming of the WCST, which is the close correlation between the number of concepts attained and the number of perseverative responses made. The CCST, by comparison, allows problem solving to be broken down into constituent processes that are, in theory, more independent. The examination, therefore, provides separate assessments of concept generation, concept identification and concept execution, in addition to various measures of perseveration. Comparing the performances of MS patients on the WCST and the CCST has shown that the primary difficulty faced by MS patients when it comes to problem solving is difficulty with identifying concepts, rather than perseveration (Beatty and Monson 1996).

More recently, the CCST has been modified and is now known as the Sorting Test. It has been incorporated into a series of cognitive tests called the Delis–Kaplan Executive Function System (Delis *et al.*, 2001). Because it allows the examiner to tease out the components of concept formation and perseveration, it is preferred to the WCST for use in MS patients (Benedict *et al.*, 2002). Another advantage is that, unlike the WCST, it has two forms, thereby facilitating serial testing.

Theories of executive dysfunction have long been linked to observations of patients with frontal lobe pathology. However, as the neural networks underpinning various aspects of executive function have been teased out, it has become clear that this association is more complex. An example pertains to the WCST, where normal performance was generally thought to be a function of an intact dorso lateral prefrontal cortex. Data linking abnormalities on the WCST in MS patients (Arnett *et al.*, 1994) to a significant frontal lesion load were in tune with observations from other disorders, such as schizophrenia, where poor performance on the task correlated with hypoperfusion of the dorso lateral prefrontal cortex as demonstrated by positron emission tomography during task activation (Weinberger *et al.*, 1986). Compelling as these findings were, they did not fit well with data from patients with non-frontal lesions, whose performance on the WCST was equally poor (Anderson *et al.*, 1991). Knowledge of discrete anatomical circuits that link areas of the prefrontal cortex (i.e. dorso lateral prefrontal cortex, orbito frontal cortex and anterior cingulate) with the basal ganglia and thalamus resolved what were initially thought to be contradictory results (Cummings, 1993). The functional implications of these findings are that lesions remote from the prefrontal cortex may produce behavioral syndromes and cognitive difficulties (such as impairment on the WCST) that are identical to those associated with lesions localized to prefrontal areas. Empirical evidence that difficulties with abstract thinking (and perseverative responses) are also indicative of generalized cerebral dysfunction comes from Mendozzi *et al.* (1993). Although they noted that approximately a third of MS patients were impaired on the WCST relative to a healthy control group, performance on the WCST could not predict performance on other aspects of frontal lobe function as assessed by the Luria–Nebraska Neuropsychological Battery.[1]

Memory and multiple sclerosis

A substantial number of MS patients have memory impairment. Staples and Lincoln (1979) reported a figure of 60% in a sample with advanced disease, while Rao *et al.* (1984) confining their investigation to patients with a chronic–progressive (CP) disease course, found 21% with moderate to severe memory impairment, 43% with mild deficits and 36% with no evidence of memory loss. These results are supported by community-based studies with a more representative patient sample. Rao *et al.* (1991) noted that a quarter to a third of 100 community-based MS patients performed poorly on tests of recent memory, a figure replicated by McIntosh-Michaelis *et al.* (1991). In a study that randomly selected patients from the community and an inpatient neurological service, 30% of MS patients were severely memory impaired, 30% had moderate impairment while only 40% had little or no impairment (Minden *et al.*, 1990). Given the frequency of memory impairment in MS, this area has been more extensively studied that any other aspect of cognition.

As with the IQ data, generalizations can obscure a more complex picture. Memory is a broad rubric and what these all-embracing statistics fail to convey is that the degree of impairment differs considerably depending on the type of memory examined. Adding to the potential for confusion, neuropsychologists differ when it comes to the classification of memory (Squire, 1987; Schacter and Tulving, 1994). This chapter will not attempt to clarify an often obtuse taxonomy, but for the sake of clarity a working system is needed to organize a plethora of terms. Hence the following schema. A broad division cleaves memory into explicit (also known as declarative) and implicit (also called procedural). The main distinction between the two is that the former is conscious (or effortful) whereas the latter is not (which makes it automatic). Much of the research into memory impairments in MS patients has focussed on explicit memory, which, in turn, has been split into discreet categories, such as short-term memory, working memory

---

[1] For a detailed review of the relationship between the frontal lobes and cognition, see Stuss and Levine (2002).

and long-term memory. The last may be further subdivided according in to episodic and semantic subtypes.

Short-term memory

Short-term memory is a limited capacity, temporary memory store that is best defined by a simple Digit Span test. Here numbers are presented to the subject at the rate of one a second. A normal digit span is seven digits repeated forwards and five digits repeated backwards. Studies comparing performance on the Digit Span test in MS patients and healthy controls have either found no abnormalities (Jambor, 1969; Rao *et al.*, 1984; Heaton *et al.*, 1985) or mild impairment (Lyon-Caen *et al.*, 1986; Huber *et al.*, 1987; Fischer, 1988; Kujala *et al.*, 1996). This is reflected in the results of a meta-analysis of short-term memory deficits in MS, which produced a weak effect size of 0.351 (Thornton and Raz, 1997). While MS patients have greater difficulty with the "digits backwards" component (Rao *et al.*, 1991; Feinstein *et al.*, 1997), the relative insensitivity of this task has led researchers to jettison its use in MS studies of cognition.

Working memory

Working memory refers to a cognitive system that is responsible for the short-term maintenance and manipulation of information necessary for the performance of tasks such as learning, comprehension and reasoning (Baddeley, 2003). When MS patients are probed on how they use and manipulate this fund of briefly stored and frequently updated information, a different picture emerges from that obtained with the Digit Span test. In a meta-analytic review of cognitive dysfunction in MS, deficits in working memory had an effect size of 0.724 (Thornton and Raz, 1997). A useful computer analogy is to consider working memory as that information which is held on-line. Working memory may be divided into three subcomponents: the phonological (or articulatory loop), the visuospatial sketchpad and the central executive. The first is responsible for the recollection of words, numbers and melodies, while the sketchpad is confined to the recall of spatial information. Both components are controlled by a central executive that regulates the distribution of limited attentional resources and controls cognitive processing when novel tasks are presented or existing habits need to be overridden (Baddeley, 1986). The gist of working memory, therefore, is a cognitive process reliant on the integrated functioning of the central executive and the speed and accuracy with which information is processed from short-term stores in the articulatory loop and visuospatial sketch pad.

D'Esposito *et al.* (1996) have attributed abnormalities in working memory in MS patients to dysfunction within the central executive system. For example, MS patients displayed more deficits than healthy controls on a primary task during a dual task paradigm, particularly when the complexity of the secondary task was increased. This result, which correlated with performance on the PASAT, may be interpreted as an inability of the central executive to provide sufficient attentional resources required to process multiple tasks simultaneously. The PASAT, which was described and discussed earlier in this chapter (p. 119) may, therefore, be considered a sensitive test of working memory as well, even as it straddles more than one cognitive domain, challenging short-term storage of data, processing speed and sustained, divided attention.

Another way of probing working memory is with the Brown–Petersen task. This investigates a subject's ability to store information while counting backwards. Certain studies have revealed normal performance in MS subjects (Litvan *et al.* 1988b; Beatty *et al.*, 1989b; Rao *et al.*, 1989, 1991) although performances may become impaired in the presence of disease exacerbations (Grant *et al.*, 1984) or if the disease course becomes CP (Beatty *et al.*, 1988).

Long-term memory

Long-term memory refers to tasks that exceed the capacity of short-term memory. Many studies have demonstrated deficits in this cognitive domain in MS patients, using both verbal and non-verbal paradigms (Staples and Lincoln, 1979; Grant *et al.*, 1984; Rao *et al.*, 1984, 1991; Caine *et al.*, 1986; Beatty *et al.*, 1988).

Memory deficits are more readily discernible on tests of recall as opposed to recognition (Rao, 1986). This discrepancy suggests the problem is mainly one of *retrieval* and not the encoding of new information. Further evidence of retrieval problems is illustrated by difficulties MS patients have with verbal fluency (Beatty *et al.*, 1988; Rao *et al.*, 1991), indicative of a retrograde memory loss. More recently, evidence highlighting difficulties with memory *acquisition* have been reported too. Although, the ability to learn with repeated presentation of stimuli (i.e. multi-trial learning) may vary considerably between MS patients, both Rao *et al.* (1984) and Fischer *et al.* (1992) were able to separate patients according to three patterns of performance: normal rate of learning, impairment on the first trial with a subsequent normal rate of learning and impaired initial and subsequent learning. These findings were supported, in part, by DeLuca *et al.* (1994), who demonstrated that MS patients required significantly more trials to learn a task initially relative to healthy controls, but once they had learnt it, their performance did not differ from healthy controls in delayed recall or recognition.

In a subsequent study, these conclusions were modified (DeLuca *et al.*, 1998). Data showed that MS patients had a different pattern of deficits depending on whether the task was verbal or visual. Forty MS patients and 20 healthy controls rehearsed a word list (a modified version of the selective reminding test) and checkerboard (modified 7/24 visual memory test) pattern until two error free trials were reached. Recall and recognition for the verbal and visual material was assessed 30 and 90 minutes later. The results revealed that MS patients took significantly longer than the healthy controls to acquire the information. When the test switched to measures of recall and recognition at 30 and 90 minutes, there were no between-group differences on the verbal test. However, MS patients performed significantly less well on visual recognition and recall across the two delay periods. These differences persisted on a test of forced recognition as well, and led the authors to conclude that acquisition, storage and retrieval of information from long-term memory was differentially affected in MS patients. For verbal information, the problem was essentially one of encoding, whereas for visual tasks, storage and acquisition were impaired. This result was partially replicated by Demaree et al. (2000), who also found that MS patients took longer than healthy controls to acquire verbal and visual information. However, no differences were found when it came to verbal recall and facial recognition 30 and 90 minutes after stimulus presentation. From this, they concluded that MS-related memory difficulties were primarily acquisition, rather than retrieval based. Notably, repetition in isolation may not help MS patients to acquire new information. This is because the more trials required to reach perfect acquisition, the less information is recalled later (Chiaravalloti et al., 2003). Consequently, if practice is to have any rehabilitative benefit, it should be incorporated with other strategies that help to organize how the information is acquired.

Some studies have approached memory deficits by focussing not on how much information can be remembered but rather on methods employed for remembering, in particular the ability of MS patients to attach meaning to what they learn (i.e. semantically encode and retrieve verbal material). An early study (Carroll et al., 1984) demonstrated that semantic processing did aid recall, but the process itself had the potential to confuse MS patients. These findings were extended by Goldstein et al. (1992), who found that semantic processing involving gist recall (i.e. memory for the more important aspects of the information) was intact in MS patients. Therefore, while MS patients recalled fewer items than healthy control subjects, the items they remembered were of greater importance. Other data, however, painted a different picture, with deficits in semantic memory attributed to the impaired ability of MS patients to understand conceptual meanings (Laatu et al., 1999).

MS patients also display deficits on tests of *autobiographical memory*.[2] Kenealy et al. (2002) administered the Autobiographical Memory Interview (AMI) to

---

[2] To neuropsychologists like Endel Tulving (1983, 2002), this refers to the conscious (i.e. effortful) recollection of unique past events that are personally experienced. He considers the term synonymous with episodic memory, hence a degree of taxonomical confusion.

30 MS patients. The information collected came from two subscales, namely the Autobiographical Incidents Schedule (AIS) and the Personal Semantic Schedule (PSS) and spanned three life stages; childhood, early adult life and recent life. The results showed that 60% and 63% of the sample were classified as abnormal on the AIS and PSS, respectively. A temporal gradient, reported in patients with Alzheimer's disease, was found here too, in that memory for recent rather than distant (childhood and early adulthood) events was more impaired. Informative as these data are, care must be taken before extrapolating too widely because the sample was skewed towards severely disabled patients (mean EDSS 8.4) living in residential care. This caution appears justified when the results of an earlier MS study that also used the AMI are examined (Paul *et al.*, 1997). Here, patients had considerably less physical morbidity and were community dwelling, factors that explain the milder nature of episodic memory deficits and the maintenance of a normal temporal sequence of remembering (i.e. recent events were better recalled than more remote ones). But despite this more promising picture, MS patients had not escaped completely unscathed. Abnormalities were still documented in personal semantic, but not personal episodic, memory.

Another aspect of long-term memory, namely *remote memory*, has been studied in MS patients by challenging their recall and recognition of famous faces and events from the past. Deficits recorded in remote memory support a problem with retrieval, but here results have been equivocal, with some (Beatty *et al.*, 1988, 1989b; Beatty and Monson, 1991), but not others (Rao *et al.*, 1991) noting abnormalities.

The relationship between short-term, working and long-term memory in multiple sclerosis

A notable finding from the meta-analytical study of memory impairment in MS was the similar effect size found for working (0.724) and long-term (0.756) memory (Thornton and Raz, 1997). This begs a question, as yet incompletely answered, whether long-term memory problems are a consequence of defects in working memory. Litvan *et al.* (1988b) teased out deficits in the articulatory loop component of working memory and reported a link with long-term memory impairment. This finding has since been disputed (Grafman *et al.*, 1990; Rao *et al.*, 1993). However, a complementary stand of evidence connecting the two memory systems emerged from a study that found a correlation between poor performances on the PASAT (as an index of working memory) and tests of long-term memory (DeLuca *et al.*, 1994). Thornton and Raz (1997), in their meta-analysis, favor the naysayers, preferring to invoke divergent, independent neural mechanisms subserving each aspect of memory. Whether this disagreement is a reflection on true differences or a by-product of disagreements in defining working memory remains unclear.

Implicit memory (procedural memory)

Implicit memory refers to memory that is not reliant on conscious recall and encompasses motor skills, conditioning and priming. It differs from explicit (or declarative) memory, which is accessed through conscious effort. There is a consensus that MS patients perform normally on tests of motor skill (Beatty *et al.*, 1990a) and priming (stem completion; Beatty and Monson, 1990). Similarly, Grafman *et al.* (1991) found that MS patients performed normally on tasks that required automatic, but not effortful, processing.

Metamemory

The ability of MS patients to appraise their own memory accurately (termed metamemory), particularly with respect to newly acquired information, is also compromised (Beatty and Monson, 1991). This observation, in the absence of clinically significant depression, is important clinically for it implies that patients' self-reports of memory impairment are likely to be inaccurate. Metamemory may be, in part, a function of the prefrontal cortex. Taylor (1990) compared objective evidence of cognitive ability (neuropsychological test performance) with patients' subjective assessments of their cognitive function and found discrepancies. The association was closer when informants' ratings of the subjects' impairment were compared with the objective evidence. Consistent with the view of Beatty and Monson (1991) of metamemory as a function of frontal integrity, Taylor noted that the greatest discrepancies in his sample occurred in patients who did poorly on frontal lobe tests.

In a related study, Sullivan *et al.* (1990) canvassed 25 000 Canadians many of whom had MS. Using the Perceived Deficits Questionnaire, subjects were asked to rate their cognitive performance on four indices: attention, retrospective memory, prospective memory and planning/organizational skills. Within this sample, 38% considered themselves cognitively impaired in at least one area, a figure that approximates those from two community-based neuropsychological studies (McIntosh-Michaelis *et al.*, 1991; Rao *et al.*, 1991). Whether the two assessment procedures are identifying the same group of patients must, however, be open to doubt given the documented evidence of metamemory problems in MS patients. The study by Sullivan *et al.* (1990) was unable to provide the answer because objective assessment procedures were not undertaken. McIntosh-Michaelis *et al.*, (1991), however, demonstrated convincingly that MS patients tended to substantially overestimate their perceptions of memory impairment and difficulties with attention. Possible reasons for this include depression masquerading as cognitive deficits (Randolph *et al.*, 2004), patients misattributing problems in attention and executive function to memory impairment, and lower education status (Randolph *et al.*, 2001).

In contrast to these findings, Kujala *et al.* (1996) found that MS patients with early cognitive decline were able to appraise their memory deficits accurately, which may indicate that metamemory is, in part, related to the overall severity of cognitive deficits. Further evidence of this comes from Marrie *et al.* (2005), who found that cognitive complaints were less common in patients whose cognition was either intact or severely impaired.

Visuospatial deficits in multiple sclerosis

In the often cited cognitive study of MS patients living in the community (Rao *et al.*, 1991), deficits in visuospatial skills were elicited across a range of tasks that included visual organization, facial recognition, line orientation and discrimination of visual form. Almost one in five patients were impaired on one or more of the tests. Other studies have replicated this finding (Laatu *et al.*, 2001) and have shown that visuospatial problems can occur in a subset of patients independently of impaired visual acuity or neurological disability (Vleugels *et al.*, 2001).

Language

Aphasia is unusual in MS patients, but this should not obscure the fact that a minority of MS patients (approximately 9%) perform poorly on tests of language, such as the Boston Naming Test (Rao *et al.*, 1991). Furthermore, abnormalities are almost three time more likely to be elicited on the COWAT (Benton and Hamsher, 1976), which is a measure not only of language but also of sustained attention and lexical memory (Rao *et al.*, 1991). The COWAT has been widely used in studying MS patients. It consists of three word naming trials and the letters most frequently used are F, A and S (hence FAS scores). Subjects are asked to generate as many words as they can think of beginning with the chosen letter, excluding proper nouns, numbers and the same word with a different suffix. A minute is allowed for each letter and the total score represents the summation of all words generated in the three minute period. Published normative data are available for comparisons. A similar paradigm, the Category Fluency Test, gets patients to name as many four-legged animals as they can in one minute.[3] The test has been regarded as a sensitive indicator of brain dysfunction, in particular dominant frontal lobe pathology (Miceli *et al.*, 1981), although Benton (1968) found that bilateral frontal lesions produced the most impaired scores. However, like many good cognitive screening instruments, the COWAT taps more than a single aspect of cognition and is, therefore, likely to defy easy localization.

---

[3] A parallel version, the Supermarket Fluency Test, asks patients to name items in a supermarket.

Crawford *et al.* (1992) demonstrated that scores correlated significantly with premorbid IQ as measured by a reading test such as the the ANART. This observation has generated data that allows the neuropsychiatrist to predict FAS scores on the basis of estimates of premorbid IQ (Crawford *et al.*, 1992). Discrepancies between actual and predicted scores are a useful, albeit indirect, measure of general decline in intellect.

The poor performance of MS patients on the COWAT (Caine *et al.*, 1986; Beatty *et al.*, 1989b, Rao *et al.*, 1991) has led to the test's inclusion in brief cognitive screening procedures for MS (Rao *et al.*, 1991; Basso *et al.*, 1996) and a more comprehensive cognitive battery endorsed by consensus opinion among MS researchers (Benedict *et al.*, 2002).

The relationship of cognition to other aspects of multiple sclerosis

Depression

Early MS studies that investigated the role of depression in cognitive dysfunction failed to find an association (Rao *et al.*, 1989, 1991; Minden *et al.*, 1990; Grafman *et al.*, 1991; Schiffer and Caine, 1991; Good *et al.*, 1992; Krupp *et al.*, 1994; Möller *et al.*, 1994). There were, however, a number of methodological problems associated with these data. These included small sample size, the use of depression rating scales that failed to reduce the confounding diagnostic effects of a vegetative symptom such as fatigue, and cognitive tests that lacked sensitivity. Furthermore, some studies restricted enrollment to patients with mild depression, thereby missing a putative threshold effect that links cognitive difficulties to more severe depressive symptomatology.

The reports that failed to find an association between depression and cognitive dysfunction have been partly offset by results from two studies, one of which also contained significant flaws. Gilchrist and Creed (1994) reported that depressed MS patients were more likely than euthymic MS patients to show significant cognitive deficits, but they failed to control for the effects of age on their findings. More impressive results emerged from a meta-analysis of 10 studies that contained data on depression and performance on two measures of working memory, namely the PASAT and the Brown Petersen Test (Thornton and Raz, 1997). A Spearman's correlation of 0.6 ($p < .05$) emerged, suggesting that depression slowed the speed of information processing and/or impaired working memory. A subsequent series of studies explored this relationship further, in particular the idea that depression may lead to a reduction in cognitive capacity, thereby making fewer attentional resources available for patients performing capacity-demanding tasks.

Pursuing this line of thinking Arnett *et al.* (1999a,b) demonstrated that clinically significant depression may lead to impaired cognitive and attentional capacity, which may be further refined as deficits in working memory and, more specifically, an executive dysfunction. Thus, the deleterious cognitive effects of low mood appear linked to a dysexecutive syndrome. A threshold effect is also apparent in depressed patients in that the more severe the mood disturbance the more likely cognitive deficits will manifest (Demaree et al., 2003).

The depression–cognition data raise an interesting, clinically relevant question. If depression was treated, would there be cognitive improvement as well? To date there are no MS data addressing this, but results from another neuropsychiatric condition are encouraging. Depressed patients with a traumatic brain injury showed improvements in tests of attention, information processing speed and executive function after anti-depressant medication successfully alleviated the low mood (Fann et al., 2001).

Medication

To what extent psychotropic medication may influence cognitive performance is an important consideration and one of practical importance given the high psychiatric morbidity associated with MS. In a study of 92 community-based MS patients, one third were taking tranquilizers, 7% were using either antidepressants or neuroleptics and 2% were taking morphine. Twenty one percent used medication that was non-sedative and only a third of patients were medication free (Stenager et al., 1994). However, when tested with an array of neuropsychological tests, including the Symbol–Digit Modality Test as a measure of information processing speed, no association was found between cognitive performance and the use of sedative medication. Lack of a specific association between medication effects and cognitive performance has also been reported by Rao et al. (1991).

Physical disability

Study of the relationship between cognitive dysfunction and physical disability has yielded contradictory findings (Heaton et al., 1985; Rao et al., 1991). In a study designed specifically to address this relationship, Marsh (1980) found that disability as measured by the Kurtzke Disability Scale (KDS; Kurtzke, 1970) correlated only with duration of illness, but not with verbal, performance or full-scale IQ on the WAIS. A failure to find any association between KDS (Kurtzke, 1970) scores and cognitive function has also been reported by others (Peyser et al., 1980; Rao et al., 1985; Lyon-Caen et al., 1986). Alternative procedures for assessing physical disability such as the Activities of Daily Living Test (Howarth and Hollings, 1979) have given similar results (Ron et al., 1991).

There are, however, exceptions to the above (Huber et al., 1987; Stenager et al., 1989), while indirect support has also come from Beatty and Gange (1977), who used five measures of motor impairment and found a correlation with memory deficits. An epidemiological study investigating the frequency, patterns and predictors of cognitive dysfunction (Rao *et al.*, 1991) noted a weak but significant correlation with disability.

Failure to find an association may be an artefact of research methodology that relies on a biased rating assessment procedure. Thus, while cognitive deficits are attributable to cerebral atrophy and plaques in the cerebral white matter, physical disability as measured by the scales such as the KDS (Kurtzke, 1970) or EDSS (Kurtzke, 1983) is weighted towards the presence of lesions in the spinal cord, posterior fossa and cerebellum, causing mainly motor effects. (See Ch. 1 for a critique of the Kurtzke scales.) A further problem in interpreting these data is that physical disability may be linked to variables such as age, exacerbation, disease duration and disease course. Consequently, more disabled patients have tended to be older, with disease of longer duration and a CP course. To separate these potentially confounding effects, Beatty *et al.* (1990b) undertook a longitudinal study during which patients underwent neurological examination every six months for a two year period. Multiple regression techniques did not elicit demographic or clinical predictors of cognitive performance.

Duration of illness

The majority of studies have failed to find an association between disease duration and cognitive dysfunction (Ivnik, 1978; Rao *et al.*, 1984, 1985, 1991). Marsh (1980), although reporting a link between disease duration and disability, found that neither duration nor disability correlated with cognition. The reason for this can be traced to the fact that patients with illnesses of similar durations may differ greatly with respect to disease activity, ranging from quiescent ("benign") to rapidly progressive. Controlling for confounding effects such as age and disease course, Beatty *et al.* (1990b) also failed to demonstrate such a relationship.

There are, however, a few studies that have reported different results. Ron *et al.* (1991) noted a positive association with a modest correlation coefficient (0.30), albeit significant at a 1% level, while Grant *et al.* (1984) showed that disturbance in short-term memory, learning and recall of verbal and non-verbal information were associated with the number of years of "active disease." They defined this concept as the "number of years in which the patient reported at least one week's duration of symptoms," which is open to criticism, not least because MRI studies have shown that clinical relapses do not often mirror the development of new brain lesions, the latter occurring at least seven times more often (Thompson *et al.*, 1992).

Disease course

Initial evidence suggested that cognitive deficits were more marked in patients with CP as opposed to relapsing–remitting (RR) MS. Heaton *et al.* (1985) studied

100 patients (57 with RR and 43 with CP MS) who were consecutive admissions to a neurological ward, and a similar number of healthy controls. Patients were clinically stable at the time of testing. Both the CP and RR groups were more cognitively impaired than the healthy controls and the patients with CP MS were, in turn, more cognitively impaired than those with RR MS on most measures. These differences were not related to greater sensory or motor impairment in the CP group and persisted when the duration of disease (longer in the CP group) was controlled for.

This result was confirmed by Rao *et al.* (1987), who compared the performances of MS patients with RR and CP disease and a control group of back pain sufferers using the WCST. While no differences were apparent between the RR group and control subjects, patients with CP MS differed from both in terms of the number of perseverative errors made and fewer categories achieved. A stepwise regression analysis suggested these differences were independent of physical disability or disease duration. Indirect evidence supporting disease course as an important predictor of cognitive dysfunction has also come from studies confined to *one* of the subgroups. For example, in a study of RR MS patients only, Anzola *et al.* (1990) reported a mild global cognitive impairment, while Beatty *et al.* (1989b) observed that cognitive deficits in their RR MS patients were less severe than those previously documented in subjects with a CP course. Studies limited to patients with CP disease have reported that three quarters were impaired on tests of information processing speed (Beatty *et al.*, 1988) and that memory was significantly compromised in over half (Rao *et al.*, 1984).

However, all these findings linking cognition to a CP disease course were reported prior to longitudinal studies being undertaken. Follow-up studies have revealed a different picture (Jennekens-Schinkel *et al.*, 1990) with brain lesion load (Feinstein *et al.*, 1992b; 1993; Hohol *et al.*, 1997; Sperling *et al.*, 2001) and brain atrophy (Amato *et al.*, 2004), not disease course, determining a patient's cognitive status. While a CP course may be associated with more extensive brain plaques, this is not invariably so. In addition, if the lesion burden falls predominantly within the spinal cord, disease course becomes less relevant with respect to cognition. Longitudinal studies have also called into question assumptions that the course of MS runs true once established. In a follow-up study over one to five years of 254 patients with definite MS (mean 2.6 years), Goodkin *et al.* (1989) found that approximately a third of patients became stable while slightly fewer (20%) RR patients deteriorated to a CP course. It should be noted, however, that no patients reverted from a CP to a RR course.

More recently, comparisons between two subgroups of patients with CP MS have been completed: those with primary progressive MS (PPMS) and secondary progressive MS (SPMS). Comi *et al.* (1995) undertook detailed neuropsychological assessments and brain MRI in 14 patients with PPMS and 17 with SPMS. The two groups were matched for age and EDSS, but the SPMS group had had the disease for longer. Cognitive impairment was seven times more common in patients with SPMS (7% versus 53%) and appeared linked to demonstrably higher lesion loads in multiple brain regions. This result received a modicum of support from Gaudino *et al.* (2001), who noted greater verbal learning problems in patients with PPMS and SPMS than in those with RR MS, with a trend for the SPMS group to have the most extensive deficits. However, Foong *et al.* (2000) described a different cognitive picture, once more in samples of modest size, but this time matched for all demographic and illness variables including duration of symptoms. In addition a group of healthy controls were tested. The only cognitive difference to emerge was subtle: patients with SPMS performed more poorly than the PPMS group on a spatial memory task, with the performance of both patient groups inferior to that in the healthy controls across all cognitive domains. Once more, lesion load was much higher in the SPMS group, but this time did not correlate with any of the neuropsychological results in either of the patient groups. The reason for the discrepant findings between the various studies is unclear. The mismatch in disease duration reported by Comi *et al.* (1995) may have introduced a degree of bias into their study, but this cannot explain why the studies differed so fundamentally in their reported pattern of brain–behavior correlations.

Before concluding this section, some comment is needed on how patients with a benign disease course fare cognitively. This area has received scant attention, presumably because the descriptor "benign" suggests an illness that is mild and without ill effect. One study investigated whether the tacit assumption held up to psychometric inquiry. Defining benign as a disease duration of 15 years or more with an EDSS of 3.0 or less, Amato *et al.* (2006) showed that 45% of patients were cognitively impaired, 54% were depressed and 49% had significant fatigue. The EDSS emerged as the only significant predictor of cognitive dysfunction, notwithstanding the limited range. This result is a salutary wake-up call to clinicians.

Genetics

Substantial evidence links polymorphism of the gene for apolipoprotein E (*APOE*) to the pathogenesis of Alzheimer's disease (Bales *et al.*, 2002) and a poor outcome following traumatic brain injury (Teasdale *et al.*, 1997; Chiang *et al.*, 2003). Of the three common alleles, (ε2, ε3 and ε4) *APOE*-ε4 wields the greatest adverse influence. It has also been implicated in some poor outcome measures in patients with MS.

In a study of 614 MS patients from 379 families, *APOE*-ε4 carriers had more severe disease (Schmidt *et al.*, 2002), although others have suggested this applies selectively to women with MS (Kantarci *et al.*, 2004). In a 40 year follow-up study, this allele also emerged as a major predictor of neurological disability in both genders (Chapman *et al.*, 2001). Moreover, it has been associated with a rapid progression of disease and a higher annual relapse rate (Fazekas *et al.*, 2001). It has also been postulated that the presence of *APOE-ε4* leads to more extensive tissue destruction compounded by less-efficient tissue repair. Data from a MRI study lends support to this theory (Fazekas *et al.*, 2000). Both MRI scans and genetic data were obtained in 83 patients with MS. The MRI comparisons were undertaken between 19 subjects with the *APOE-ε3/ε4* genotype and 64 with the *APOE-ε2/ε3* genotype. While the *ε3/ε4* group showed a non-significant trend for more lesions on proton density scans, they had a significantly higher "black hole" ratio, defined as T_1/T_2 lesion load $\times$ 100. The presence of more T_1 weighted lesions in the *ε3/ε4* group was taken as evidence of greater tissue damage and fits with the theory of genetically modulated tissue damage and repair.

Given the consistency in the MS *APOE-ε4* data as outlined above, it is surprising that the two studies looking for cognitive correlates of *APOE-ε4* have revealed, at best, equivocal findings. In the first of these, it can be persuasively argued that the negative result reflected the study's problematic methodology (Olvieri *et al.*, 1999). First, the sample size was 89 patients, of whom only 12 subjects had at least one *APOE-ε4* allele. This raises the distinct possibility of a type II error. Second, the brief cognitive battery was idiosyncratic. There was also no neuroimaging component to this study. In a second study, cognitive decline was identified in 56% of 503 MS patients and, in male patients only, was associated with the presence of the *APOE-ε4* allele (Savettieri *et al.*, 2004). No adequate explanation was given for this gender divide, which may have been an artefact of the sample selection. For example, male patients in general were found to have greater cognitive difficulties, which were linked to higher EDSS scores, longer disease duration and lower levels of education. No such associations were present in female patients.

Based on the results from these two studies, it is premature to arrive at any definite conclusions concerning the role of *APOE-ε4* in the cognitive functioning of MS patients. So far the clear association between the *APOE-ε4* allele and abnormal brain imaging indices has not been replicated when it comes to cognitive dysfunction. What is needed to clarify this issue is a study with greater statistical power, a valid neuropsychological assessment and MRI that can delineate variables such as lesion and regional brain volumes.

Multiple sclerosis and dementia: a summation of cognitive abnormalities

Dementia is defined by the Diagnostic and Statistical Manual of the American Psychiatric Association (1994) as memory impairment (impaired ability to learn new information or to recall previously learned information) plus one or more of the following cognitive disturbances: aphasia, apraxia, agnosia and disturbances in executive function (i.e. planning, organizing, sequencing, abstracting). No mention is made of delayed information processing speed, considered the hallmark cognitive deficit in MS patients. Even with the omission of a crucial cognitive deficit, data from a prospectively collected sample of 291 patients revealed that 22% of patients met the DSM-IV criteria for dementia (R. H. B. Benedict, personal communication). This is lower than the 40% figure for cognitive impairment that researchers quote, but nonetheless represents an important clinical observation.

Summary

- The prevalence of cognitive dysfunction in a representative, community-based sample of MS patients is approximately 40%.
- Decline in intellect (IQ) does occur, but as a group, MS patients' scores remain within the normal range.
- The hallmark of cognitive dysfunction is a reduction in speed of information processing.
- Memory function has been well studied and reveals deficits in working memory and long-term memory. Verbal and non-verbal memory are adversely affected and the mechanism probably involves failures at the acquisition, storage and retrieval stages.
- Metamemory is impaired.
- Implicit memory is spared.
- Well-described deficits are present on tests of executive function, where the predominant problem may be generating concepts as opposed to perseverative responses.
- The correlations between cognitive dysfunction and physical disability, disease duration and disease course are either weak or absent.
- The relationship between cognitive dysfunction and depression is complex. Patients who complain of cognitive dysfunction are more likely to have depression than objective evidence of cognitive difficulties. However, not all subjective cognitive complaints can be attributed to depression. Data have linked depression with deficits in working memory and executive function.

References

Amato MP, Bartolozzi ML, Zipoli V, *et al.* (2004) Neocortical volume decrease in relapsing-remitting MS patients with mild cognitive impairment. *Neurology*, **63**, 80–93.

Amato MP, Zipoli V, Goretti B, *et al.* (2006) Benign multiple sclerosis: cognitive, psychological and social aspects in a clinical cohort. *Journal of Neurology*, **253**, 1054–1059.

American Psychiatric Association (1994) *Diagnostic and Statistical Manual of Mental Disorders*, 4th edn. Washington: American Psychiatric Press.

Anderson SW, Damasio H, Jones RD, Tranel D. (1991) Wisconsin Card Sorting Test performance as a measure of frontal lobe damage. *Journal of Clinical and Experimental Neuropsychology*, **13**, 909–922.

Anzola GP, Bevilacqua L, Cappa SF, *et al.* (1990) Neuropsychological assessment in patients with relapsing–remitting multiple sclerosis and mild functional impairment: correlation with magnetic resonance imaging. *Journal of Neurology, Neurosurgery and Psychiatry*, **53**, 142–145.

Arnett PA, Rao SM, Bernardin L, *et al.* (1994) Relationship between frontal lobe lesions and Wisconsin Card Sort Test performance in patients with multiple sclerosis. *Neurology*, **44**, 420–425.

Arnett PA, Higginson CI, Voss WD, *et al.* (1999a) Depressed mood in multiple sclerosis: relationship to capacity-demanding memory and attentional functioning. *Neuropsychology*, **13**, 434–446.

Arnett PA, Higginson CI, Voss WD, *et al.* (1999b) Depression in multiple sclerosis: relationship to working memory. *Neuropsychology*, **13**, 546–556.

Baddeley A. (1986) *Working Memory*. New York: Oxford University Press.

Baddeley A. (2003) Working memory: looking back and looking forward. *Nature Reviews/Neuroscience*, **4**, 829–839.

Bales KR, Dodart JC, DeMattos RB, Holtzman DM, Paul SM. (2002) Apolipoprotein E, amyloid and Alzheimer's disease. *Molecular Interventions*, **2**, 363–375.

Basso MR, Beason-Hazen S, Lynn J, Rammohan K, Bornstein RA. (1996) Screening for cognitive dysfunction in multiple sclerosis. *Archives of Neurology*, **53**, 980–984.

Beatty PA, Gange JJ. (1977) Neuropsychological aspects of multiple sclerosis. *Journal of Nervous and Mental Disease*, **164**, 42–50.

Beatty WW (1993) Memory and "frontal lobe" dysfunction in multiple sclerosis. *Journal of the Neurological Sciences*, **115**(Suppl.), 38–41.

Beatty WW, Goodkin DE. (1990) Screening for cognitive impairment in multiple sclerosis. An evaluation of the mini-mental state examination. *Archives of Neurology*, **47**, 297–301.

Beatty WW, Monson N. (1990) Semantic priming in multiple sclerosis. *Bulletin of the Psychonomic Society*, **28**, 397–400.

Beatty WW, Monson N. (1991) Metamemory in multiple sclerosis. *Journal of Clinical and Experimental Neuropsychology*, **13**, 309–327.

Beatty WW, Monson N. (1996) Problem solving by patients with multiple sclerosis: Comparison of performance on the Wisconsin and California card sorting tests. *Journal of the International Neuropsychological Society*, **2**, 134–140.

Beatty WW, Goodkin DE, Monson N, Beatty PA, Hertsgaard D. (1988) Anterograde and retrograde amnesia in patients with chronic–progressive multiple sclerosis. *Archives of Neurology*, **45**, 611–619.

Beatty WW, Goodkin DE, Beatty PA, Monson N. (1989a) Frontal lobe dysfunction and memory impairment in patients with chronic–progressive multiple sclerosis. *Brain and Cognition*, **11**, 73–86.

Beatty WW, Goodkin DE, Monson N, Beatty PA. (1989b) Cognitive disturbance in patients with relapsing–remitting multiple sclerosis. *Archives of Neurology*, **46**, 1113–1119.

Beatty WW, Goodkin DE, Monson N, Beatty PA. (1990a) Implicit learning in patients with chronic–progressive multiple sclerosis. *International Journal of Clinical Neuropsychology*, **12**, 153–162.

Beatty WW, Goodkin DE, Hertsgaard D, Monson N. (1990b) Clinical and demographic predictors of cognitive performance in MS. Do diagnostic type, disease duration and disability matter? *Archives of Neurology*, **47**, 305–308.

Beatty WW, Paul RH, Wilbanks SL, *et al.* (1995a) Identifying multiple sclerosis patients with mild or global cognitive impairments using the Screening Examination for Cognitive Impairment (SEFCI). *Neurology*, **45**, 718–723.

Beatty WW, Hames KA, Blanco CR, Paul RH, Wilbanks SL (1995b) Verbal abstraction deficit in multiple sclerosis. *Neuropsychology*, **9**, 198–205.

Benedict RHB, Fischer JS, Archibald CJ, *et al.* (2002) Minimal neuropsychological assessment of MS patients: a consensus approach. *The Clinical Neuropsychologist*, **16**, 381–397.

Benedict RHB, Weinstock-Guttman B, Fishman I, Sharma J, Tjoa CW. (2004) Prediction of neuropsychological impairment in multiple sclerosis. Comparison of conventional magnetic resonance imaging measures of atrophy and lesion burden. *Archives of Neurology*, **61**, 226–230.

Benton AL. (1968) Differential behavioral effects of frontal lobe disease. *Neuropsychologia*, **6**, 53–60.

Benton AL, Hamsher K de S. (1976) *Multilingual Aphasia Examination*. Iowa City, IA: University of Iowa Press.

Berg EAA. (1948) A simple objective test for measuring flexibility in thinking. *Journal of General Psychology*, **39**, 15–22.

Bobholz JA, Rao SM. (2003) Cognitive dysfunction in multiple sclerosis: a review of recent developments. *Current Opinion in Neurology*, **16**, 283–288.

Caine ED, Bamford KA, Schiffer RB, Shoulson I, Levy S. (1986) A controlled neuropsychological comparison of Huntington's disease and multiple sclerosis. *Archives of Neurology*, **43**, 249–254.

Canter AH (1951) Direct and indirect measures of psychological deficit in multiple sclerosis. Part 1. *Journal of General Psychology*, **44**, 3–25.

Carroll M, Gates R, Roldan F. (1984) Memory impairment in multiple sclerosis. *Neuropsychologia*, **22**, 297–302.

Chapman J, Vinokurov S, Achiron A, *et al.* (2001). APOE genotype is a major predictor of long-term progression of disability in MS. *Neurology*, **56**, 312–316.

Charcot J-M. (1877) *Lectures on the Diseases of the Nervous System delivered at La Salpetriere*. London: New Sydenham Society, pp. 194–195.

Chiang MF, Chang JG, Hu CJ. (2003) Association between apolipoprotein E genotype and outcome of traumatic brain injury. *Acta Neurochirurgica*, **145**, 649–654.

Chiaravalloti ND, Demaree H, Gaudino EA, DeLuca L. (2003) Can the repetition effect maximise learning in multiple sclerosis. *Clinical Rehabilitation*, **17**, 58–68.

Christodoulou C, Krupp LB, Liang Z, *et al.* (2003) Cognitive performance and MTR markers of cerebral injury in cognitively impaired MS patients. *Neurology*, **60**, 1793–1798.

Comi G, Filippi M, Martinelli V, *et al.* (1995) Brain MRI correlates of cognitive impairment in primary and secondary progressive multiple sclerosis. *Journal of the Neurological Sciences*, **132**, 222–227.

Cottrell SS, Wilson SAK (1926) The affective symptomatology of disseminated multiple sclerosis. *Journal of Neurological Psychopathology*, **7**, 1–30.

Crawford JR, Moore JW, Cameron IM. (1992) Verbal fluency: a NART-based equation for the estimation of premorbid performance. *British Journal of Clinical Psychology*, **31**, 327–329.

Cummings JL. (1986) Subcortical dementia. Neuropsychology, neuropsychiatry, and pathophysiology. *British Journal of Psychiatry*, **149**, 682–697.

Cummings JL (1993) Frontal subcortical circuits and human behaviour. *Archives of Neurology*, **50**, 873–80.

Delis DC, Kaplan E, Kramer JH. (2001) *D-KEFS Executive Function System. Technical Manual.* San Antonio TX: Psychological Corporation.

DeLuca J, Barbieri-Berger S, Johnson SK. (1994) The nature of memory impairment in multiple sclerosis: acquisition versus retrieval. *Journal of Clinical and Experimental Neuropsychology*, **16**, 183–189.

DeLuca J, Gaudino EA, Diamond BJ, Christodoulou C, Engel RA. (1998) Acquisition and storage deficits in multiple sclerosis. *Journal of Clinical and Experimental Neuropsychology*, **20**, 376–390.

Demaree HA, Gaudino EA, DeLuca J, Ricker JH. (2000) Learning impairment is associated with recall ability in multiple sclerosis. *Journal of Clinical and Experimental Neuropsychology*, **22**, 865–873.

Demaree HA, Gaudino E, DeLuca J. (2003) The relationship between depressive symptoms and cognitive dysfunction in multiple sclerosis. *Cognitive Neuropsychiatry*, **8**, 161–171.

Denney DR, Lynch SG, Parmenter BA, Horne N. (2004) Cognitive impairment in relapsing and primary progressive multiple sclerosis: mostly a matter of speed. *Journal of the International Neuropsychological Society*, **10**, 948–956.

D'Esposito M, Onishi K, Thompson H, *et al.* (1996) Working memory impairments in multiple sclerosis: Evidence from a dual-task paradigm. *Neuropsychology*, **10**, 51–56.

Elsass P, Zeeberg I. (1983) Reaction time deficit in multiple sclerosis. *Acta Neurologica Scandinavica*, **68**, 257–261.

Fann JR, Uomoto JM, Katon WJ. (2001) Cognitive improvement with treatment of depression following mild traumatic brain injury. *Psychosomatics*, **42**, 48–54.

Fazekas F, Strasser-Fuchs S, Schmidt H, *et al.* (2000). Apoliprotein E genotype related differences in brain lesions of multiple sclerosis. *Journal of Neurology, Neurosurgery and Psychiatry*, **69**, 25–28.

Fazekas F, Strasser-Fuchs S, Kollegger H, *et. al.* (2001). Apolipoprotein E ε4 is associated with rapid progression of multiple sclerosis. *Neurology*, **57**, 853–857.

Feinstein A, Youl B, Ron M. (1992a) Acute optic neuritis. A cognitive and magnetic resonance imaging study. *Brain*, **115**, 1403–1415.

Feinstein A, Kartsounis L, Miller D, Youl B, Ron M. (1992b) Clinically isolated lesions of the type seen in multiple sclerosis followed up: a cognitive, psychiatric and MRI study. *Journal of Neurology, Neurosurgery and Psychiatry*, **55**, 869–876.

Feinstein A, Ron M, Thompson A. (1993) A serial study of psychometric and magnetic resonance imaging changes in multiple sclerosis. *Brain*, **116**, 569–602.

Feinstein A, Feinstein KJ, Gray T, O'Connor P. (1997) Neurobehavioral correlates of pathological crying and laughing in multiple sclerosis. *Archives of Neurology*, **54**, 1116–1121.

Fischer J. (1988) Using the Wechsler Memory Scale-Revised to detect and characterize memory deficits in multiple sclerosis. *Clinical Neuropsychology*, **2**, 149–172.

Fischer J, Kawczak K, Daughtry MM, *et al.* (1992). Unmasking subtypes of verbal memory impairment in multiple sclerosis. *Journal of Clinical and Experimental Neuropsychology*, **14**, 32.

Fisk JD, Archibald CJ (2001) Limitations of the Paced Auditory Serial Addition Test as a measure of working memory in patients with multiple sclerosis. *Journal of the International Neuropsychological Society*, **7**, 363–372.

Folstein MF, Folstein SE, McHugh PR. (1975) "Mini-Mental State": a practical method for grading the cognitive state of patients for the clinician. *Journal of Psychiatric Research*, **12**, 189–198.

Foong J, Rozewicz L, Chong WK, *et al.* (2000) A comparison of neuropsychological deficits in primary and secondary multiple sclerosis. *Journal of Neurology*, **247**, 97–101.

Franklin GM, Heaton RK, Nelson LM, Filley CM, Seibert C. (1988) Correlation of neuropsychological and MRI findings in chronic–progressive multiple sclerosis. *Neurology*, **38**, 1826–1829.

Gaudino EA, Chiaravalloti ND, DeLuca J, Diamond BJ. (2001) A comparison of memory performance in relapsing–remitting, primary progressive and secondary progressive multiple sclerosis. *Neuropsychiatry, Neuropsychology and Behavioral Neurology*, **14**, 32–44.

Gilchrist AC, Creed FH. (1994) Depression, cognitive impairment and social stress in multiple sclerosis. *Journal of Psychosomatic Research*, **38**, 193–201.

Goldstein FC, McKendall RR, Haut MC. (1992) Gist recall in multiple sclerosis. *Archives of Neurology*, **49**, 1060–1064.

Good K, Clark CM, Oger J, Paty, Klonoff H. (1992) Cognitive impairment and depression in mild multiple sclerosis. *Journal of Nervous and Mental Disease*, **180**, 730–732.

Goodkin DE, Hertsgaard D, Rudick RA. (1989) Exacerbation rates and adherence to disease type in a prospectively followed-up population with multiple sclerosis. *Archives of Neurology*, **46**, 1107–1112.

Grafman J, Rao SM, Litvan I. (1990) Disorders of memory. In *Neurobehavioural Aspects of Multiple Sclerosis*, ed. S. Rao New York: Oxford University Press, pp. 102–117.

Grafman J. Rao S, Bernardin L, Leo GJ. (1991) Automatic memory processes in patients with multiple sclerosis. *Archives of Neurology*, **48**, 1072–1075.

Grant I, McDonald WI, Trimble MR, Smith E, Reed R. (1984) Deficient learning and memory in early and middle phases of multiple sclerosis. *Journal of Neurology, Neurosurgery and Psychiatry*, **47**, 25–55.

Gronwall DMA, Wrightson P. (1974) Delayed recovery of intellectual function after minor head injury. *Lancet*, **i**, 605–609.

Heaton RK (1981) *Wisconsin Card Sorting Test Manual*. Odessa, Fl: Psychological Assessment Resources.

Heaton RK, Nelson LM, Thompson DS, Burk JS, Franklin GM. (1985) Neuropsychological findings in relapsing–remitting and chronic–progressive multiple sclerosis. *Journal of Consulting and Clinical Psychology*, **53**, 103–110.

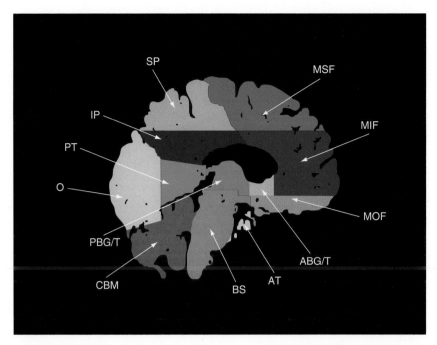

Plate 1.   MRI sagittal (medial) view demonstrating semi-automated brain region extraction (SABRE)-generated brain regions. MIF, medial inferior frontal; MOF, medial orbital frontal; MSF, medial superior frontal; SP, superior parietal; IP, inferior parietal; AT, anterior temporal; PT, posterior temporal; ABG/T, anterior basal ganglia/thalamus; PBG/T, posterior basal ganglia/thalamus; O, occipital; BS, brainstem; CBM, cerebellum.

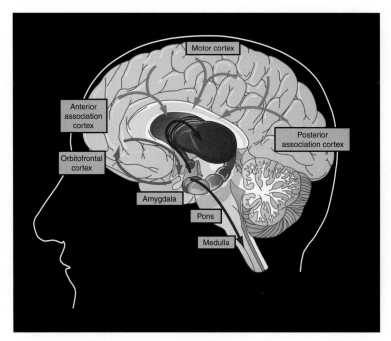

Plate 2a.　Neural circuits processing unconscious/visceral emotion. (By permission of the American Geriatric Society and with thanks to Joshua Grill.)

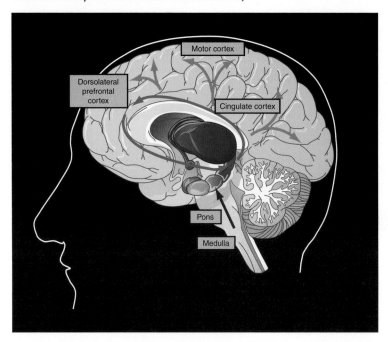

Plate 2b.　Neural circuit processing conscious/cognitive emotion. (By permission of the American Geriatric Society and with thanks to Joshua Grill.)

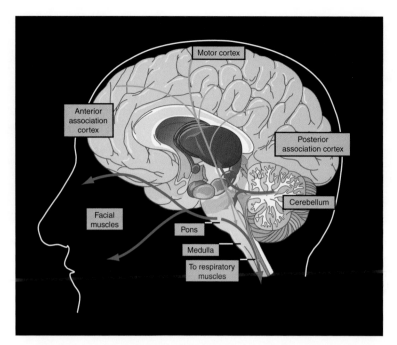

Plate 3a.   The cortico-ponto-cerebellar circuit processing emotion. (By permission of the American Geriatric Society and with thanks to Joshua Grill.)

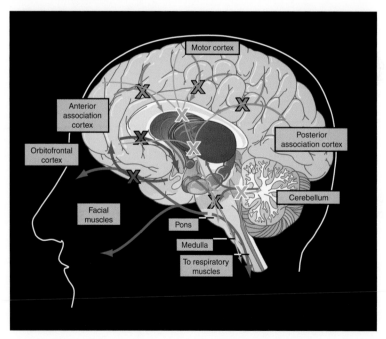

Plate 3b.   Pseudobulbar affect associated with lesions at multiple anatomical sites. (By permission of the American Geriatric Society and with thanks to Joshua Grill.)

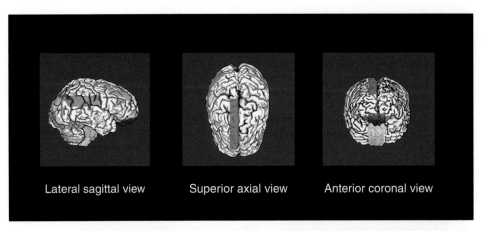

Plate 4.   Brain regions implicated in pseudobulbar affect demarcated by MRI. Yellow, brainstem; red, medial inferior frontal; green, inferior parietal; blue, medial superior frontal (R).

Hohol MJ, Guttmann CRG, Orav GA, *et al.* (1997) Serial neuropsychological assessment and magnetic resonance imaging analysis in multiple sclerosis. *Archives of Neurology*, **54**, 1018–1025.

Howarth RJ, Hollings EM. (1979) Are hospital assessments of daily living activities valid? *International Rehabilitation Medicine*, **1**, 59–62.

Huber SJ, Paulsen GW, Suttleworth EC, *et al.* (1987) Magnetic resonance imaging correlates of dementia in multiple sclerosis. *Archives of Neurology*, **44**, 732–736.

Ivnik RJ. (1978) Neuropsychological test performance as a function of the duration of MS related symptomatology. *Journal of Clinical Psychiatry*, **46**, 304–312.

Jambor KL. (1969) Cognitive functioning in multiple sclerosis. *British Journal of Psychiatry*, **115**, 765–775.

Jennekens-Schinkel A, Sanders EACM, Lanser JBK, van der Velde EA. (1988a) Reaction time in ambulant multiple sclerosis patients. Part 1. Influence of prolonged cognitive effort. *Journal of the Neurological Sciences*, **85**, 173–186.

Jennekens-Schinkel A, Sanders EACM, Lanser JBK, van der Velde EA. (1988b) Reaction time in ambulant multiple sclerosis patients. Part II. Influence of task complexity. *Journal of the Neurological Sciences*, **85**, 187–196.

Jennekens-Schinkel A, Laboyrie PM, Lanser JBK, van der Velde EA. (1990) Cognition in patients with multiple sclerosis after 4 years. *Journal of the Neurological Sciences*, **99**, 229–247.

Kantarci OH, Hebrink DD, Achenbach SJ, *et al.* (2004). Association of APOE polymorphisms with disease severity in MS is limited to women. *Neurology*, **62**, 811–814.

Kenealy PM, Beaumont JG, Lintern TC, Murrell RC. (2002) Autobiographical memory in advanced multiple sclerosis: assessment of episodic and personal semantic memory across three time spans. *Journal of the International Neuropsychological Society*, **8**, 855–860.

Kurtzke JF. (1970) Neurologic impairment in multiple sclerosis and the Disability Status Score. *Acta Neurologica Scandinavica*, **46**, 493–512.

Kurtzke JF (1983) Rating neurologic impairment in multiple sclerosis: an expanded disability scale. *Neurology*, **33**, 1444–1452.

Krupp LB, Alvarez LA, LaRocca N, Scheinberg LC. (1988) Fatigue in multiple sclerosis. *Archives of Neurology*, **45**, 435–437.

Krupp LB, Sliwinski M, Masur DM, Friedberg F, Coyle PK. (1994) Cognitive functioning and depression in patients with chronic fatigue syndrome. *Archives of Neurology*, **51**, 705–710.

Kujala P, Portin R, Revonsuo A, Ruutiainen J. (1994) Automatic and controlled information processing in multiple sclerosis. *Brain*, **117**, 1115–1126.

Kujala P, Portin R, Revonsuo A, Ruutiaïnen J. (1995) Attention related performance in two cognitively different subgroups of patients with multiple sclerosis. *Journal of Neurology, Neurosurgery and Psychiatry*, **59**, 77–82.

Kujala P, Portin R, Ruutiainen J. (1996) Memory deficits and early cognitve deterioration in MS. *Acta Neurologica Scandinavica*, **93**, 329–335.

Laatu S, Hamäläinen P, Revonsuo A, Portin RV, Ruutiainen J. (1999) Semantic memory deficit in multiple sclerosis: impaired understanding of conceptual meanings. *Journal of the Neurological Sciences*, **162**, 152–161.

Laatu S, Revonsuo A, Hamäläinen P, Ojanen V, Ruutiainen J. (2001) Visual object recognition in multiple sclerosis. *Journal of the Neurological Sciences*, **185**, 77–88.

Litvan I, Grafman J, Vendrell P, Martinez JM. (1988a) Slowed information processing speed in multiple sclerosis. *Archives of Neurology*, **45**, 281–285.

Litvan I, Grafman J, Vendrell P, *et al.* (1988b) Multiple memory deficits in patients with multiple sclerosis. Exploring the working memory system. *Archives of Neurology*, **45**, 607–610.

Lyon-Caen O, Jouvent R, Hauser S, *et al.* (1986) Cognitive function in recent onset demyelinating diseases. *Archives of Neurology*, **43**, 1138–1141.

Marrie RA, Chelune GJ, Miller DM, Cohen JA. (2005) Subjective cognitive complaints relate to mild impairment of cognition in multiple sclerosis. *Multiple Sclerosis*, **11**, 69–75.

Marsh GG (1980) Disability and intellectual function in multiple sclerosis patients. *Journal of Nervous and Mental Disease*, **168**, 758–762.

McIntosh-Michaelis SA, Wilkinson SM, Diamond ID, *et al.* (1991) The prevalence of cognitive impairment in a community survey of multiple sclerosis. *British Journal of Clinical Psychology*, **30**, 333–348.

Mendozzi L, Pugnetti L, Saccani M, Motta A. (1993) Frontal lobe dysfunction in multiple sclerosis as assessed by means of Lurian tasks: effects of age of onset. *Journal of the Neurological Sciences*, **115**(Suppl.), S42–S50.

Miceli G, Caltagirone C, Gainotti G, Masullo C, Silveri MC. (1981) Neuropsychological correlates of localised cerebral lesions in non-aphasic brain damaged patients. *Journal of Clinical Neuropsychology*, **3**, 53–63.

Minden SL, Moes EJ, Orav J, Kaplan E, Reich P. (1990) Memory impairment in multiple sclerosis. *Journal of Clinical and Experimental Neuropsychology*, **12**, 566–586.

Möller A, Wiedemann G, Rohde U, Backmund H, Sonntag A. (1994) Correlates of cognitive impairment and depressive mood disorder in multiple sclerosis. *Acta Psychiatrica Scandinavica*, **89**, 117–121.

Nelson HE (1982) *National Adult Reading Test: Manual.* Windsor: NFER-Nelson.

Oliveri RL, Cittadella R, Sibilia G, *et al.* (1999) APOE and the risk of cognitive impairment in multiple sclerosis. *Acta Neurologica Scandinavica*, **100**, 290–295.

Paul RH, Blanco CR, Hames KA, Beatty WW. (1997) Autobiographical memory in multiple sclerosis. *Journal of the International Neuropsychological Society*, **3**, 246–251.

Parsons OA, Stewart KD, Arenberg D. (1957) Impairment of abstracting ability in multiple sclerosis. *Journal of Nervous and Mental Disease*, **125**, 221–225.

Peyser JM, Edwards KR, Poser CM, Filskov SB. (1980) Cognitive function in patients with multiple sclerosis. *Archives of Neurology*, **37**, 577–579.

Peyser JM, Rao SM, LaRocca NG, Kaplan E. (1990) Guidelines for neuropsychological research in multiple sclerosis. *Archives of Neurology*, **47**, 94–97.

Randolph JJ, Arnett PA. Higginson CI. (2001) Metamemory and tested cognitive functioning in multiple sclerosis. *The Clinical Psychologist*, **15**, 357–368.

Randolph JJ, Arnett PA, Freske P. (2004) Metamemory in multiple sclerosis: exploring affective and executive contributors. *Archives of Clinical Neuropsychology*, **19**, 259–279.

Rao SM (1986) Neuropsychology of multiple sclerosis. A critical review. *Journal of Clinical and Experimental Neuropsychology*, **8**, 503–542.

Rao SM, Hammeke TA, McQuillen MP, Khatri BO, Lloyd D. (1984) Memory disturbance in chronic–progressive multiple sclerosis. *Archives of Neurology*, **41**, 625–631.

Rao SM, Glatt S, Hammeke TA, *et al.* (1985) Chronic–progressive multiple sclerosis: relationship between cerebral ventricular size and neuropsychological impairment. *Archives of Neurology*, **42**, 678–682.

Rao SM, Hammeke TA, Speech TJ (1987) Wisconsin Card Sort Test performance in relapsing–remitting and chronic–progressive multiple sclerosis. *Journal of Consulting and Clinical Psychology*, **55**, 263–265.

Rao SM, Leo GJ, St. Aubin-Flaubert P. (1989) On the nature of memory disturbance in multiple sclerosis. *Journal of Clinical and Experimental Neuropsychology*, **11**, 699–712.

Rao SM, Leo GJ, Bernardin L, Unverzagt F. (1991) Cognitive dysfunction in multiple sclerosis. 1. Frequency, patterns and prediction. *Neurology*, **41**, 685–691.

Rao SM, Grafman J, DiGiulio D, *et al.* (1993) Memory dysfunction in multiple sclerosis: its relation to working memory, semantic encoding, and implicit learning. *Neuropsychology*, **7**, 364–374.

Reitan RM, Reed JC, Dyken ML. (1971) Cognitive, psychomotor and motor correlates of multiple sclerosis. *Journal of Nervous and Mental Disease*, **153**, 218–224.

Ron MA, Callanan MM, Warrington EK. (1991) Cognitive abnormalities in multiple sclerosis. a psychometric and MRI study. *Psychological Medicine*, **21**, 59–68.

Savettieri G, Messina D, Andreoli V, *et al.* (2004) Gender related effect of clinical and genetic variables on the cognitive impairment in multiple sclerosis. *Journal of Neurology*, **251**, 1208–1214.

Schacter DL, Tulving E. (1994) *Memory Systems*. Cambridge, MA: MIT Press.

Schiffer RB, Caine ED. (1991) The interaction between depressive affective disorder and neuropsychological test performance in multiple sclerosis. *Journal of Neuropsychiatry and Clinical Neurosciences*, **3**, 28–32.

Schmidt S, Barcellos LF, DeSombre K, *et al.* (2002) Association of polymorphisms in the apolipoprotein E region with susceptibility to and progression of multiple sclerosis. *American Journal of Human Genetics*, **70**, 708–717.

Smith A. (1982) *Symbol digit modalities test: Manual*. Los Angeles, CA: Western Psychological Services.

Sperling RA, Guttmann C, Hohol MJ, *et al.* (2001) Regional magnetic resonance imaging lesion burden and cognitive function in multiple sclerosis: a longitudinal study. *Archives of Neurology*, **58**, 115–121.

Squire LR. (1987) *Memory and Brain*. New York: Oxford University Press.

Staples D, Lincoln NB. (1979) Intellectual impairment in multiple sclerosis and its relation to functional abilities. *Rheumatology and Rehabilitation*, **18**, 153–160.

Stenager E, Knudsen L, Jensen K. (1989) Correlation of Beck depression inventory score, Kurtzke disability status and cognitive functioning in multiple sclerosis. In *Current Problems in Neurology* 10: *Mental Disorders and Cognitive Deficits in Multiple Sclerosis*, Ed. K Jensen, L Knudsen, E Stenager, I Grant. London: John Libbey, pp. 147–152.

Stenager E, Knudsen L, Jensen K. (1994) Multiple sclerosis: methodological aspects of cognitive testing. *Acta Neurologica Belgica*, **94**, 53–56.

Stuss DT, Levine B. (2002) Adult clinical neuropsychology: lessons learned from the frontal lobes. *Annual Review of Psychology*, **53**, 401–433.

Sullivan MJL, Edgley K, Dehoux E. (1990) A survey of multiple sclerosis. Part 1: Perceived cognitive problems and compensatory strategy use. *Canadian Journal of Rehabilitation*, **4**, 99–105.

Taylor R. (1990) Relationships between cognitive test performance and everyday cognitive difficulties in multiple sclerosis. *British Journal of Clinical Psychology*, **29**, 251–252.

Teasdale GM, Nicoll JA, Murray G, Fiddes M. (1997) Association of apolipoprotein E polymorphism with outcome after head injury. *Lancet*, **350**, 1069–1071.

Thompson AJ, Miller D, Youl B, *et al.* (1992) Serial gadolinium enhanced MRI in relapsing remitting multiple sclerosis of varying disease duration. *Neurology*, **42**, 60–63.

Thornton AE, Raz N. (1997) Memory impairment in multiple sclerosis. *Neuropsychology*, **11**, 357–366.

Tulving E. (1983) *Elements of Episodic Memory*, Oxford: Clarendon Press.

Tulving E. (2002) Episodic memory: From mind to brain. *Annual Review of Psychology*, **53**, 1–25.

van den Burg W, van Zomeren AH, Minderhoud JM, Prange AJA, Meijer NSA (1987) Cognitive impairment in patients with multiple sclerosis and mild physical disability. *Archives of Neurology*, **44**, 494–501.

Vleugels L, Lafosse C, van Nunen A, *et al.* (2001) Visuoperceptual impairment in multiple sclerosis patients: nature and possible neural origins. *Multiple Sclerosis*, **7**, 389–401.

Weinberger DR, Berman KF, Zec RF (1986) Physiologic dysfunction of the dorsolateral prefrontal cortex in schizophrenia. *Archives of General Psychiatry*, **43**, 114–124.

Wishart H, Sharpe D. (1997) Neuropsychological aspects of multiple sclerosis: a quantitative review. *Journal of Clinical and Experimental Neuropsychology*, **19**, 810–824.

8

The natural history of cognitive change in multiple sclerosis

The initial cognitive studies in MS were concerned with establishing the prevalence and nature of the deficits. Once these objectives had largely been attained, attention could be directed at other areas such as the pathogenesis, natural history, clinical significance and treatment of cognitive difficulties. This chapter will review the findings relating to one of these aspects, namely the natural history of cognitive decline in MS, and attempt to answer the following questions. How early in the illness does cognitive dysfunction become apparent? How do these changes progress over the years or, indeed, do they progress? With MS frequently running a relapsing–remitting course characterized by disease exacerbations and variable degrees of recovery, how do these changes affect cognition?

The onset of cognitive dysfunction

Canter (1951) had shown that a general decline in intellect occurred within four years of developing MS. However, it was unclear whether cognitive decline coincided with the onset of neurological symptoms or at some point thereafter. In addition, the limited scope of his psychometric battery and the paucity of objective measures of neurological disease curtails the study's conclusions.

Clinically isolated syndromes of the type seen in multiple sclerosis

In order to assess how early cognitive abnormalities become apparent, research has been directed at patients with clinically isolated syndromes (CIS) of the type seen in MS. These syndromes may present as optic neuritis, brainstem or spinal cord syndromes (Ch. 1). Given that CIS are frequently the harbinger of MS, the search for cognitive abnormalities in these patients may indicate how early in the disease process intellectual deficits begin. Callanan et al. (1989) studied a heterogeneous group of 48 patients with CIS composed almost equally of optic neuritis, brainstem and spinal cord presentations. The mean duration of symptoms was 2.2 years and performance of the group on a number of cognitive indices was compared with a control group with physically disabling conditions sparing brain involvement (i.e. rheumatoid arthritis). The CIS group was found to have a greater decline in IQ and more deficits on tests of auditory attention than the control group. Eighty one percent of the CIS patients had abnormalities on brain MRI, which correlated significantly with indices of cognitive dysfunction. The high number of patients with cerebral lesions is, however, unusual for a sample of patients with CIS and probably reflects the mean two year duration of neurological symptoms prior to MR imaging.

The study replicated the results of earlier work by Lyon-Caen *et al.* (1986), who investigated the presence of cognitive and psychiatric abnormalities in nine patients with optic neuritis and 21 patients with definite or probable MS of less than 2 years' duration. In comparison with a control group with neurological disorders such as headache, epilepsy and facial palsy, the study group showed cognitive deficits in 60%. The patients with optic neuritis were less cognitively impaired than the MS group, but both groups had deficits on a number of the subscales of the Wechsler Adult Intelligence Scale and the Wechsler Memory Scale.

While both the above studies pointed towards the development of cognitive dysfunction early in the disease process, neither could say whether cognitive changes were present when patients first became symptomatic. This was addressed by Feinstein *et al.* (1992a) in a study of 42 patients with acute optic neuritis, whose mean duration of symptoms was 14 days. No subject had a duration of symptoms greater than five weeks and subjects were excluded if the vision in the affected eye was less than 6/6. A battery of psychometric tests including an estimate of premorbid IQ, Purdue Pegboard Test, a short version of the Raven Progressive Matrices, Stroop Colour Word Test, Symbol-Digit Modalities Test, the Paced Auditory Serial Addition Task (PASAT), the Paced Visual Serial Addition Task (PVSAT), and tests of Simple Reaction Times and Choice Reaction Times were given to patients and a demographically matched group of healthy subjects. Subjects also underwent MRI of the brain and abnormalities noted in 55% of the sample.

A three-way cognitive comparison was undertaken between patients with optic neuritis with and without brain lesions and the healthy control group. The results are displayed in Table 8.1 and illustrate that significant deficits in the pegboard performance and auditory (PASAT) and visual (PVSAT) attention were present in the optic neuritis group, particularly if brain lesions were present. The failure of the optic neuritis group with brain involvement to perform adequately on the serial addition tasks reflects not only difficulties with attention but also abnormalities in speed or efficiency of information processing, considered hallmark

Table 8.1. Comparisons in cognition between healthy controls and patients with optic neuritis with and without brain lesions on MRI

	Group 1: controls (n = 36) (mean [SD] or median [range])	Group 2: ON with normal MRI (n = 19) (mean [SD] or median [range])	Group 3: ON with abnormal MRI (n = 23) (mean [SD] or median [range])	Oneway ANOVA/Kruskal–Wallis	Significance	1 vs 2	1 vs 3	2 vs 3
Pegboard test	41.8 (4.4)	37.3 (4.6)	37.7 (4.6)	$F = 9.0$	$p < 0.0001$	+	+	.
Raven's matrices	11.4 (3.)	10.5 (2.5)	10.1 (2.6)	$F = 1.9$	NS	.	.	.
Stroop test	22.4 (4.8)	22.1 (4.9)	25.1 (7.0)	$F = 2.1$	NS	.	.	.
SDMT	11.8 (1.8)	12.0 (1.0)	12.9 (1.9)	$F = 3.0$	$p < 0.06$	.	.	.
PASAT (4 s)	2.0 (0–8.0)	1.0 (0–7.0)	3.0 (0–14.0)	$x^2 = 7.3$	$p < 0.03$	.	+	+
PASAT (2 s)	7.9 (3.7)	8.1 (4.4)	11.2 (5.4)	$F = 4.3$	$p < 0.01$	.	+	.
PVSAT (4 s)	0.5 (0–6.0)	0 (0–5.0)	1.0 (0–15.0)	$x^2 = 0.14$	NS	.	.	.
PVSAT (2 s)	4.8 (3.4)	5.9 (4.6)	7.8 (4.6)	$F = 3.7$	$p < 0.03$	.	+	.

SDMT, Symbol-Digit Modalities Test; PASAT, Paced Auditory Serial Addition Task; PVSAT, Paced Visual Serial Addition Task; s, time in seconds between the stimulus presentation; SD, standard deviation. The Stroop and SDMT scores are times (in seconds).

Source: From Feinstein *et al.* (1992a) by permission of Oxford University Press.

cognitive deficits in patients with a confirmed diagnosis of MS (Ch. 7). Tasks like the PASAT also tap into a number of different cognitive processes including retrieval from short-term memory, thereby making it a sensitive discriminator of cognitive speed between brain-damaged patients and controls, particularly when stimuli are presented more quickly (Litvan *et al.*, 1988). This too was noted in the optic neuritis sample with brain lesions.

Studies of cognitive change

Studies investigating cognitive change over time in MS have adopted one of two strategies. The first has taken a cross-sectional approach with the patient sample stratified according to disease duration. The second method has been to follow patients longitudinally with serial measurements of various cognitive indices.

Cross-sectional studies

Evidence from cross-sectional studies supporting a progression of deficits has been equivocal. Ivnik (1978a) studied 36 patients with MS divided into triads on the basis of the number of years they had MS symptoms (1–5, 6–10 and >10 years). The three groups were matched for sex, education and age of onset of symptoms. No cognitive differences were found between the three groups and only in tests dependent on intact tactile perception did the group with the longer duration perform more poorly. Halligan *et al.* (1988) divided 60 MS patients into three equal groups with differing durations of illness (<5, 5–15 and >15 years) and found that a mild decline in abstracting and memory functions were present in the group with the longest duration of illness. However, other cognitive functions were intact and occupational and social functioning appeared unrelated to duration. Finally, Achiron *et al.* (2005) tested 150 MS patients to look for correlations between disease duration and indices of cognitive impairment. They concluded that there was a temporal sequence to cognitive decline, deficits in verbal fluency and verbal memory manifesting before visuospatial impairments, which, in turn, preceded problems with attention and information processing speed.

Longitudinal studies
Follow-up studies of patients with clinically isolated syndromes

A cognitive, psychiatric and MRI follow-up study of the original cohort of patients with CIS seen by Callanan *et al.* (1989) was undertaken by Feinstein *et al.* (1992b). Subjects were reassessed after a mean interval of 4.5 years (range, 42 to 67 months), by which time the sample size had decreased to 44 because the passage of time and reexamination of medical records made it clear that four patients had been incorrectly diagnosed. One patient was rediagnosed with motor neurone disease, another with a presenile dementia of the Alzheimer type and two were reassessed as having had MS not CIS at their index examination. Of the remaining 44 subjects, 35 (80%) were prepared to return to hospital and undergo a repeat battery of cognitive tests and a second brain MRI. Psychometric testing examined the following areas: IQ deficit, verbal and visual recognition memory, verbal recall memory, abstracting ability, visual and auditory attention, and naming ability.

At follow-up, half the subjects had developed MS, with two thirds following a relapsing–remitting course and the remainder in a chronic–progressive phase. As a group, the MS patients' cognitive performance had deteriorated significantly only with respect to visual memory, but when a three-way comparison was undertaken, the patients with a chronic–progressive course were more impaired on tests of verbal recall memory and auditory attention and were also significantly more depressed. They also had a greater lesion load on MRI and this correlated significantly with the degree of cognitive impairment. A noticeable finding was the marked individual variability that characterized cognitive change. If a patient's disease status remained unchanged (i.e. CIS at follow-up), there was no change in cognitive function or mood status. Similarly, even if the disease had progressed from CIS to relapsing–remitting MS, no significant cognitive decline was discernible. The critical variable that determined intellectual deterioration was the degree to which the brain total lesion load had increased (Ch. 10).

Short-term (up to one year) follow-up of patients with multiple sclerosis

Rapidly progressive dementia in which MS patients experience profound physical and mental deterioration over the course of a few months has been described. Bergin (1957) reported two such cases, both young women, in one of whom the diagnosis was made only at postmortem. Cognitive decline was inexorable and rapid. Such reports are, however, rare. Also unusual are cases in which cognition deteriorated as part of a clinical exacerbation, only to recover once neurological improvement occurred (Bieliauskas *et al.*, 1980; Rozewicz *et al.*, 1996).

In order to improve understanding of short-term fluctuations in cognition, Feinstein *et al.* (1993) studied two patient groups: five patients with early relapsing–remitting disease (group A) and five patients with benign MS (group B). Each patient was individually matched with a healthy control in terms of age, sex and premorbid IQ. The testing protocol called for patients to undergo contrast-enhanced MRI, neurological examination (including EDSS ratings) and neuropsychological evaluation at two (group A) and four (group B) week intervals. Apart from the Purdue Pegboard Test, all psychometric tests were computerized to remove or minimize a motor component to testing and confined primarily to tests of attention and information processing speed, as they were thought to be less affected by practice than other aspects of cognition. To minimise the practice effects still further, parallel versions of the tests were employed.

The results indicated that patients as a group performed more poorly than controls on all psychometric tests, although both groups tended to improve over the six month period at a comparable rate. In patients with a relatively stable lesion load throughout the six months of the study, no consistent changes in test performance were noted, other than those attributable to practice effects (i.e. performances improved). However, those patients in whom lesion load had significantly increased displayed less uniform results. Some exhibited decline in test performance while others did not. The individual matching of patient with healthy control highlighted the marked individual variability in the performance of MS subjects. By grouping together all the subjects, these individual differences were obscured.

Medium-term (one to four years) follow-up of patients with multiple sclerosis

An early study by Fink and Houser (1966) noted that MS patients often had problems completing the performance subscale of the WAIS. They, therefore, confined their one year longitudinal study to an analysis of verbal measures and reported that poor performance on tests such as Digit Span and Similarities correlated inversely with physical disability: the greater the physical disability, the lower the verbal score. Notwithstanding this observation, an overall four point improvement in verbal IQ was found. A relative preservation of verbal skills at the expense of psychomotor performance was also noted by Ivnik (1978b) in a three year follow-up study of 14 patients with MS. Similarly, Canter (1951), in a six month follow-up of 47 MS patients and 38 healthy controls, noted that, while deterioration was present on all but two of the Wechsler-Bellevue Scales, it was again the performance IQ that was most affected.

In the first wide-ranging longitudinal study of medium-term cognitive change, Filley *et al.* (1990) retested a group of 46 MS patients with the expanded Halsteid–Reitan Battery after an interval of one to two years. The study was significant because it took into account many factors omitted from earlier studies (i.e. disease course and exacerbations, physical disability ratings and disease duration). The sample was divided at the outset into three categories: stable relapsing–remitting, exacerbating relapsing–remitting and chronic progressive. Although the last group were initially more cognitively impaired, confirming the original observation on the same sample (Heaton *et al.*, 1985), disease course and disease exacerbation were not strongly predictive of cognitive change. Furthermore, group data did not reveal a significant cognitive decline, with deterioration noted only on 6 of 36 test measures. In some cases, the scores on summary measures such as performance IQ improved, which was put down to practice effects. It was, however, difficult to interpret these changes without recourse to comparisons with healthy control subjects, a major limitation of the study. This left the results uncertain and no firm conclusions could be reached about cognitive stability over a one to two year period.

Subsequent medium-term longitudinal studies avoided this pitfall, incorporated control subjects and generally arrived at confluent findings. Jennekens-Schinkel *et al.* (1990) found that, although MS patients as a group were initially more cognitively impaired than a healthy control group, three quarters of their sample did not show cognitive further decline after a four year follow-up period. In some patients, improvement occurred, but whether this was related to the effects of practice or a direct improvement in brain function was less clear for neuroimaging was not undertaken. The authors commented on some of the difficulties inherent in longitudinal studies of MS patients and cautioned that psychomotor deterioration (such as a patient's ability to assess visual information rapidly and respond accordingly) was not commensurate with a deterioration in other cognitive areas. They concluded that cognitive change showed considerable individual variation. This was also characteristic of variables such as disease course and physical disability, confirming their unreliability as predictors of cognitive decline.

A similar conclusion was reached by Amato *et al.* (1995) in a four year follow-up study of 50 patients with recent-onset MS and 70 healthy control subjects. Deficits in verbal memory and abstract reasoning in the MS group, present at the index assessment, had generally not progressed. However, some new deficits had become apparent, namely problems with word fluency and verbal comprehension. Once again, disease course, physical disability and duration of illness could not predict a patient's cognitive status, but the situation with respect to disease activity was more equivocal. Although no association was reported between cognitive impairment and the annual relapse rate, this variable measures the frequency, but not the severity, of relapses and the result may thus have been misleading.

Kujala *et al.* (1997) employed a different methodology in assessing cognitive change over a three year period. Three groups of subjects were examined with an extensive array of cognitive tests: cognitively impaired MS patients (n = 22; mean EDSS = 5.5 [SD, 1.3]), cognitively intact MS patients (n = 23; EDSS = 5.1 [SD, 1.7]) and healthy controls (n = 35). Drop-out rate was low at 5%. The most notable findings were as follows: cognitively intact MS patients remained unchanged and their performances matched the healthy controls at both test points. The cognitively impaired group, however, continued to deteriorate over time, showing not only new deficits but also more extensive deficits in domains first identified as impaired. In keeping with previous studies (Ivnik, 1978b; Feinstein *et al.*, 1992b; Amato *et al.*, 1995), no associations were found between cognitive decline and MS disease-related variables. The marked deterioration in the one group's cognition was attributed to more extensive brain pathology, even though MRI analyses were not part of the study. Nevertheless, such an assumption seems justified in light of data from a series of imaging studies attesting to just such an association (Mariani *et al.*, 1991; Hohol *et al.*, 1997; Patti *et al.*, 1998; Sperling *et al.*, 2001; see Ch. 10 for a review of longitudinal MRI and cognitive studies).

Long-term (over 10 years) follow-up of patients with multiple sclerosis

The importance of following patients over a more extended period of time was illustrated by Amato *et al.* (2001) in a study that re-examined cognitive and neurological outcomes in their original group of 50 MS patients (and 70 healthy controls) 10 years after a baseline assessment. Sample size had decreased to 45 patients (three deceased, two drop-outs) and 65 (five drop-outs) controls. Over the course of a decade, conclusions that had been reached with a more abbreviated follow-up period were now shown to be incorrect. For example, substantially more patients developed cognitive difficulties with the passage of time. By 10 years, 56% of patients were considered impaired relative to their healthy control group. Moreover, some of the patients initially deemed mildly impaired at the four year mark had deteriorated further and were now considered moderately impaired. The range of cognitive impairment also increased, with deficits in attention and short-term spatial memory added to earlier problems noted with verbal memory, abstract thinking and language. But the most striking result from an extended follow-up period was that disease and demographic variables first considered unrelated to cognition now assumed a predictive value. For example, a deteriorating EDSS, a progressive disease course, be it primary or secondary, and age were associated with further cognitive decline. The ecological validity of these results were reinforced when correlates were sought with markers of employment and social difficulties. The EDSS emerged as the best predictor of handicap in both spheres, followed by the number of cognitive tests failed. A more detailed look at the statistics are informative: 68% of patients with mild to moderate cognitive impairment had to stop or modify their work activities, whereas a slightly higher percentage required a considerable degree of help in their personal lives (defined as three or more hours of assistance daily). The corresponding figure for patients found to be cognitively intact was 10%. The authors concluded that over a time span of 10 years cognitive and neurological impairments increased in tandem, with impaired cognition exerting an independent, deleterious effect on patients' abilities to work and socialize.

Summary

- Subtle evidence of cognitive change may occur in patients with clinically isolated syndromes of the type seen in MS. Therefore, cognitive decline can be one of the earliest manifestations of demyelination.

- Rapidly progressive cases of dementia are exceedingly rare. Similarly, it is unusual for cognition to deteriorate with a disease exacerbation only to recover with disease remission.
- Further cognitive decline over the medium term (one to four years) is characterized by considerable individual variability, with disease-related variables such as course of illness and EDSS correlating poorly with cognitive performance.
- Long-term follow-up (10 or more years) reveals a different picture, in which cognitive dysfunction becomes more frequent, affecting more cognitive domains and now linked more closely to markers of physical disability (EDSS) and social dysfunction.

References

Achiron A, Polliack M, Rao SM, *et al.* (2005) Cognitive patterns and progression in multiple sclerosis: Construction and validation of percentile curves. *Journal of Neurology, Neurosurgery and Psychiatry*, **76**, 744–749.

Amato MP, Ponziani G, Pracucci G, *et al.* (1995) Cognitive impairment in early-onset multiple sclerosis. *Archives of Neurology*, **52**, 168–172.

Amato MP, Ponziani G, Siracusa G, Sorbi S. (2001) Cognitive dysfunction in early-onset multiple sclerosis: a reappraisal after 10 years. *Archives of Neurology*, **58**, 1602–1608.

Bergin JD. (1957) Rapidly progressive dementia in disseminated sclerosis. *Journal of Neurology, Neurosurgery and Psychiatry*, **20**, 285–292.

Bieliauskas LA, Topel J, Huckman MS. (1980) Cognitive, neurologic and radiologic test data in a changing lesion pattern. *Journal of Clinical Neuropsychology*, **2**, 217–230.

Callanan MM, Logsdail SJ, Ron M, Warrington EK. (1989) Cognitive impairment in patients with clinically isolated lesions of the type seen in multiple sclerosis. *Brain*, **112**, 361–374.

Canter AH. (1951) Direct and indirect measures of psychological deficit in multiple sclerosis. Part 1. *Journal of General Psychology*, **44**, 3–50.

Feinstein A, Youl B, Ron M. (1992a) Acute optic neuritis. A cognitive and magnetic resonance imaging study. *Brain*, **115**, 1403–1415.

Feinstein A, Kartsounis L., Miller D, Youl B, Ron M. (1992b) Clinically isolated lesions of the type seen in multiple sclerosis followed up. *Journal of Neurology, Neurosurgery and Psychiatry*, **55**, 869–876.

Feinstein A, Ron M, Thompson A.(1993) A serial study of psychometric and magnetic resonance imaging changes in multiple sclerosis. *Brain*, **116**, 569–602.

Filley CM, Heaton RK, Thompson LL, Nelson LM, Franklin GM. (1990) Effects of disease course on neuropsychological functioning. In Neurobehavioural Aspects of Multiple Sclerosis, ed. SM Rao. New York: Oxford University Press, pp. 136–148.

Fink SL, Houser HB. (1966) An investigation of physical and intellectual changes in multiple sclerosis. *Archives of Physical Medicine and Rehabilitation*, **2**, 56–61.

Halligan FR, Reznikoff M, Friedman HP, La Rocca NG. (1988) Cognitive dysfunction and change in multiple sclerosis. *Journal of Clinical Psychology*, **44**, 540–548.

Heaton RK, Nelson LM, Thompson DS, Burk JS, Franklin GM. (1985) Neuropsychological findings in relapsing–remitting and chronic–progressive multiple sclerosis. *Journal of Consulting and Clinical Psychology*, **53**, 103–110.

Hohol MJ, Guttmann CRG, Orav J, *et al.* (1997) Serial neuropsychological assessment and magnetic resonance imaging analysis in multiple sclerosis. *Archives of Neurology*, **54**, 1018–1025.

Ivnik RJ. (1978a) Neuropsychological test performance as a duration of MS-related symptomatology. *Journal of Clinical Psychiatry*, **39**, 304–312.

Ivnik RJ. (1978b) Neuropsychological stability in multiple sclerosis. *Journal of Consulting and Clinical Psychology*, **46**, 913–923.

Jennekens-Schinkel A, Laboyrie PM, Lanser JBK, van der Velde EA. (1990) Cognition in patients with multiple sclerosis after four years. *Journal of the Neurological Sciences*, **99**, 229–247.

Kujala P, Portin R, Ruutianen J. (1997) The progress of cognitive decline in multiple sclerosis. A controlled 3 year follow-up study. *Brain*, **120**, 289–297.

Litran I, Grafman J, Vendrell P, Martinez JM. (1988) Slowed information processing in multiple sclerosis. *Archives of Neurology*, **45**, 281–285.

Lyon-Caen O, Jouvent R, Hauser S, Lhermitte F. (1986) Cognitive function in recent onset demyelinating diseases. *Archives of Neurology*, **43**, 1138–1141.

Mariani C, Farina E, Cappa SF, *et al.* (1991). Neuropsychological assessment in multiple sclerosis: a follow-up study with magnetic resonance imaging. *Journal of Neurology*, **238**, 395–400.

Patti F, Failla G, Ciancio MR, L'Episcopo MR, Reggio A. (1998) Neuropsychological, neuro-radiological and clinical findings in multiple sclerosis: A 3 year follow-up study. *European Journal of Neurology*, **5**, 283–286.

Rozewicz L, Langdon DW, Davie CA, Thompson A, Ron M. (1996) Resolution of left hemisphere cognitive dysfunction in multiple sclerosis with magnetic resonance correlates: a case report. *Cognitive Neuropsychiatry*, **1**, 17–25.

Sperling RA, Guttmann C, Hohol MJ, *et al.* (2001) Regional magnetic resonance imaging lesion burden and cognitive function in multiple sclerosis: a longitudinal study. *Archives of Neurology*, **58**, 115–121.

9

Cognitive impairment in multiple sclerosis: detection, management and significance

With the recognition that cognitive impairment affects approximately 40% of patients with MS, new challenges have presented themselves. Among them is a need to detect cognitive abnormalities accurately in a time-efficient, cost-effective way. Almost one in two patients with cognitive dysfunction will be missed during the routine neurological examination, indicating that neurological impairment is not a reliable predictor of deficits (Peyser *et al.*, 1980). While there is no alternative to neuropsychological testing in this regard, the procedure is time consuming, expensive and may not be readily available in many centers.

This has prompted a search for a brief, reliable and easy to score method for eliciting deficits that may also lend itself to repeat testing for documenting cognitive change over time. As a result, the efficacy of existing cognitive screening procedures, such as the Mini-Mental State Examination (MMSE; Folstein *et al.*, 1975), have been assessed in patients with MS, while efforts at developing new measures specifically targeting this population continue. This chapter will critically review progress to date. A discussion on treatment options for the compromised patient will follow and the chapter will conclude with a brief overview of studies that reveal the real-world challenges faced by cognitively impaired MS patients.

When discussing the possibility of cognitive decline with MS patients, considerable tact is required. Many patients are young and may still be working. Many are in the process of coming to terms either with the diagnosis of MS and the loss of some neurological function. These factors alone demand psychological resilience. Introducing the specter of dementia may prove emotionally overwhelming. It may also prove unfounded. In addressing patients' fears on this score, one approach is to point out that the majority of MS patients (approximately 60%) do *not* have cognitive decline and in those who do, deficits may not be progressive. At the same time, it is doing patients a disservice to downplay abnormalities when present. As this chapter will make clear, cognitive testing is not mandatory in every MS subject. It is up to the clinician to decide on the judicious use of this investigation according to the individual merits of each case. Guidelines in this regard are provided.

The Mini-Mental State Examination

The MMSE (Folstein *et al.*, 1975) was developed to provide a quick, standardized method for assessing cognition. The test examines orientation to time and place, attention (serial subtractions or reverse spelling), short-term memory, constructional ability and language; the individual scores are summed to give a total out of 30. Initially, a cut-off score of <20 was used to signify dementia (Folstein *et al.*, 1975), but this has subsequently been raised to <24 (DePaulo and Folstein, 1978). The MMSE takes approximately 5–10 minutes to complete and is now widely used in a variety of clinical and research settings. Although not formulated for disorders with substantial subcortical white matter involvement, the MMSE has been used for cognitive screening of patients with MS, prompting queries about its validity.

Studies have found the MMSE helpful in a MS research setting, but a closer look at the raw data raises questions about the clinical usefulness of the results. In particular, the frequent ability of cognitively impaired MS patients to score well within the normal range suggests major deficiencies when the instrument is applied to this population. Huber *et al.* (1987) and Rao *et al.* (1991a) found important statistically significant differences between patients with MS and healthy controls, but in both studies the mean MMSE scores for the MS samples were well above the cut-off point for dementia. Similarly, Rao *et al.* (1989) found that cognitively impaired MS patients had significantly lower MMSE scores than cognitively intact MS patients, but the means scores for both groups were again >27. A similar situation pertains to another brief screening instrument, the Cognitive Capacity Screening Examination (CCSE; Jacobs *et al.*, 1977). This instrument assesses orientation, short-term memory (after a brief distraction), attention, calculation, delayed recall and verbal reasoning (similarities and opposites). Like the MMSE, a score out of 30 is obtained and anything less than 20 is considered impaired. Heaton *et al.* (1990) demonstrated that the CCSE was better than the MMSE in differentiating MS patients from healthy controls, but scores on the CCSE were also within the upper normal range, thereby compromising clinical utility.

Despite these failings, the MMSE has remained a potentially attractive option to researchers and clinicians alike owing to its brevity and wide usage in a neurological setting. It has also stimulated a number of comparisons with other more comprehensive methods of cognitive assessment. Franklin *et al.* (1988) looked at the effectiveness of the MMSE versus a 45 minute comprehensive neuropsychological battery in detecting cognitive impairment in a group of 60 patients with clinically definite, chronic–progressive MS. A cut-off point of 24 on the MMSE was used and no MS patient scored below this, although 83% of the same sample (60% when motor deficits were factored out) were found to be impaired on the more detailed testing. Attempts to apply a different cut-off score to the MMSE based on results from the neuropsychological battery were equally problematic and managed to identify only 20% of the cognitively impaired sample.

Prompted by this demonstration of poor sensitivity in the study of Franklin *et al.* (1988), but cognizant of the need for brevity, Beatty and Goodkin (1990) investigated ways of improving the efficacy of the MMSE. A limited battery of cognitive tests were given to a sample of 85 MS patients evenly divided between a relapsing–remitting and chronic–progressive course. The tests included the Boston Naming Test (i.e. total number correct, uncued), the Wisconsin Card Sort Test (WCST) (i.e. number of categories achieved out of six), speed of information processing (measured either by a test of verbal fluency [FAS test] or the Symbol–Digit Modality Test [SDMT]) and various memory paradigms (i.e. recognition and recall for both short- and long-term memory). Dementia was defined as impairment (i.e. scores at or below the 5th percentile relative to healthy control subjects) on three of the four functions tested. In addition, a modified version of the MMSE, controlling for possible motor difficulties, was completed by all subjects.

The results confirmed the deficiencies of the MMSE when used in this population. Of the 35 patients with a 100% MMSE score, 34% were impaired on the SDMT, 23.5% scored below the 5th percentile on the FAS test and a test of long-term recognition memory, while the percentage of patients demonstrating impaired performance on the remainder of the tests varied from 9.4% to 20%. With a MMSE score indicating dementia (i.e. <24), all subjects were impaired on every cognitive test. Of the nine tests in the battery, the SDMT was found to be the most sensitive, followed by the WCST and a test of immediate recall. Most tellingly, a quarter of patients with a MMSE score in the normal range were impaired on all tests. Raising the cut-off score did not help either. A score of 27 still missed too many impaired individuals while a score of 28 produced an unacceptably high number of false positives.

Adding the Boston Naming Test or the SDMT to the MMSE, or increasing the number of recall items from three to seven, have been suggested as ways to improve sensitivity. Of the three, the SDMT was the most sensitive and Beatty and Goodkin (1990) advocated incorporating it in all screening procedures. The test, which takes only a few minutes to complete, can be presented in a computerized form, thereby preventing difficulties with writing from obscuring true cognitive deficits. Feinstein *et al.* (1992) have demonstrated that the SDMT is a sensitive indicator of cognitive difficulties even when disease is in the clinically isolated syndrome phase of demyelination.

Finally, in a comprehensive study of the clinical utility of the MMSE in MS, further compelling evidence was found that the instrument lacks sensitivity (Swirsky-Sacchetti *et al.*, 1992). The relationship between MMSE scores and a host of variables, such as brain lesion area on MRI, physical disability as measured by the EDSS (Kurtzke, 1983) and Scripps neurological rating scale (Sipe *et al.*, 1984), and cognition assessed by detailed neuropsychological testing, was investigated. The neuropsychological tests were chosen to minimize a sensorimotor component and included indices of abstract/conceptual reasoning, language, memory, visuoperceptual skills and processing speed. A subject was considered demented if the performance was impaired relative to normative data on 50% or more of the 11 neuropsychological tests.

The mean MMSE score for the 56 MS patients was 26.51 (SD, 3.51) and 16% of patients performed below the cut-off point of 24. The 72% false-negative rate fell to 9% if the cut-off was raised to 27/30, but false positives then rose to an unacceptably high 30%. The MMSE was the only cognitive index that did not correlate significantly with total lesion area in the brain. Significant correlations, however, were present between scores on the MMSE and the EDSS and Cripps scales, suggesting the MMSE may be more reflective of overall disease severity, including physical disability, than a measure of subtle cognitive impairment. The study underscored the point made by earlier reports that the MMSE was not a suitable cognitive screening measure in MS.

Brief screening batteries for patients with multiple sclerosis

In a frequently cited study, Rao *et al.* (1991a) reported that 43% of a community-based sample of MS patients had cognitive impairment. They arrived at this conclusion using a battery of 22 neuropsychological tests and then went on to determine which of the tests were the most sensitive detectors of impairment. The result was the development of a cognitive screening measure, the Neuropsychological Screening Battery for MS (NPSBMS), that takes 20–25 minutes to complete and comprises four tests; Consistent Long-Term Retrieval (CLTR) from the Buschke Selective Reminding Test, Total Recall from the 7/24 Spatial Recall Test, the Controlled Oral Word Association Test (COWAT) and the Paced Auditory Serial Addition Test (PASAT), the last using stimuli presented at three and two seconds. Taking impairment on any two tests relative to normative data as a sign of cognitive dysfunction, the NPSBMS had a 71% sensitivity and a 94% specificity, a considerable improvement compared with the MMSE.

A variant of this test was also developed for serial testing. It comprised the four tests mentioned above with the Spatial Recall Test made more challenging by increasing the amount of visual material to be learnt (10/36 items instead of the original 7/24). A fifth test was also added, namely the SDMT. These five tests are known as the Brief Repeatable Neuropsychological Battery (BRNB; Rao, 1990). There are 15 alternative, equivalent versions to facilitate the longitudinal study of the natural history of cognitive change and possible cognitive responses in treatment trials. Normative data, corrected for age, gender and education, have been acquired from 140 healthy subjects using two parallel versions of the BRNB (Boringa *et al.*, 2001).

To investigate the effectiveness of the BRNB in a serial setting, Bever *et al.* (1995) tested a group of 19 MS patients at 60 day intervals for four months. In keeping with longitudinal studies using more comprehensive cognitive batteries (Ch. 8), they noted individual variability over time and the ability of patients to benefit from practice. This finding was robustly replicated by Hohol *et al.* (1997) in a serial MRI study that used the original four item Rao battery to assess cognition at entry to the study and one year later. Not only did the BRNB detect cognitive change, but results correlated significantly with changes in brain lesion load, thereby supplying a further marker of validity.

The BRNB has been investigated as a specific screening instrument for *memory* problems in MS, with mixed results (Dent and Lincoln, 2000). The Wechsler Memory Scale-revised (WMS-R) was chosen as the marker of memory function against which the five tests of the BRNB were compared. Based on receiver operating curves, two of the BRNB tests (the SDMT and immediate recall on the 10/36 Spatial Recall Test) emerged as predictors of memory impairment. However, the 93% sensitivity was offset by a poor (48%) specificity.

Although an improvement on the MMSE, the four (NPSBMS) and five (BRNB) item screening procedures have been criticized for the high false-negative rate and the narrow range of cognitive abilities assessed. Attempting to overcome these limitations Basso *et al.* (1996) developed a 35–50 minute cognitive screen that retained some of the cognitive indices recommended by Rao and colleagues, but added others. The two batteries have in common measures of auditory attention (Seashore Rhythm Test [Basso] versus PASAT [Rao]), verbal fluency (COWAT in both) and verbal learning (Logical Memory Saving Score [Basso] and the CLTR from the Selective Reminding Test [Rao]). However, the Rao battery included another measure of memory, namely a non-verbal short-term recall test while Basso introduced tests of graphesthesia and astereognosis. The last two are surprising inclusions given the infrequency with which such abnormalities have been reported in MS patients. Nevertheless, their addition contributed to a screening procedure with a 100% sensitivity and a 80% specificity. As a result, the Basso battery detects more cognitively impaired patients but at the expense of over-diagnosis, compared with the Rao battery. Whether this is a meaningful improvement depends on individual perspective. The advantages of improved detection are self-evident, but false positives bring their own potential problems, such as engendering anxiety and depression in a group that is known to be prone to mood disorders. Furthermore, the Basso battery takes longer to administer, which may offset any advantage. The 35–50 minute duration places it alongside other intermediate length instruments.

A third choice available to clinicians and researchers is the Screening Examination for Cognitive Impairment (SEFCI; Beatty *et al.*, 1995). This 25 minute battery, which boasts an impressive 86% sensitivity and a 90% specificity, consists of the SDMT, measures of learning and delayed verbal recall, and tests of vocabulary and verbal abstraction taken from the Shipley Institute of Living Scale. In a study of 103 MS subjects, the SEFCI was compared with a two hour neuro-psychological battery made up of tests known to be sensitive to cognitive difficulties in MS patients. It was able to identify 100% of subjects who had impairments on at least three of the cognitive domains measured by the more comprehensive battery.

Currently faced with three different screening batteries that have similar sensitivities and specificities, clinicians and researchers now have the dilemma posed by choice. A couple of studies have tried to provide pointers in this regard. Solari *et al.* (2002) compared the BRNB and the SEFCI in a sample of 213 Italian MS patients matched to the same number of healthy control subjects. Scores on any of the cognitive tests were deemed impaired if they fell below the fifth percentile relevant to the healthy control data. The first observation was that the SEFCI is significantly quicker to administer both in MS and control subjects. Average test durations for the MS cohort were 40.8 (SD, 5.6) minutes for the BRNB and 29.7 (SD, 4.5) minutes for the SEFCI. The MS patients did significantly less well than healthy controls on both cognitive batteries. Sensitivity to global cognitive impairment, however, varied according to definitions. For example, if failure on a single cognitive measure was taken as a overall marker of impairment, the BRNB had a sensitivity of 41.9% and the SEFCI 31.5%. If failure on two tests was used as the threshold, the sensitivity of the BRNB was 16.2% and that of the SECI 18.5%. Focussing down on individual tests, the Buschke Selective Reminding Test and PASAT from the BRNB and the SDMT from the SEFCI emerged as the most sensitive. The authors concluded their comparison with the salient observation that the slightly longer duration of administration of the BRNB was counterbalanced by the advantage of having serial versions available, an attribute the SEFCI lacks.

The NPSBMS and SEFCI went head to head in a three-way comparison that also included the Repeatable Battery for the Assessment of Neuropsychological Status

(Auperle *et al.*, 2002). Surprisingly, the last battery, which consists of 12 short tests probing immediate memory, visuospatial and construction skills, language, attention, and delayed memory, fared poorly as a cognitive screen, with a sensitivity similar to that of the MMSE. Of the two remaining batteries, the SEFCI once again was quicker to administer. There was, however, little to choose with respect to sensitivity. Among the 64 MS patients who completed all the tests, 56.6% failed one or more tests on the SEFCI versus 61.3% on the NPSBMS, while 43.8% failed two or more tests on the SEFCI versus 36% on the NPSBMS.

To the uninitiated, these multiple acronyms may be confusing, if not irritating. So, in summarizing the data, the full names of the test batteries will be given once more. Two stand out as the pick of the bunch: the Neuropsychological Screening Battery (NPSBMS; Rao *et al.*, 1991a), which also has a serial version called the Brief Repeatable Neuropsychological Battery (BRNB), and the Screening Examination for Cognitive Impairment (SEFCI; Beatty *et al.*, 1995). Given the statistics, it is a little surprising that the latter languishes in relative obscurity having long since ceded pride of place to the former. Perhaps the dominance of the BRNB can be traced to the following factors. First, although slightly longer to administer, there are serial versions making it useful for longitudinal research. Second, the BRNB appeared five years before the SEFCI, so that by the time the latter was published, a substantial database was already in place. Which meant that if researchers wanted a yardstick by which to compare their newly minted data sets, the BRNB and NPSBMS could provide it. Consequently, in an effort to speak the same language as it were, the Rao batteries, *de facto*, became the chosen cognitive screen. And here it remains, cited eight times more often than its less popular, but equally worthy, alternative (total citations as of April 2006).

Both the batteries described above are easy to administer, but they do require some advance training before they can be reliably administered. To clinicians in a busy, solo practice, this can present obstacles. Hence the search for a reductionist approach: a cognitive probe that is so straightforward and quick to administer it can be integrated easily into any basic neurological examination. The Clock Drawing Test offers this possibility, with some preliminary data suggesting it may be useful as a cognitive screen in MS patients (Barak *et al.*, 2002).

Cognitive screening procedures of intermediate length

What is meant by "intermediate" is arbitrary, but one safe definition is to include all those batteries whose length of administration falls between the day-long duration, as typified by the Expanded Halstead-Reitan Battery on the one hand, and brief measures such as the MMSE (5–10 minutes) and the BRNB (approximately 20 minutes) on the other. A number of such intermediate length procedures have been developed, ranging from an 18 item battery (Heaton *et al.*, 1990) to a core battery of neuropsychological tests recommended by the National Multiple Sclerosis Society that may take up to two hours (Peyser *et al.*, 1990). The advantage to this approach compared with the brief screening measures is that it supplies a more comprehensive analysis of a patient's cognitive deficiencies and strengths, both of which are important when it comes to management. This point deserves emphasising. While researchers may disagree on the exact composition of what constitutes the most effective screening instrument, they all concur that an important function of screening patients within a clinical setting is to identify those who may require a more comprehensive assessment, without which it is impossible to gain a complete understanding of the scope and degree of the intellectual difficulties.

Faced with a plethora of cognitive tests with variable applicability to MS patients, a group of neuropsychologists from the USA, Canada, the UK and Australia convened with the aim of providing some guidance as to the best choice of instruments (Benedict *et al.*, 2002). A consensus document identified a series of tests that takes approximately 90 minutes to administer and is considered the minimum assessment required by MS patients. The Minimal Assessment of Cognitive Function in MS (MACFIMS), assesses cognition in the following domains (with the test names/abbreviations added in parentheses): Processing speed/working memory (PASAT, SDMT), learning and memory (California Verbal Learning Test-II, Brief Visuospatial Memory Test-Revised), executive function (D-KEFS Sorting Test), visual perception/spatial processing (Judgement of Line Orientation Test), language/other (COWAT). For inclusion, the tests had to satisfy a series of checks that included standardized stimulus materials and administration, normative data, adequate range of results, reliability, criterion validity (i.e. the ability to distinguish MS patients, even those with mild impairment, from healthy controls), alternative forms and practical to administer. In addition to these cognitive measures, the group recommended that an index of premorbid abilities should be obtained at the initial assessment: the National Adult Reading Test (or its North American version) and the Wide Ranging Achievement Test were suggested options. Finally, the authors felt that prior to beginning the cognitive battery, measures of fatigue (Fatigue Impact Scale), depression (Chicago Multiscale Depression Inventory) and motor dexterity (9 Hole Peg Test) should be obtained at each test session.

The MACFIMS occupies an important niche in the MS–cognition literature. Not only does it provide clinicians and researchers with a clear, practical framework for cognitive testing, it also establishes a means for comparing data between research centers. One of the unfortunate consequences of a burgeoning area of research coupled with a multiplicity of assessment procedures has been a 'tower of Babel' effect: researchers clamoring to be heard but talking past one another.

A Self-Report instrument of cognitive dysfunction

A theme common to all the test batteries reviewed so far is that the cognitive assessment is based on objective data, that is, data ascertained by a psychometrician using validated tests. But what of MS patients' subjective complaints of cognitive difficulties? How accurate are these? And can they be used as an index of cognitive dysfunction? To explore these questions, Benedict *et al.* (2003) developed a 15 item self-administered screening instrument for cognitive impairment, the Multiple Sclerosis Neuropsychological Questionnaire (MSNQ). Two versions of the questionnaire need to be completed, one by the patient and one by an informant who is well acquainted with the patient. To assess the validity of these two measures, 50 MS patients completed a detailed neuropsychological battery. The same patients and their informants also answered the questionnaires. The most notable findings to emerge were as follows. Patients' subjective cognitive complaints did not match the objective neuropsychological evidence but rather correlated more closely with their depression scores. Conversely, the informants' assessment matched the objective neuropsychological data, but not the patients' depression scores. A cut-off score of 27 on the informant questionnaire was found to be the most accurate predictor of cognitive impairment in patients, with a sensitivity of 83% and a specificity of 97%.

These impressive figures, surpassing those from the BRNB and the SEFCI, must be viewed with cautious optimizm. The data were collected from MS patients with a short duration of illness and normal or mildly impaired cognitive function. In addition, sample size was modest. Aware of these shortcomings, the authors undertook a second study with a different methodology (Benedict *et al.*, 2004). The MSNQ was given to 85 MS patients and 40 demographically matched normal controls. All subjects underwent detailed neuropsychological testing in addition to completing the MSNQ. Thirty four MS patients completed the MSNQ again one week later and the results revealed a good test–retest reliability. Some of the other findings, however, differed from the first study. For example, with a cut-off score of 24, the patients' subjective assessment of their cognitive abilities turned out to be correct in over two thirds of patients. If one removed depressed patients from these data, the percentage correctly classified rose to 74%. Figures for the informant-based MSNQ were lower than first reported but still remained impressive: a decline from 94% to 85% in those correctly classified. Once again, an association was noted between depression and patients' perceptions of their cognitive function, and as in the first report, informants were more accurate than patients in their assessment of cognitive dysfunction. With a sensitivity of 87% and a specificity of 84%, the informant-based MSNQ once again outperformed the BRBN and was on a par with the SEFCI. Having made these points, it is still premature to conclude that 15 simple questions asked of a concerned relative or friend trumps the BRNB and SEFCI. This promising questionnaire, nevertheless, deserves a place in the clinical care of MS patients, where it can provide a quick and valid assessment of patients' global cognitive abilities. This, is turn, may indicate the need for a more detailed neuropsychological assessment.

Indications for comprehensive testing

Under what circumstances should cognitive testing be completed and how should this be done? Does the patient require a brief or a comprehensive assessment? How should the patient be approached with a view to suggesting an assessment, and when completed, how should the results be presented back to the patient? Answers to some of these will be dictated by circumstances. For example, not every neurologist will have access to a neuropsychologist who can undertake the testing, and for some patients in countries without universal health coverage, such a service may not be affordable.

Even before deciding to refer a patient for cognitive testing, the neurologist or neuropsychiatrist may have a high index of suspicion that deficits are present based on clinical and neuroimaging findings. Most MS patients will have had a brain MRI as part of their initial work-up. Given the association between brain MRI changes and cognition, a large lesion load and/or atrophy often signals intellectual compromise. The importance of listening to what family members have to say is emphasised, because MS patients, with possible impairment in metamemory (Ch. 7), may not be the best judge of their own difficulties. The presence of frontal release signs is also a predictor of cognitive dysfunction (Franklin *et al.*, 1990). Under these circumstances, screening patients as a preliminary procedure would be indicated.

Some further guidelines about when to test and whether to use a modest screening test or proceed to more detailed testing have been provided by Franklin *et al.* (1990). Indications for neuropsychological assessment include the patient who complains that cognitive difficulties affect functioning at home or at work, the patient whose employer reports a fall-off in work performance, the patient seeking vocational counselling to obtain employment matched to his or her disability, the patient in rehabilitation whose suspected cognitive dysfunction may be impeding the progress of treatment, the patient entering a treatment trial where a pretreatment cognitive baseline is required and the patient with a treatment-resistant depression masquerading as a dementia. Should any of these situations arise in the context of an MRI displaying a heavy lesion load or significant atrophy, either generalized or confined to the third ventricle, the argument for neuropsychological testing becomes compelling.

Conversely, situations where testing is not required include the patient who denies cognitive difficulties (without objective evidence to dispute his or her claim) and the patient who is significantly physically disabled, in a low demand environment and in whom a cognitive assessment is unlikely to furnish fresh insights or lead to a change in patient care.

Counselling the patient pre- and post-testing is important in dealing with the attendant anxieties and the implications pertaining to the findings.

Management strategies

Little has been written about therapy for cognitive difficulties in MS. Approaches may be divided into two broad categories, namely restorative or compensatory (Sohlberg and Mateer, 1989). Restorative refers to a process whereby cognitive deficits are identified and specific remedial therapies are introduced with the aim of increasing performance in that area. In contrast to this, compensatory strategies do not try to bring about a recovery of function. Rather, attempts are made to maximize the abilities a patient retains. The latter approach has received the most attention in MS research.

Compensatory strategies

Before describing therapy to develop compensatory strategies, it is worth noting that MS patients who perceive themselves as cognitively impaired often spontaneously adopt strategies that are compensatory in nature (Sullivan *et al.*, 1990).

Compensatory strategies are based on three tenets: structuring, scheduling and recording. The underlying principle is to bring as much structure and stability to the patient's environment. This, in turn, ensures a measure of predictability, thereby reducing demands on planning, organization and memory (Sullivan *et al.*, 1989). A first step in the process is to assess the individual's current cognitive strengths and weaknesses through neuropsychological testing. An estimate of premorbid IQ via the vocabulary subtest on the WAIS is useful as an approximate marker of what the patient was capable of intellectually prior to the onset of MS. An assessment of the patient's environment is also mandatory for this provides information on the daily demands that must be confronted. With all this information, the therapist can identify those areas of daily functioning that are most affected by cognitive difficulties, and these are discussed with the patient before a specific plan is implemented. Consultations with family members at this point are helpful because any changes that need to be implemented may require their cooperation.

Once this stage is complete, implementation can begin. The use of a day calender as an aide mémoire for patients with memory difficulties could be tried. It is not enough just to suggest patients go out and buy the day calender, because they will also require help in deciding when to use it and what kinds of information need to be recorded (Sullivan *et al.*, 1989). When it comes to difficulties with planning and organization, whether at home or at work, attempts could be made to manipulate the environment to provide greater structure. By using a day planner, patients are reminded that a specified task should be carried out at a set time each day, using items that should always be kept in the same place. Depending on a patient's cognitive ability, this structure may be applied to factors ranging from work-related tasks to the more mundane activities of daily living such as meal preparation, grocery shopping, cleaning, transportation and personal safety issues (Bennett *et al.*, 1991).

Remedial strategies

Remedial cognitive strategies in MS, unlike the situation in traumatic brain injury, have received little attention (Grafman, 1984).The reasons probably relate to the nature of cognitive dysfunction in MS. In stroke and head injury, the insult is sudden and is followed by a period of expected, albeit variable, recovery. MS-related cognitive change follows an altogether different course. The onset may be insidious, and deterioration, if it is to occur over time, is unlikely to be interrupted by periods of cognitive improvement. For this reason, compensatory strategies in MS are considered more useful (Minden and Moes, 1990).

Despite a preference for compensatory approaches, remediation has been tried in MS patients. A process of graded practice for improving memory using computer programs has been implemented in at least one MS rehabilitation setting (LaRocca, 1990). In a study that randomly assigned 40 MS patients to one of two groups, remediation plus compensation versus non-specific, diffuse mental stimulation, the former was found to be more effective, with improvements reported in some memory functions after a six month follow-up (Jonsson *et al.*, 1993). Results from two subsequent studies have not, however, been so encouraging (Lincoln *et al.*, 2002; Solari *et al.*, 2004). In particular, the negative result reported by Solari *et al.* (2004) is disappointing given the strength of their randomized, double-blind study design, the intensity and duration of treatment (16 sessions over eight weeks), the good sample size ($n = 82$), and the emphasis on computer-assisted training focussing on memory and attention, aspects of cognition known to be impaired in MS patients.

A variant of remedial therapy has been developed specifically to target communication skills in MS patients (Foley *et al.*, 1994). Here cognitive difficulties are framed according to their effects on interpersonal communication, such as the ability to listen accurately, the capacity to display empathy, the ability to compromise, make requests and give feedback to others about the impact of their behavior. The authors identified three phases to this treatment: education, rehearsal and application. In the first stage, interviews with the patients and informants together with neuropsychological assessments provide pointers to the way in which the patients communicate. In the rehearsal phase, remedial skills that target communication problems are rehearsed with help from the therapist. In the final stage, the newfound communication abilities are applied by the patients in day to day, real-life situations. Given that communication deficits are invariably accompanied by other cognitive problems, the psycho-remediation principles described here are bolstered by compensatory strategies that focus on memory. For example, using an aide mémoire the patients are encouraged to document daily interpersonal situations and the emotions associated with them. This way patients can keep a record of their personal lives and feelings, which become more fully integrated with the attempts at communication remediation. This program is well thought out and is backed by promising anecdotal reports, but as yet no empirically based treatment trials.

Physicians and allied health workers need to show flexibility in their choice of a rehabilitation strategy. As the report by Foley and colleagues (1994) makes clear, mixing and matching remedial and compensatory approaches can work where indicated. What must not be overlooked, irrespective of the strategy selected, is that cognitive rehabilitation should not take place in isolation. It is just one part of a comprehensive treatment plan that begins at the moment of diagnosis. This broad-based approach focuses primarily on the patient but also includes family members when relevant. It embraces cognitive strategies, treatment for neurological symptoms (e.g. the interferon drugs), psychopathology (antidepressant and anxiolytic medication, psychotherapy) and help for psychosocial difficulties.

Medication strategies to help cognition

There is now a small literature devoted to medications that may assist cognition. These drugs may be divided into three broad categories: cholinergic-enhancing agents, disease-modifying treatments (Ch. 11) and a miscellaneous group of symptomatic agents.

Cholinergic drugs

The cholinergic drugs have been used primarily in the treatment of Alzheimer's disease. The principle behind treatment is to enhance the amount of acetylcholine available in the brain. Donepezil hydrochloride, the most widely used of these agents, does this by reversibly inhibiting the enzyme acetylcholinesterase. A early pilot study in four MS subjects suggested that the medication may have some cognitive benefits (Krupp *et al.*, 1999). Three subsequent studies have examined this question in a more substantial manner. In an open label 12 week trial,

17 cognitively impaired MS patients (MMSE ≤ 25) were given four weeks of 5 mg donepezil daily followed by eight weeks of 10 mg daily (Greene *et al.*, 2000). Serial cognitive, neurological and behavioral assessments were undertaken at baseline and at 4 and 12 weeks. Improvement over time was reported in tests such as the Digit Span, Boston Naming Test, COWAT, and the Mattis Dementia Rating Scale. Similarly, behavioral improvement was noted over time in a neuropsychiatric inventory that recorded diverse symptoms such as delusions, depression, euphoria, apathy, disinhibition, irritability and appetite. The medication was generally well tolerated, with a case of spasticity the only medical side effect potentially linked to treatment. The study, however, had some major limitations. The lack of a control group made it difficult to tease out the cognitively enhancing effects of practice from actual drug benefits. In this regard, the behavioral improvements that were noted carry added weight even if the open label design introduced a bias. Finally, the findings derived from a small group of patients with dementia living in a long-term care facility cannot be applied to MS patients in general. Because of these problems, which the authors themselves duly noted, the main value of this study lies not in the empirical data, which were possibly flawed, but in the broader introduction of an idea that drugs developed for one disease, i.e., Alzheimer's disease, may be beneficial in another, i.e., MS. It has been left to other studies to determine whether this is in fact so.

Krupp *et al.* (2004) have provided weightier evidence in support of donepezil as a treatment for cognitive dysfunction in MS patients. In a double-blind placebo-controlled trial, 69 MS patients were randomly assigned to either 10 mg donepezil or placebo daily over a 24 week period. Subjects were limited to an age range of 18 to 55 years. Overall neurological disability was moderate and the average duration of disease approached 10 years. Of the 35 MS patients taking donepezil, two thirds had relapsing–remitting disease, which differed significantly from the placebo group, where two thirds had a chronic–progressive course. Apart from this variable, drug and placebo groups were well matched demographically and on measures of depression and premorbid intelligence. Equal numbers of patients in both groups were taking interferon beta treatments. The cognitive battery comprised the BRNB (described above) supplemented by a test of executive function, the Tower of Hanoi task. The primary outcome measure was the change in score in the Selective Reminding Test over the 24 weeks. Secondary outcome measures included change in the other cognitive domains tested, plus patients' and their neurologists' subjective assessments of cognitive change.

The results revealed that patients treated with donepezil showed a significant improvement on the primary outcome measure; that is change in total recall in the Selective Reminding Test. A trend towards improvement on the PASAT was also noted in patients taking donepezil. Donepezil did not, however, improve cognition in other domains. Patients on placebo did not improve cognitively on any measure. In addition, patients on donepezil rather than placebo were significantly more likely to rate their cognition as improved, a finding that was matched by the neurologists' clinical impression. By 24 weeks, however, patients taking donepezil, but not placebo, were more likely to guess their medication status, which may have biased their subjective response of cognitive improvement. Neurologists by comparison, were no more likely to guess medication status. Donepezil was generally well tolerated, with over 80% of patients remaining on treatment for the study's duration.

This well-conducted study is important because it provides evidence, in the laboratory at least, that donepezil may enhance memory in cognitively impaired MS patients. Whether this modest statistical effect translates into meaningful improvement for patients in their day to day lives cannot, however, be answered, as yet. Important as this result is, it is also sobering to note the failure of donepezil to assist aspects of cognition other than verbal memory. Whether this is a function of small sample size or an indication of the drug's limitations must still be elucidated. Finally, the significance of the mismatch in disease course remains unclear. More donepezil patients had relapsing–remitting disease, which may have conferred a cognitive advantage compared with the placebo group with its preponderance of patients with chronic–progressive disease.

This cautiously optimistic finding is contradicted by a smaller, randomized, double-blind placebo-controlled crossover trial; this failed to find any cognitive benefits after six weeks of treatment (Rorie et al., 2001). Small sample size (32 in total with 25 subjects completing the trial) and a short duration of treatment limit the interpretation of data.

A second cholinergic-enhancing agent, rivastigmine, has been used in five MS patients in conjunction with functional MRI (fMRI). This was not a treatment trial. The emphasis was on fMRI-demonstrable brain changes in relation to cognition. As an aside, however, the few patients receiving medication showed improvement on the Stroop test that correlated with functional imaging changes. (Parry et al., 2003; see Ch. 10 for a more detailed account of the study).

Of note are two earlier reports of physostigmine used to treat cognitive dysfunction in MS. Tentative evidence from a pilot study of four subjects suggested that *intravenous* physostigmine at a higher dose (1.0 mg) when combined with lecithin brought about some improvement in memory as measured by the Selective Reminding Test (Leo and Rao, 1988). The data were replicated in eight patients using *oral* physostigmine in a double-blind, placebo-controlled design (Unverzagt et al., 1991). The advent of acetylcholinesterase inhibitor drugs meant that this line of pharmacological inquiry was not pursued, but physostigmine did presage the appearance and use of donepezil in this population.

Disease-modifying drugs

The potential cognitive benefits of disease-modifying drugs, interferon beta-1b, interferon beta-1a (Rebif and Avonex) and glatiramir acetate are reviewed in Ch. 11. The best cognitive evidence to date favors interferon beta-1a, but it needs to be emphasised that studies are few and methodologies are not always sound.

Symptomatic drug treatments

Many MS patients receive *steroids* for a relapse with little consideration as to the effects, either deleterious or restorative, on cognition. Details are provided in Ch. 10 of a patient with a severe relapse, who, on receiving intravenous steroids, showed a dramatic and quick improvement in neurological function matched by cognitive improvements and positive changes on brain MRI and spectroscopy (Rozewicz *et al.*, 1996). From this isolated case, it can be inferred that steroids may in certain cases help cognition. But this finding must be counterbalanced by the potentially injurious effects of more long-standing steroid use (Keenan *et al.*, 1996).

Oliveri *et al.* (1998) investigated the effects of pulsed methylprednisolone on memory function in 14 patients with relapsing–remitting MS experiencing a relapse. Neuropsychological data were collected before treatment with steroids and thereafter at 7 and 60 days post-treatment. There were three intravenous steroid treatment regimens: 2.5 g over five days ($n = 4$), 5 g over seven days ($n = 5$) and 10 g over five days ($n = 5$). Cognitive data were also collected from 12 healthy controls. The MS patients performed more poorly than controls on a number of cognitive tasks, most notably on indices of verbal learning. In addition, intravenous steroids irrespective of dosing produced a short-term fall-off in performance on tests of explicit memory (immediate and delayed Rey Auditory Verbal Learning). By 60 days post-treatment, this feature had recovered completely to baseline levels, which were still impaired relative to healthy controls. This result was replicated by Uttner *et al.* (2005), who used doses of 500 and 2000 mg over a five day period and cognitively tested their sample before treatment and on days 6 and 60. The conclusions to be drawn from these studies are that pulsed steroids do not appear to have any long-term adverse cognitive sequelae and, in isolated cases involving catastrophic physical relapse, steroids may restore, in part, cognition alongside neurological function.

Fatigue, a virtually ubiquitous symptom in MS, may be ameliorated by a number of medications, one of which is *amantadine*. Whether this medication has some additional beneficial cognitive properties was investigated in a group of 24 MS patients (Sailer *et al.*, 2000). In a randomized double-blind placebo-controlled design, a reaction time test was the sole measure of cognition to complement a number of electrophysiological measurements. Amantadine was found to increase the speed of reaction time, but only in patients with disease of longer duration, defined here as more than seven years. No convincing explanation was put forward to account for this finding, other than the unlikely suggestion that with longer disease duration cognition becomes increasingly impaired, thereby allowing amantadine to exert a more noticeable effect. In an earlier placebo-controlled crossover trial that primarily focussed on fatigue, with cognitive tests as secondary outcome measures, amantadine did bring about an improvement in performance on the Stroop test (Cohen and Fisher, 1989). Similarly, in a three-way comparison of amantadine, pemoline and placebo, only amantadine led to improved scores on the SDMT (Geisler et al., 1996).

A second line of inquiry has focussed on 4-aminopyridine, a potassium channel blocker that has been reported to bring some symptomatic relief in MS (van Diemen et al., 1992). To assess the effects on cognition, Smits et al. (1994) undertook a randomized, double-blind, placebo-controlled, crossover study in 20 MS patients using serial neuropsychological testing. Although there was a trend for patients to show cognitive improvement on some tests, the results were not promising, an impression subsequently confirmed by Rossini et al. (2001). A double-blind placebo-controlled trial of 3,4-diaminopyridine that evaluated cognition alongside physical symptoms also failed to report benefits (Bever et al. 1996).

Finally, there are some preliminary data suggesting cyclophosphamide may help cognition in patients with chronic–progressive (primary and secondary) MS (Zéphir et al., 2005). Of 30 patients, 24 finished a one year trial of monthly perfusions of cyclophosphamide combined with methylprednisolone. Although cognitive improvements were noted at the 6 and 12 month test sessions across a wide array of tests (Verbal IQ, Digit Span, Stroop, Wechsler Memory Scale, among others), the absence of a control group makes data interpretation problematic. Consequently, it could not be ascertained how much of the improvement was due to practice alone, or practice plus cyclophosphamide or cyclophosphamide plus steroids. Nevertheless, these data offer a semblance of optimizm in the rather bleak landscape of effective treatments for chronic–progressive MS.

The clinical significance of cognitive impairment

Cognitive impairment may affect the results of a rehabilitation program (Langdon and Thompson, 1999). In a study of 28 patients with considerable neurological disability (mean EDSS; 7.5 [range, 5.0–9.0]), the authors identified deficits on the WAIS-Vocabulary score and cerebellar dysfunction as major impediments to rehabilitation. Presumably the problems patients had with vocabulary interfered with their verbal communication, thereby adding another hurdle to rehabilitation.

Evidence that cognitive dysfunction exerts an adverse effect on social functioning for MS patients comes from the community study of 100 patients by Rao *et al.* (1991b); the patients were almost evenly divided on the basis of detailed neuropsychological testing into cognitively intact and impaired groups. The two groups, who were closely matched on demographic and disease-related characteristics, were compared across a number of different parameters that included measures of physical disability, an occupational therapy assessment, self-report measures of depression, anxiety and sickness-related disability and an informant's (relative or friend) rating of the subject's emotional adjustment. The cognitively impaired patients were found to be at a considerable social disadvantage, with difficulties spanning work, relationships, vocational activities, sexual function and activities of daily living. The study was, however, cross-sectional and the authors, therefore, cautioned against drawing direct etiological inferences. Although longitudinal data are awaited, there appears sound preliminary evidence linking cognitive impairment in MS patients to a compromised quality of life.

The many difficulties cognitively impaired MS patients confront have been confirmed with respect to employment (Benedict, 2005), displaying appropriate social skills (Knight *et al.*, 1997) and driving a motor vehicle (Schulteis *et al.*, 2001, 2002).

Summary

- The routine neurological examination and mental state assessment will miss detecting cognitive dysfunction in the majority of MS patients, hence the need for sensitive, brief screening procedures.
- The Mini-Mental State Examination is not useful in screening patients with MS for cognitive impairment.
- Brief cognitive screening batteries have been developed specifically for patients with MS. The most widely used is the Neuropsychological Screening Battery for MS (NPSBMS), which takes 20–25 minutes to complete and comprises four tests; Consistent Long-Term Retrieval (CLTR) from the Buschke Selective Reminding Test, the Total Recall from the 7/24 Spatial Recall Test, the Controlled Oral Word Association Test (COWAT) and the Paced Auditory Serial Addition Test (PASAT). A repeatable version of the NPSBMS that has the Symbol–Digit Modalities Test added, is available and useful in longitudinal studies.
- Cognitive batteries of intermediate length provide more detailed information on a patient's deficits and residual strengths. The Minimal Assessment of Cognitive Function in MS (MACFIMS) is the method of choice for MS patients

and takes 90 minutes to complete. It arose from a consensus meeting of neuro-psychologists with expertise in testing MS patients.

- For those clinicians without access to neuropsychological expertise or who do not have the time to complete formal screening batteries such as the NPSBMS, there is a validated 15 item self-report questionnaire, the Multiple Sclerosis Neuropsychological Questionnaire (MSNQ), which provides accurate information on cognitive status. In particular, informants' rather than patients' ratings correlate well with cognitive deficits. Patients' subjective cognitive complaints appear more closely linked to depression.
- Rehabilitation generally follows a compensatory rather than a remedial approach. The aim is to enhance a patient's occupational or psychosocial functioning (both, if relevant) by utilizing residual cognitive strengths and planning around them.
- Preliminary data suggest medication may help with cognitive deficits. Trials with anticholinesterase inhibitors such as donepezil hydrochloride and psycho-stimulants such as amantadine have reported favorable results. The ecological validity of these studies has yet to be determined.
- There are empirical data demonstrating that cognitive dysfunction exerts an adverse effect on a patient's quality of life in many different spheres, ranging from the workplace to relationships to such basic aspects as the activities of daily living.

References

Auperle RL, Beatty WW, Shelton F, Gontkovsky ST. (2002) Three screening batteries to detect cognitive impairment in multiple sclerosis. *Multiple Sclerosis*, **8**, 382–389.

Barak Y, Lavie M, Achiron A. (2002) Screening for early cognitive impairment in multiple sclerosis patients using the clock drawing test. *Journal of Clinical Neurosciences*, **9**, 629–632.

Basso MR, Beason-Hazen S, Lynn J, Rammohan K, Bornstein RA. (1996) Screening for cognitive dysfunction in multiple sclerosis. *Archives of Neurology*, **53**, 980–984.

Beatty WW, Goodkin DE. (1990) Screening for cognitive impairment in multiple sclerosis. An evaluation of the Mini-Mental State Examination. *Archives of Neurology*, **47**, 297–301.

Beatty WW, Paul RH, Wilbanks SL, *et al.* (1995) Identifying multiple sclerosis patients with mild or global cognitive impairments using the Screening Examination for Cognitive Impairment (SEFCI). *Neurology*, **45**, 718–723.

Benedict RHB (2005) Integrating cognitive function screening and assessment into the routine care of multiple sclerosis patients. (2005) *CNS Spectrums*, **10**, 384–391.

Benedict RHB, Fischer JS, Archibald CJ, *et al.* (2002) Minimal neuropsychological assessment of MS patients: a consensus approach. *The Clinical Neuropsychologist*, **16**, 381–397.

Benedict RHB, Munschauer F, Linn R, *et al.* (2003) Screening for multiple sclerosis cognitive impairment using a self-adminsitered 15-item questionnaire. *Multiple Sclerosis*, **9**, 95–101.

Benedict RHB, Cox D, Thompson LL, *et al.* (2004) Reliable screening for neuropsychological impairment in multiple sclerosis. *Multiple Sclerosis*, **10**, 675–678.

Bennett T, Dittmar C, Raubach S. (1991) Multiple Sclerosis: cognitive deficits and rehabilitation strategies. *Cognitive Rehabilitation*, **9**, 18–23.

Bever CT, Grattan L, Panitch HS, Johnson KP. (1995) A brief repeatable battery of neuropsychological tests for multiple sclerosis: a preliminary serial study. *Multiple Sclerosis*, **1**, 165–169.

Bever CT, Andersen PA, Leslie J, *et al.* (1996) Treatment with oral 3,4 diaminopyridine improves leg strength in multiple sclerosis patients: results of a randomized, double-blind, placebo-controlled, crossover trial. *Neurology*, **47**, 1457–1462.

Boringa JB, Lazeron RHC, Reuling IEW, *et al.* (2001) The Brief Repeatable Battery of Neuropsychological Tests: normative values allow application in multiple sclerosis practice. *Multiple Sclerosis*, **7**, 263–267.

Cohen RA, Fisher M. (1989) Amantadine treatment of fatigue associated with multiple sclerosis. *Archives of Neurology*, **46**, 676–680.

Dent A, Lincoln NB. (2000) Screening for memory impairment in multiple sclerosis. *British Journal of Clinical Psychology*, **39**, 311–315.

DePaulo JR, Folstein MF. (1978) Psychiatric disturbance in neurological patients: detection, recognition, and hospital course. *Annals of Neurology*, **4**, 225–228.

Feinstein A, Youl B, Ron M. (1992) Acute optic neuritis. A cognitive and magnetic resonance imaging study. *Brain*, **115**, 1403–1415.

Foley FW, Dince WM, Bedell JR, *et al.* (1994) Psychoremediation of communication skills for cognitively impaired persons with multiple sclerosis. *Journal of Neurological Rehabilitation*, **8**, 165–176.

Folstein MF, Folstein SE, McHugh PR. (1975) Mini-Mental State: a practical method for grading the cognitive state of patients for the clinician. *Journal of Psychiatric Research*, **12**, 189–198.

Franklin GM, Heaton RK, Nelson LM, Filley CM, Seibert C. (1988) Correlation of neuropsychological and MRI findings in chronic–progressive multiple sclerosis. *Neurology*, **38**, 1826–1829.

Franklin GM, Nelson LM, Heaton RK, Filley CM. (1990) Clinical perspectives in the identification of cognitive impairment. In *Neurobehavioral Aspects of Multiple Sclerosis*, ed. SM Rao. New York: Oxford University Press, pp. 161–174.

Geisler MW, Sliwinski M, Coyle PK, *et al.* (1996) The effects of amantadine and pemoline on cognitive functioning in multiple sclerosis. *Archives of Neurology*, **53**, 185–188.

Grafman J. (1984) Memory assessment and remediation. In *Behavioral Assessment and Rehabilitation of the Traumatically Brain Damaged*, ed. BA Edelstein, ET Couture. New York: Plenum Press, pp 151–189.

Greene YM, Tariot PN, Wishart H, *et al.* (2000) A 12-week open trial of donepezil hydrochloride in patients with multiple sclerosis and associated cognitive impairment. *Journal of Clinical Psychopharmacology*, **20**, 350–356.

Heaton RK, Thompson LL, Nelson LM, Filley CM, Franklin GM. (1990) Brief and intermediate length screening of neuropsychological impairment in multiple sclerosis. In *Neurobehavioral Aspects of Multiple Sclerosis*, ed. SM Rao. New York: Oxford University Press, pp. 149–160.

Hohol MJ, Guttmann CRG, Orav J, *et al.* (1997) Serial neuropsychological assessment and magnetic resonance imaging analysis in multiple sclerosis. *Archives of Neurology*, **54**, 1018–1025.

Huber SJ, Paulson GW, Shuttleworth EC, *et al.* (1987) Magnetic resonance imaging correlates of dementia in multiple sclerosis. *Archives of Neurology*, **44**, 732–736.

Jacobs JW, Bernhard MR, Delgado A, Strain JJ. (1977) Screening for organic mental symptoms in the medically ill. *Annals of Internal Medicine*, **86**, 40–46.

Jonsson A, Korfitzen EM, Heltberg A, Ravnborg MH, Byskoz-Ottosen E. (1993) Effects of neuropsychological treatment in patients with multiple sclerosis. *Acta Neurologica Scandinavica*, **88**, 394–400.

Keenan PA, Jacobson MW, Soleymani RM, *et al.* (1996) The effect on memory of chronic prednisone treatment in patients with systemic disease. *Neurology* **47**, 1396–1402.

Knight RG, Devereux RC, Godfrey HP. (1997) Psychosocial consequences of caring for a spouse with multiple sclerosis. *Journal of Clinical and Experimental Neuropsychology*, **19**, 7–19.

Krupp LB, Elkins LE, Scott SR, *et al.* (1999) Donepezil for the treatment of memory impairments in multiple sclerosis. *Neurology*, **52**(Suppl. 2), A137.

Krupp LB, Christodoulou C, Melville P, *et al.* (2004) Donepezil improved memory in multiple sclerosis in a randomized clinical trial. *Neurology*, **63**, 1579–1585.

Kurtzke JF. (1983) Rating neurologic impairment in multiple sclerosis: an expanded disability status scale. *Neurology* (Cleveland), **33**, 1444–1452.

Langdon DW, Thompson AJ. (1999) Multiple sclerosis: a preliminary study of selected variables affecting rehabilitation outcome. *Multiple Sclerosis*, **5**, 94–100.

LaRocca N. (1990) Management of neurobehavioral dysfunction. A rehabilitation perspective. In *Neurobehavioral Aspects of Multiple Sclerosis*, ed. SM Rao. New York: Oxford University Press, pp. 215–229.

Leo GJ, Rao SM. (1988) Effects of intravenous physostigmine and lecithin on memory loss in multiple sclerosis: report of a pilot study. *Journal of Neurological Rehabilitation*, **2**, 123–129.

Lincoln NB, Dent J, Hardig N, *et al.* (2002) Evaluations of cognitive assessment and cognitive intervention for people with multiple sclerosis. *Journal of Neurology, Neurosurgery and Psychiatry*, **72**, 93–98.

Minden S, Moes E. (1990) Management of neurobehavioral dysfunction. A psychiatric perspective. In *Neurobehavioral Aspects of Multiple Sclerosis*, ed. SM Rao. New York: Oxford University Press, pp. 230–250.

Oliveri RL, Sibilia G, Valentino P, *et al.* (1998), Pulsed methylprednisolone induces a reversible impairment of memory in patients with relapsing–remitting multiple sclerosis. *Acta Neurologica Scandinavica*, **97**, 366–369.

Parry AMM, Scott RB, Palace J, Smith S, Mathews PM. (2003) Potentially adaptive functional changes in cognitive processing for patients with multiple sclerosis and their acute modulation by rivastigmine. *Brain*, **126**, 2750–2760.

Peyser JM, Edwards KR, Poser CM, Filskov SB. (1980) Cognitive function in patients with multiple sclerosis. *Archives of Neurology*, **37**, 577–579.

Peyser JM Rao SM, LaRocca NG, Kaplan E. (1990) Guidelines for neuropsychological research in multiple sclerosis. *Archives of Neurology*, **47**, 94–97.

Rao SM, for the Cognitive Function Study Group of the National Multiple Sclerosis Society. (1990) *A Manual for the Brief Repeatable Battery of Neuropsychological Tests in Multiple Sclerosis.* New York: National Multiple Sclerosis Society.

Rao SM, Leo GJ, Haughton VM, St. Aubin-Faubert P, Bernardin L. (1989) Correlation of magnetic resonance imaging with neuropsychological testing in multiple sclerosis. *Neurology,* **39**, 161–166.

Rao SM, Leo GJ, Bernardin L, Unverzagt F. (1991a) Cognitive dysfunction in multiple sclerosis. 1. Frequency, patterns, and prediction. *Neurology,* **41**, 685–691.

Rao SM, Leo GJ, Ellington L, *et al.* (1991b) Cognitive dysfunction in multiple sclerosis. 11. Impact on employment and social functioning. *Neurology,* **41**, 692–696.

Rorie KD, Stump DA, Jeffery DR,. Winston-Salem NC. (2001) Effects of donepezil on cognitive function in patients with multiple slcerosis. *Neurology,* **56**(Suppl. 3), A99.

Rossini PM, Pasqualetti P, Pozzilli C, *et al.* (2001) Fatigue in progressive multiple sclerosis: results of a randomized, double-blind, placebo-controlled crossover trial of oral 4-amino-pyridine. *Multiple Sclerosis,* **7**, 354–358.

Rozewicz L, Langdon DW, Davie CA, Thompson AJ, Ron MA. (1996) Resolution of left hemisphere cognitive dysfunction in multiple sclerosis with magnetic resonance correlates: a case report. *Cognitive Neuropsychiatry,* **1**, 17–25.

Sailer M, Heinze H-J, Schoenfeld MA, Hauser U, Smid HGOM. (2000) Amantadine influences cognitive processing in patients with multiple sclerosis. *Pharmacopsychiatry,* **33**, 28–37.

Schultheis MT, Garay E, DeLuca J. (2001) The influence of cognitive impairment on driving performance in multiple sclerosis. *Neurology,* **56**, 1089–1094.

Schultheis MT, Garay E, Millis SR, DeLuca J. (2002) Motor vehicle creashes and violations among drivers with multiple sclerosis. *Archives of Physical Medicine and Rehabilitation,* **83**, 1175–1178.

Sipe JC, Knobler RL, Breheny SL, *et al.* (1984) A neurologic rating scale (NRS) for use in multiple sclerosis. *Neurology* **34**, 1368–1372.

Smits RCF, Emmen HH, Bertelsmann FW, *et al.* (1994) The effects of 4-aminopyridine on cognitive function in patients with multiple sclerosis: a pilot study. *Neurology,* **44**, 1701–1705.

Sohlberg M, Mateer C. (1989) Introduction to cognitive rehabilitation. *Theory and Practice.* New York: Guildford.

Solari A, Mancuso L, Motta A, Mendozzi L, Serrati C. (2002) Comparison of two brief neuro-psychological batteries in people with multiple sclerosis. *Multiple Sclerosis,* **8**, 169–176.

Solari A, Motta L, Mendozzi E, *et al.* (2004) CRIMS trial: Computer-aided retraining of memory and attention in people with multiple sclerosis: randomized double-blind controlled trial. *Journal of the Neurological Sciences,* **222**, 99–104.

Sullivan MJL, Dehoux E, Buchanan DC. (1989) An approach to cognitive rehabilitation in multiple sclerosis. *Canadian Journal of Rehabilitation,* **3**, 77–85.

Sullivan MJL, Edgley K, Dehoux E. (1990) A survey of multiple sclerosis. Part 1: perceived cognitive problems and compensatory strategy use. *Canadian Journal of Rehabilitation,* **4**, 99–105.

Swirsky-Sacchetti T, Field HL, Mitchell DR, *et al.* (1992) The sensitivity of the Mini-Mental State Examination in the white matter dementia of multiple sclerosis. *Journal of Clinical Psychology,* **48**, 779–786.

Unverzagt FW, Rao SM, Antuono PG. (1991) Oral physostigmine in the treatment of memory loss in multiple sclerosis. *Journal of Clinical Experimental Neuroppsychology*, **13**, 74.

Uttner I, Muller S, Zinser C, *et al.* (2005) Reversible impaired memory induced my pulsed methylprednisolone in patients with MS. *Neurology*, **64**, 1971–1973.

van Diemen HAM, Polman CH, van Dongen TMMM, *et al.* (1992) The effect of 4-amino-pyridine on clinical signs in multiple sclerosis: a randomised, placebo-controlled, double-blind, cross-over study. *Annals of Neurology*, **32**, 123–130.

Zéphir H, de Seze J, Dujardin K, *et al.* (2005) One-year cyclophosphamide treatment combined with methylprednisolone improves cognitive function in progressive forms of multiple sclerosis. *Multiple Sclerosis*, **11**, 360–363.

10

Neuroimaging correlates of cognitive dysfunction

This chapter will review structural and functional brain imaging correlates of cognitive dysfunction. The emphasis will be on MRI given the sensitivity of this technique in demonstrating MS pathology in the brain. It is no coincidence that the renewed interest shown by researchers in the neurobehavioral sequelae of MS dates from the advent of MRI as a research and clinical tool in the 1980s. The use of MRI provides a window into the brain of MS patients and offers an unprecedented opportunity to delineate the cerebral correlates of cognitive dysfunction. While MRI–cognitive studies initially largely focussed on lesion detection and the quantification of lesion volume, attention has shifted more recently to markers of cerebral atrophy as potentially more powerful correlates of cognitive dysfunction. In addition, newer MRI techniques such as diffusion tensor imaging (DTI) and magnetization transfer ratios (MTR), which provide information on normal appearing brain tissue have offered clues concerning the pathogenesis of impaired cognition. These data are complemented by those from a small literature devoted to nuclear magnetic resonance (NMR) spectroscopy and the findings pertaining to cognition will also be reviewed. Finally, insights into cognitive dysfunction derived from functional brain imaging will be discussed. Here too there has been a recent shift in emphasis, this time away from positron emission tomography (PET) and single photon emission computed tomography (SPECT) scanning to the rapidly evolving modality of functional MRI (fMRI).

Computed axial tomography

Abnormalities on computed axial tomography (CT) in the brains of patients with MS were first reported in the mid 1970s (Glydenstedt, 1976; Warren *et al.*, 1976). Although high-resolution scanners, contrast enhancement and delayed scanning have all led to greater sensitivity in detecting MS lesions (Spiegel *et al.*, 1985), the yield is still low. It is, nevertheless, of value in demonstrating sulcal widening and ventricular dilatation, usually present in well-established, severe disease. Depending on the sample under study, these abnormalities have been found in 20–60% of MS subjects (Rao, 1990).

Given the lack of sensitivity of CT in detecting specific MS pathology, it is not surprising that correlations between imaging and cognitive measurements have been weak. No study has attempted to correlate the extent of lesion involvement in the brain with cognitive abnormalities, preferring to concentrate on parameters of cerebral atrophy instead, with varying degrees of success (Brooks *et al.*, 1984; Rao *et al.*, 1985; Rabins *et al.*, 1986; Rao, 1990).

The use of CT in MS has largely been superseded by MRI, and it is generally only in centers without ready access to MRI that CT scanning still takes place. The reasons are that comparisons between MRI and CT in MS have shown that the former detects many more lesions (Young *et al.*, 1981) and in cases where the diagnosis cannot be made with clinical criteria alone, MRI significantly increases the diagnostic yield over CT (Paty *et al.*, 1988). A comparison of the sensitivity of CT and MRI, the latter with and without contrast enhancement, in detecting MS brain lesions is shown in Fig. 10.1.

Magnetic resonance imaging

Monographs on MRI are available (Young, 1984; Andrew *et al.*, 1990) for the reader looking for a detailed description of the principles and techniques. However, a brief explanation is included to set in place the clinical–MRI correlations that follow.

Technique

The MRI technique creates images of objects such as the brain using the magnetic resonance of protons in the atomic nucleus. In body tissues, before the application of a magnetic field, the magnetic moments of the protons (^{1}H) are randomly aligned and have zero net magnetization (M_0). When an external field is applied (produced by the magnet of the MRI system), the individual magnetic moments align parallel or anti-parallel with the applied magnetic field. There are slightly more parallel than anti-parallel protons, resulting in a slight net magnetization.

In a static magnetic field, the energy required to stimulate or excite the low-energy parallel protons to higher energy anti-parallel protons is supplied by electromagnetic radiofrequency waves. When radio waves of the right frequency are passed through the sample, some parallel protons will absorb energy and be excited to a higher energy state in the anti-parallel direction. The amount of energy required to flip a proton from a parallel to an anti-parallel orientation (and thus a higher energy state)

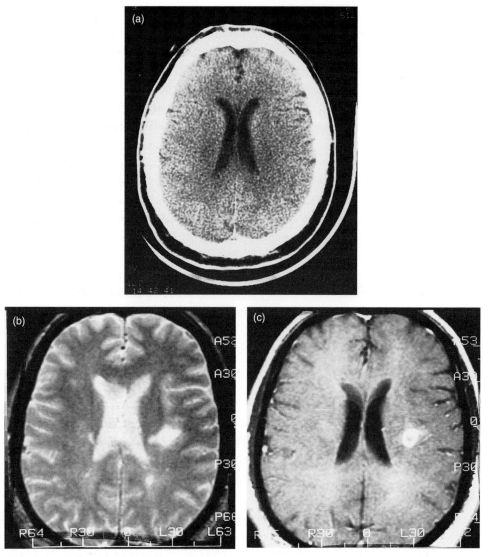

Fig. 10.1.　A comparison of images derived from computed tomography (CT) (a), magnetic resonance imaging (MRI) (b), and MRI with contrast enhancement (c) in one patient with multiple sclerosis (MS). The scans were performed within a day of each other and the sequences seen here are at the same anatomical level. (a) Axial CT scan without evidence of MS plaques. (b) Axial MRI scan in the same patient showing lesions of varying sizes in both hemispheres. (c) Axial T_1 weighted gadolinium–DTPA-enhanced MRI scan demonstrating the presence of a single, discrete contrast-enhanced lesion corresponding with one of the plaques shown on the previous T_2 weighted image. Note that the other lesions shown in (b) are no longer visible.

is dependent on the strength of the magnetic field. The high-energy protons are then observed as they return (relax) to their low energy state. In doing so, they emit electromagnetic energy of the same frequency as the radiofrequency source and this is detected using a sensitive radio receiver. It is this signal that eventually generates the image to be viewed. The size or magnitude of the signal is proportional to the number of protons (proton density) in the tissue under study.

In principle, the procedure is confined to those nuclei that possess an odd number of protons, neutrons or both (e.g. ^{1}H, ^{13}C, ^{19}F, ^{23}Na and ^{31}P), although, in practice, imaging utilizes ^{1}H nuclei because of their high concentration (principally in water) and high NMR sensitivity.

Relaxation times as weighted images

Three principle properties of a substance can be measured: density of nuclear species (e.g. protons) and two relaxation times (T_1 and T_2). "Relaxation time" refers to the time required for the net tissue magnetization vectors to come to equilibrium in a static external magnetic field. In the absence of an applied radiofrequency, transverse magnetization decays exponentially towards zero with a time constant T_2 and the longitudinal magnetization returns exponentially towards the equilibrium value (M_0) with a characteristic time constant T_1. Relaxation times supply valuable information concerning the physical state of a sample and can detect pathological changes in tissues that appear macroscopically normal. Their values increase as the amount of free water in the sample increases, as in edema.

By varying the scanning parameters (i.e. using combinations of radiofrequency pulses), a predominantly T_1, or proton density, or T_2 weighted image can be obtained. The different physical properties of normal (e.g. air, fat, etc.) and abnormal (infarct, blood, tumor, MS plaque) tissue enables them to be differentiated (Tables 10.1 and 10.2). In general, a T_1 weighted image displays cerebral anatomy well, whereas a T_2 weighted image is superior for detecting pathology, such as MS plaques. A useful intermediate scan, with characteristics between a T_1 and a T_2 weighted scan, is a proton density weighted sequence in which the CSF (water) shows up dark (hypointense), thereby offsetting the hyperintense MS plaque and allowing for better periventricular lesion–CSF discrimination (Fig. 10.2). The CSF can be made darker still by using a fluid attenuated inversion recovery (FLAIR) sequence, making it a particularly useful scan for detecting periventricular and juxtacortical lesions.

Diffusion tensor imaging

A recent MRI technique, DTI, is sensitive to local differences in random motion of water molecules. This molecular motion is highly dependent on its environment. For example, in healthy cerebral white matter, water diffusion occurs mainly longitudinally

Table 10.1. Characteristics of normal tissue in T_1 and T_2 weighted magnetic resonance imaging (MRI), computed tomography (CT) and X-ray radiography

	MRI		CT (X-ray)
	T_1	T_2	
Cortical bone	Very hypointense	Very hypointense	Very high density
Air	Very hypointense	Very hypointense	Very low density
Fat	Very hyperintense	Hypointense	Very low density
Water	Hypointense	Hyperintense	Low density
Brain	Gray matter = gray White matter = white	Intermediate (isointense)	Intermediate

Table 10.2. Characteristics of abnormal tissue in T_1 and T_2 weighted magnetic resonance imaging (MRI), computed tomography (CT) and X-ray radiography

	MRI		CT (X-ray)	Contrast enhancement[a]
	T_1	T_2		
Infarct	Hypointense	Hyperintense	Low density	Subacute
Blood	Very hyperintense[b]	Very hyperintense[b]	High density	No
Tumor	Hypointense	Hyperintense	Low density[c]	Yes
MS plaque	Hypointense	Hyperintense	Low density[d]	Acute

[a] Enhancement signifies breakdown of the blood–brain barrier. Contrast used for MRI is gadolinium–DTPA and for CT is iodinated material.
[b] Blood appears bright unless very fresh or very old.
[c] Tumor may appear hyperintense if calcified or hemorrhagic.
[d] MS plaque may appear isodense on CT, hence making detection difficult.

along the axons with limited movement cross-sectionally. In the presence of brain pathology, the restrictions placed on this movement are reduced and when measured provide a subtle index of structural changes occurring in lesions and normal appearing brain parenchyma. Two useful indices are obtained. Mean diffusivity, which provides a measurement of molecular motion, and fractional anisotropy, which is a reflection of the organization and integrity of cellular structures.

Magnetization transfer imaging

Tissue contrast is determined by proton density and T_1 and T_2 relaxation times in conventional MRI. Only relatively mobile or free water protons (approximately

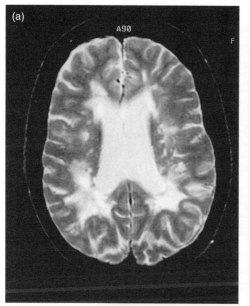

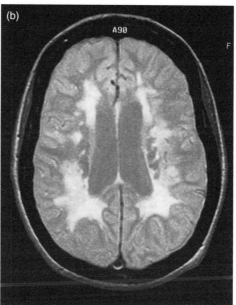

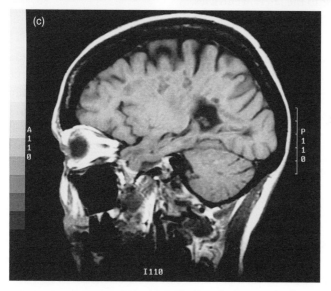

Fig. 10.2.   Magnetic resonance imaging (MRI) with varying relaxation times. (a) Axial T_2 weighted (spin echo) MRI scan demonstrating extensive periventricular lesions typical of MS. (b) Axial proton density (spin echo) MRI scan in the same patient, at the same anatomical plane. Note how the CSF now appears hypointense (dark). (c) A sagittal T_1 weighted MRI scan in the same patient demonstrating plaques that now appear hypointense (dark), as opposed to the hyperintense (bright) lesions revealed by the spin echo sequences.

80% of all the total) are visible. The remaining 20% of water protons are tightly bound to proteins and lipid membranes, have very short relaxation times and are not visible. The exchange of magnetization between the bound and unbound protons can be manipulated by altering the MR scanning techniques (for example pre-pulse saturation of the bound water). In the process, information (i.e. a magnetization transfer ratio [MTR]) is obtained that reflects the complexity of a macromolecular structure such as myelin.

Magnetic resonance imaging in multiple sclerosis

Lesions

Magnetic resonance imaging is a highly sensitive technique for demonstrating brain lesions in patients with MS. Abnormalities are present in virtually all patients with clinically definite MS (Miller *et al.*, 1988), the position of MRI lesions correlating with plaques seen at postmortem (Ormerod *et al.*, 1987). The characteristic pattern is one of multifocal white matter lesions, the majority situated adjacent to the lateral ventricles.

Relaxation times

Prolonged T_1 and T_2 relaxation times have been noted in normal appearing white matter (NAWM) in MS patients compared with healthy controls (Ormerod *et al.*, 1986) or those with systemic lupus erythematosus (Miller *et al.*, 1989), while patients with clinically isolated syndromes (e.g. optic neuritis) tend to occupy an intermediate position between MS patients and healthy controls (Ormerod *et al.*, 1986). The reasons for these changes are not entirely clear, but they probably reflect the presence of microscopic abnormalities such as perivascular inflammation in the NAWM (Allen *et al.*, 1981).

Magnetization transfer and diffusion tensor imaging

Values for MTR, fractional anisotropy and mean diffusivity can be obtained from multiple tissue compartments in the brain and spinal cord, for example lesions (hypointense, hyperintense, contrast enhancing), regions of white matter with and without (NAWM) lesions and so on. Correlations between fractional anisotropy and mean diffusivity values obtained from lesions correlate with values derived from normal appearing brain tissue (Filippi *et al.*, 2001), and the same applies to MTR data (Traboulsee *et al.*, 2003). Of note however, is that in a study of patients with relapsing–remitting MS no significant correlations emerged between brain indices derived from DTI and MTR, suggesting that these imaging techniques may supply relatively independent measures of lesion burden (Iannucci *et al.*, 2001).

In general, MTR (van Buchem *et al.*, 1998; Santos *et al.*, 2002; Traboulsee *et al.*, 2003) and DTI (Ciccarelli *et al.*, 2001) measures correlate significantly, albeit modestly, with measures of physical disability (Expanded Disability Status Scale [EDSS]) and can provide valuable clues as to the evolution of disease over time (Filippi *et al.*, 2000; Iannucci *et al.*, 2000; Santos *et al.*, 2002). They may also provide markers of response to treatment. The reader is directed to informative reviews of diffusion MRI (Goldberg-Zimring *et al.*, 2005; Rovaris *et al.*, 2005) and MT imaging (Horsfield, 2005).

Specificity

Although MRI has proved invaluable in elucidating the dynamic nature of brain changes in vivo, it is not without limitations. Small demyelinating lesions may escape detection because of restrictions on spatial resolution, although this problem may be reduced by using contiguous slices with a thin slice thickness. Another difficulty is distinguishing MS plaques from coarse vascular lesions (Ormerod *et al.*, 1984) and those seen in the vasculitides, namely systemic lupus erythematosus and Behçet's disease amongst others (Miller *et al.*, 1987). Nevertheless, there are certain lesion characteriztics relating to size, frequency and site that tilt the differential diagnosis towards MS (Barkof *et al.*, 1997; Tintoré *et al.*, 2000). More recently, the diagnostic importance of MRI in MS has become enshrined with the McDonald criteria (McDonald *et al.*, 2001), subsequently revised (Polman *et al.*, 2005) (Ch. 1). Very specific criteria now provide evidence of dissemination of disease in time and space.

Areas of high signal intensity in the cerebral white matter may also be found in healthy individuals, particularly with advancing age. The radiological appearance of these lesions is occasionally indistinguishable from that seen in MS (George *et al.*, 1986; Hachinski *et al.*, 1987; Fig. 10.3). With technology outstripping clinical knowledge, Hachinski *et al.* (1987) initially advised against prematurely attributing these brain changes to a pathological process. Searching for a suitable descriptor, they called these areas of heightened signal intensity "leukoaraiosis," a word derived from the Greek *leuko* meaning "white," and *araios* signifying "loose," and implying a diminution in density.

Early cognitive studies supported this cautionary view. Rao *et al.* (1989a) compared the neuropsychological performance of healthy, normotensive patients with ($n = 10$) and without ($n = 40$) MRI signs of leukoaraiosis. No cognitive differences were found, in accord with reports from more elderly subjects (Brandt-Zawadski *et al.*, 1985; Tupler *et al.*, 1992). A limitation in these studies, however, was the method of MRI assessment, which relied on a rating scale approach and so was unable to provide volumetric estimates. It is, therefore, significant that a study with a wide age scatter that used computerized quantification of lesion volume and functional brain imaging (PET) found significant cognitive and other radiological differences between patients with varying degrees of white matter lesions (DeCarli *et al.*, 1995). The crucial point related to threshold. A white matter hyperintensity volume in excess of 0.5% ($10\,\text{cm}^3$)

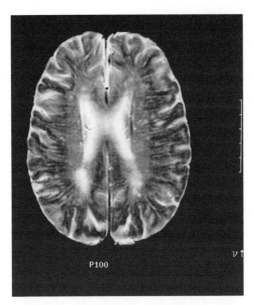

Fig. 10.3.   An axial T_2 weighted magnetic resonance image in a 71-year-old asymptomatic, normotensive male. Note the confluent periventricular and multiple discrete, small white matter hyperintensities (leukoaraiosis) together with prominent Virchow–Robbin spaces.

of intracranial volume was associated not only with cognitive impairment but also with increased ventricular volume and reduced brain volume. Despite all adults being deemed healthy prior to enrollment, a significant association emerged between increased white matter lesions and raised systolic blood pressure. The notion of lesions having to exceed a particular threshold of white matter volume before cognitive problems manifested echoed a finding in MS patients linking a total lesion area exceeding 30 cm^2 to cognitive dysfunction (Rao *et al.*, 1989b).

More recent data from large epidemiological studies of asymptomatic adults have confirmed the link between white matter hyperintensities and cognitive difficulties both in elderly (de Groot *et al.*, 2000) and middle-aged (Mosley *et al.*, 2005) adults. Furthermore, these white matter changes may be associated with increased ventricular and sulcal size, two further ominous predictors of subtle cognitive deficits in non-demented samples.

Safety and serial imaging

MRI is a safe procedure. The recognized hazards are those that the magnetic field can exert upon ferromagnetic materials such as certain aneurysm clips and pace-makers (New *et al.*, 1983; Pavlicek *et al.*, 1983). Furthermore, MRI has no measurable adverse effect on cognition (Sweetland *et al.*, 1987). The lack of unwanted effects has made serial studies with MRI possible. These have helped to chart the natural history of MS (Isaac *et al.*, 1988; Miller *et al.*, 1988; Willoughby *et al.*, 1989) and the cerebral responses to disease-modifying treatments (Martinelli *et al.*, 2004; Goodin, 2006).

The progressive nature of brain involvement in MS is illustrated by the changes in lesion load over time. While approximately 60% of patients with clinically isolated lesions have brain abnormalities at initial presentation (Ormerod *et al.*, 1987), this progresses to virtually 100% by the time they develop definite MS (Miller *et al.*, 1992). Fluctuations in both lesion size and lesion number, particularly in those with a secondary progressive type of illness, have been documented (Thompson *et al.*, 1991). The dynamic nature of the lesions plus the finding of increased disease activity in patients whose disease was thought to be quiescent (Filippi *et al.*, 1996a) illustrate the heterogeneity of inflammatory changes in MS and account for the modest correlation of neuroimaging and clinical findings (Jacobs *et al.*, 1986; Isaac *et al.*, 1988; Thompson *et al.*, 1990).

Contrast magnetic resonance imaging

The use of a contrast compound such as gadolinium–DTPA, has shed light on the pathogenesis of lesion formation, for the presence of enhancement signifies a breakdown of the blood–brain barrier (Hawkins *et al.*, 1990) and is a consistent finding in new lesions (Miller *et al.*, 1988; Thompson *et al.*, 1992; Fig. 10.4). Serial studies with gadolinium–DTPA have also demonstrated that disruption of the blood–brain barrier can precede other MRI abnormalities and clinical evidence of new lesion formation (Kermode *et al.*, 1990a,b). In over two thirds of patients, the duration of enhancement is less than six weeks (Miller *et al.*, 1988; Thompson *et al.*, 1992).

In an effort to increase the ability of MRI to detect acute lesions, the dose of gadolinium–DTPA has been trebled (i.e. to 0.3 mmol/kg body weight), without an associated increase in side effects. In a serial study of 22 patients who were first scanned with a standard dose of gadolinium–DTPA (0.1 mol/kg) followed 6 to 24 hours later with the triple dose regimen, Filippi *et al.* (1996b) reported that the number of enhancing lesions detected increased significantly from 83 (in 14 patients) to 138 (in 18 patients), a 28% increase. The total lesion area identified per patient also increased, as did the number of large enhancing lesions, both changes proving highly significant.

Cortical lesions

While MS has long been considered the quintessential white matter disease, MRI and neuropathological data have confirmed the presence of a significant number of cortical lesions. The use of a particular MRI scanning sequence, FLAIR, increases the sensitivity of spin echo sequences in detecting these MS lesions. It does so by suppressing CSF signal, thereby improving detection of lesions at CSF

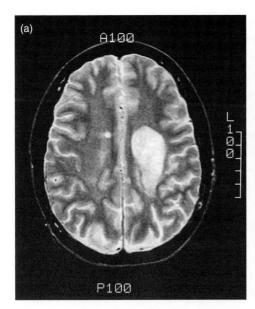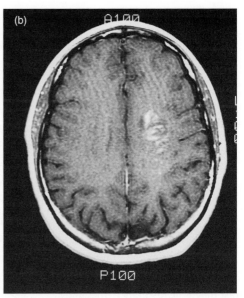

Fig. 10.4.   Magnetic resonance imaging in a patient with multiple sclerosis (MS). (a) Axial T_2 weighted image showing a large MS plaque in the left hemisphere and a smaller, circumscribed lesion in the right hemisphere. (b) Axial T_1 weighted contrast-enhanced (gadolinium–DTPA) image of the same patient showing how the large left hemisphere lesion, visible on the T_2 sequence is no longer visible and has been replaced by smaller areas of contrast enhancement, indicative of more active disease and breakdown of the blood–brain barrier. The small right hemisphere lesion visible on the T_2 weighted scan has also disappeared on the T_1 weighted image.

surfaces. In addition, it increases the contrast between lesions and normal appearing brain tissue and is particularly helpful in revealing juxtacortical lesions (De Coene *et al.*, 1992). The latter are also better visualized with contrast enhancement. For example, in a serial MRI study, the use of gadolinium–DTPA led to a 140% increase in cortical lesion detection, the majority of which was juxtacortical (i.e. at the interface of the white and gray matter) and histologically identical to those arising in the deeper white matter (Kidd *et al.*, 1999). Fully one quarter of all lesions, however, were cortical in origin and appeared intimately linked to the various types of cortical veins.

Chronic–progressive disease course

There are clear MRI differences between patients with primary progressive (PP) and secondary progressive (SP) MS. Patients with PPMS have lower lesion loads (Thompson *et al.*, 1990; Filippi *et al.*, 1995). They also have fewer contrast enhancing lesions. Over a six month period 12 patients with PPMS were compared with 12 patients with SPMS using serial gadolinium–DTPA scans. The latter group developed 109 new lesions of which 87% enhanced whereas in the former there were 20 new lesions, of which only one enhanced (Thompson *et al.*, 1991). Not only do patients with SPMS have more lesions, but these lesions have a lower magnetization ratio, suggesting a more destructive pathological process, which may include increased demyelination and axonal loss (Gass *et al.*, 1994).

Cerebral atrophy

Magnetic resonance imaging has also demonstrated cerebral atrophy in MS patients, reflecting a degenerative process that begins early in the disease. Atrophy is a sign of neuronal loss and irreversible tissue destruction. Serial brain MRI has revealed the progressive nature of parenchymal loss, which encompasses not only lesion development but also the microscopic changes affecting NAWM (Stone *et al.*, 1995; Losseff *et al.*, 1996). Furthermore, there is evidence linking a decline in cortical gray matter volume to the remote effects of white matter lesion volume, a relationship that is less clear when it comes to deep gray matter. Markers of cerebral atrophy are now considered more robust correlates of physical disability than measurements of lesion volumes (see Miller *et al.* [2002] and Bermel and Bakshi [2006] for useful reviews of cerebral atrophy associated with MS).

Relationship between magnetic resonance imaging and cognitive abnormalities

Total lesion score and cognitive dysfunction

The strength of the association detected between cognitive dysfunction and MRI lesion load has been influenced by the method used to quantify lesions. Two approaches have been followed: the use of rating scales to estimate the size and number of lesions and the direct quantification of lesion area/volume using computerized methods. Early studies relied on the former, which is considered inferior because it is prone to human error and produces a range of artificially restricted values (Rao, 1990). Nevertheless, the computated measurement of lesion volume has not yet reached routine clinical practice and remains largely the purlieu of the researcher. As such, dismissing the utility of rating scales is premature.

The majority of studies using the *rating scale approach* to MRI analysis have reported modest correlations between total lesion score and indices of cognitive dysfunction (Medaer *et al.*, 1987; Franklin *et al.*, 1988; Callanan *et al.*, 1989; Anzola *et al.*, 1990; Pozzilli *et al.*, 1991a; Ron *et al.*, 1991; Feinstein *et al.*, 1992a, 1993; Maurelli *et al.*, 1992; Comi *et al.*, 1993, 1995; Pugnetti *et al.*, 1993; Tsolaki *et al.*, 1994; Ryan *et al.*, 1996).

Evidence suggests that if a more focussed approach is adopted, for example limiting the ratings to brain regions known to be rich in cholinergic pathways, then reasonable correlations with psychometric measures of memory can be obtained.

Chamelian *et al.* (2005) applied the Cholinergic Pathways Hyperintensity Scale to the MR images of 40 MS patients who also underwent testing with the Neuropsychological Screening Battery for MS (Rao *et al.*, 1991). Patients with high lesion scores on MRI analysis performed significantly more poorly on measures of verbal and visuospatial memory. The Cholinergic Pathway Hyperintensity Scale is straightforward to use and easily applicable in a clinical setting; it also provides a cut-off score (sensitivity of 82%, specificity of 83%) beyond which cognitive dysfunction is likely.

Direct computerized quantification of total brain lesion load has strengthened the correlations with cognitive dysfunction (Rao *et al.*, 1989b; Feinstein *et al.*, 1992b; Swirsky-Sacchetti *et al.*, 1992; Camp *et al.*, 1999). An early, often cited study suggested that total hyperintense lesion area was a more robust imaging predictor of cognitive dysfunction than a measurement of brain atrophy, namely the ventricular brain ratio (Rao *et al.*, 1989b). Notable, total lesion area correlated significantly with a wide array of cognitive deficits, including measures of verbal and non-verbal memory (Selective Reminding Test, 7/24 Spatial Recall Test, Story Recall Test), abstract and conceptual reasoning (Wisconsin Card Sort Test [WCST], Ravens Matrices and Stroop Test), language abilities (COWAT, Boston Naming Test) and visuospatial skills (Hooper Visual Orientation Test, Facial Recognition Test, Visual Form Discrimination Test). The cognitive correlates of total lesion area differed from those associated with the size of the corpus callosum (see below). Overall, 25 cognitive parameters correlated with the semi-automated measurement of gross T_2 weighted lesion area, but the strength of the associations were modest, at best ($0.3 \leq r \leq 0.5$). As with the leukoaraiosis data (DeCarli *et al.*, 1995), an imaging threshold effect was found: when total lesion area exceeded $30\,\mathrm{cm}^2$, over 80% of MS patients were deemed cognitively impaired.

Localized brain abnormalities and cognitive dysfunction

Corpus callosum

The corpus callosum is composed of white matter fibers linking the hemispheres and, as such, is likely to be affected by demyelination, showing signs of atrophy and/or lesion involvement (Fig. 10.5). The cognitive deficits most closely identified with corpus callosum abnormalities have been speed of information processing and rapid problem solving (Rao *et al.*, 1989c). Furthermore, atrophy of the corpus callosum has also correlated significantly with deficits when verbal stimuli are presented dichotically, which may account for the difficulties experienced by some MS patients on tests of laterality and sustained attention and vigilance (Rao *et al.*, 1989c; Pelletier *et al.*, 1993). Other cognitive problems linked to the corpus callosum include verbal fluency deficits, which have been associated with anterior callosal pathology (Pozzilli *et al.*, 1991b), and visual retention difficulties, which have been related to lesions of the genu (Ryan *et al.*, 1996).

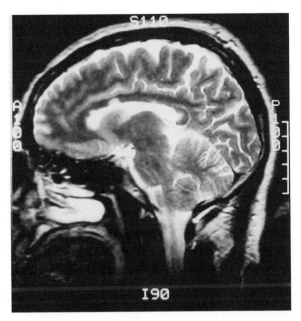

Fig. 10.5. A mid-sagittal T_2 weighted (fast spin echo) sequence showing the punched out appearance of lesions within the corpus callosum of a patient with multiple sclerosis.

Periventricular lesion load

There are reports of cognitive dysfunction, most frequently various aspects of memory, being associated with periventricular lesions (Reischies *et al.*, 1988; Izquierdo *et al.*, 1991; Pozzilli *et al.*, 1991a; Maurelli *et al.*, 1992), but these data are hard to interpret. Periventricular lesions are often confluent, making a more precise anatomical localization difficult. In addition, the propensity of MS lesions for periventricular sites will generally ensure that this lesion area correlates signifi-cantly with total lesion area. The possibility of the periventricular lesions affecting the function of more distant sites, through a process of "disconnection" (i.e., the interruption of neural circuitry by demyelination), must also be considered.

Juxtacortical lesion load

A small, but growing literature suggests juxtacortical lesions detected on FLAIR and fast FLAIR sequences may be a more robust predictor of cognitive impairment than subcortical (white matter) lesions (Moriarty *et al.*, 1999; Lazeron *et al.*, 2000; Rovaris *et al.*, 2000).

Frontal lobe lesion load

A few studies have explored the association between frontal lesion load and cognitive tasks that are dependent, in part, on the functional integrity of this region. Significant associations have been reported between a measure of frontal lesion load on the one hand and impaired performance on the WCST (Arnett *et al.*, 1994; Swirsky-Sacchetti *et al.*, 1992) and the Tower of London Task (Foong *et al.*, 1997) on the other.

Atrophy

Over the past few years, a consensus has been building that cerebral atrophy rather than lesion quantification can explain more of the variance associated with cognitive dysfunction. Different methods have been applied to the assessment of parenchymal loss, but the results have generally been consistent. Cognitive dysfunction has been linked to (a) ventricular enlargement on CT (Rao *et al.*, 1985), transcranial sonography (Berg *et al.*, 2000) and MRI (Pozzilli *et al.*, 1991a; Clark *et al.*, 1992; Comi *et al.*, 1993); (b) reductions in total white matter (Edwards *et al.*, 2001), neocortical (cortical gray matter) (Amato *et al.*, 2004) and relative parenchymal (i.e. total parenchymal/intracranial) (Lazeron *et al.*, 2005) volumes; (c) increased bicaudate ratios (i.e. the minimum intercaudate distance divided by the brain width along the same line) (Bermel *et al.*, 2002); (d) frontal cortical atrophy (Benedict *et al.*, 2002, Locatelli *et al.*, 2004).

In an effort to tease out the contribution of various indices of brain pathology to cognitive impairment, Benedict *et al.* (2004) undertook a detailed MRI brain analysis of 37 MS patients and 27 healthy controls. The MR indices included T_1 weighted hypointense lesion volume, hyperintense lesion volume measured on a FLAIR sequence, third ventricle width, bicaudate ratio and brain parenchymal fraction. The Minimal Assessment of Cognitive Function in MS cognitive battery was given to all study participants. After controlling for the potential confounding effects of age, premorbid intelligence and depression, third ventricular width emerged as the most robust MRI predictor of cognitive deficits, followed by brain parenchymal fraction. The robustness of third ventricle atrophy as a predictor of cognitive dysfunction was attributed, in part, to atrophy of the thalamus, an important relay station for cortical and subcortical neural pathways. Indirect support for this finding comes from Christodoulou *et al.* (2003), who adopted a different approach to quantifying cerebral atrophy. These authors defined an index they called central cerebral atrophy, which was the percentage of central CSF to total intracranial volume (gray and white matter, lesion and CSF volumes). This variable emerged as a stronger predictor of cognitive dysfunction than lesion volume, accounting for more than half the variance in cognitive performance (the NMR spectroscopy data in this study are discussed on p. 197).

Longitudinal studies

The safety of MRI has facilitated its use in longitudinal studies, where combined with serial measures of cognitive function it has been important in clarifying the pathogenesis and natural history of cognitive change in MS. In addition, the use of contrast-enhanced MRI has allowed the relationship between the development of acute brain lesions and their neuropsychological sequelae to be explored.

In a follow-up study of 48 patients with clinically isolated syndromes, Feinstein *et al.* (1992a) repeated MRI and a cognitive battery on average 4.5 years after initial assessment. Approximately half the subjects developed MS during the follow-up period, displaying a significantly higher lesion load in the process. These patients also developed a number of new cognitive deficits, most prominently memory impairment. The study was illuminating for two reasons. First, it demonstrated the progression of cognitive impairment first detected early in the demyelination process and, second, by controlling for a host of variables (age, gender, education, disease duration, disease course, physical disability and emotional factors such as depression and anxiety), it clearly demonstrated that the progression of brain pathology determined the pace of cognitive decline.

The same conclusions were reached in follow-up studies of patients with established MS examined over one year (Hohol *et al.*, 1997), two years (Mariani *et al.*, 1991) and four years (Sperling *et al.*, 2001). The Hohol study was the first MRI–cognition investigation to use a fully automated, three-dimensional computer-assisted method of lesion quantification. Forty four patients were assessed with MRI and the Brief Repeatable Battery of Neuropsychological Tests (BRNB) on admission to the study and after a duration of one year. At one year follow-up, group cognitive data had not declined. However, in the four patients who had cognitively deteriorated, total lesion volume increased more than ten-fold compared with those patients whose cognitive state either improved ($n = 19$) or remained constant ($n = 21$). At neither index nor follow-up appointment did physical disability (EDSS) correlate with the MRI variables, confirming that cognition was a more sensitive indicator than neurological signs of brain pathology.

These data were refined by Sperling *et al.* (2001) in their longitudinal study of 28 MS patients seen after one and four years. The cognitive battery was again the BRNB, but the MRI data were now analyzed according to brain region as well. Total lesion volume did not significantly increase over time and remained predominantly frontal. Significant correlations were found at all time points between deficits on the Paced Auditory Serial Addition Test (PASAT) and the Bushke Verbal Selective Reminding Test and lesion volume affecting frontal, parietal and whole brain regions. These brain–behavior correlations were consistent over time, essentially replicating the findings by Hohol *et al.* (1997). In other words, in the absence of further deterioration in lesion load, cognitive dysfunction likewise remained unchanged.

A longitudinal study that failed to find an association between deteriorating indices of cognition and brain lesion load was compromised by a high attrition rate over the 8.5 year follow-up period and an outdated method of MRI analysis (Piras *et al.*, 2003). More informative is a three year follow-up study in which neither lesion load nor cognition deteriorated, with both variables correlating with one another at study onset and conclusion (Patti *et al.*, 1998).

The studies cited above have helped to clarify longitudinal brain–cognition relationships over an interval spanning one to four years, but they could not elucidate whether cognition mirrored the weekly waxing and waning in size and contrast enhancement known to occur with MS lesions. To investigate this possibility, more frequent scanning and psychometric testing was required. In a serial study over six months confined to patients with relapsing–remitting MS, Feinstein *et al.* (1993) undertook gadolinium-enhanced MRI at intervals of two weeks in five patients with active disease (group A) and at intervals of four weeks in five patients with "benign" MS (group B). Neuropsychological testing preceded MRI in each subject at each session.

The study highlighted not only the variability in cognitive performance over time (Ch. 8) but also a commensurate variability in MRI brain lesion scores. In general, tests of sensorimotor function were the most sensitive to a deteriorating brain lesion score. For other cognitive functions, practice effects exerted a powerful influence, which meant patients' performances on tests such as the Stroop and PASAT continued to improve despite a constant or even a deteriorating lesion score. Finally, the hazards of predicting changes over time in the brains of MS patients was clearly demonstrated. Of the five patients in group A deemed to have "active" MS prior to enrollment, only two displayed longitudinal evidence of a worsening lesion score. This variability on so many fronts accounts for the failure of another serial gadolinium-enhanced MRI and cognitive study to report significant associations between the variables in question (Mattioli *et al.*, 1993).

Relaxation times and cognition

Brain changes that are not macroscopically discernible may also influence cognition. The T_1 and T_2 relaxation times provide one such measure as they reflect the presence of microscopic abnormalities such as perivascular inflammation, myelin breakdown and astrocyte hyperplasia (Allen *et al.*, 1981). One study has reported correlations between raised T_1 relaxation times in an area of frontal NAWM and abnormalities in tasks of abstraction, visual memory and naming (Feinstein *et al.*, 1992b). These results have not been replicated in MS patients, although similar associations have been reported in Alzheimer's disease (Besson *et al.*, 1990). The reluctance on the part of researchers in general to pursue studies of relaxation time abnormalities in MS (not only in relation to cognition) may be attributed to the emergence of newer more informative methods of brain imaging (see below).

Diffusion tensor imaging and cognition

Rovaris *et al.* (2002) undertook an exploratory examination of DTI–cognitive correlates in 34 patients with relapsing–remitting MS and mild physical disability. The cognitive battery comprised the core BRNB supplemented by the WCST, Symbol–Digit Modality Test (SDMT) and Stroop tests. Multiple MRI measurements were computed: T_1 and T_2 lesion volume, whole brain volume and mean diffusivity and fractional anisotropy. Lesions, values derived from brain tissue (i.e. parenchyma plus lesions), normal appearing brain tissue (i.e. parenchyma with lesions removed), NAWM and normal appearing gray matter. Approximately a quarter of the sample were found to have cognitive impairment and modest correlations emerged between three cognitive tests (SDMT, verbal fluency and the 10/36 Spatial Recall Test) and the following MRI variables: T_1 and T_2 lesion volumes and average mean diffusivity values for lesions, NAWM, normal appearing gray matter, normal appearing brain tissue and whole brain tissue. Unfortunately, the authors did not investigate the relative contributions of the various MRI measurements to the cognitive variance, so the reader cannot gauge whether the DTI measurements add to the lesion data. Nevertheless, the findings should be viewed alongside those from other imaging modalities that have highlighted the importance of probing normal appearing brain matter in the search for an improved understanding of the pathogenesis of cognitive dysfunction.

Magnetization transfer imaging and cognition

The technique of MTR imaging has been used more often than DTI in the search for brain–cognition correlates. In a heterogenous sample of 30 MS patients with a mix of disease courses, MTR values obtained from lesions and brain parenchyma were significantly lower in patients who were cognitively compromised (Rovaris *et al.*, 1998). Correlation coefficients were similar in magnitude to the mean diffusivity values obtained with DTI (in the range $0.45 < r < 0.59$). In a subsequent article, average cortical/subcortical MTR emerged from a multivariate regression analysis as the most robust predictor of cognitive impairment, exceeding the presence of lesions detected by T_1 and T_2 weighted imaging (Rovaris *et al.*, 2000). This finding was reinforced in a study of MS patients in the early phase of a relapsing–remitting disease course, where MTR of normal appearing brain tissue and brain parenchymal fraction (a measure of cerebral atrophy) were the only MRI variables independently correlated with cognitive impairment (Zivadinov *et al.*, 2001). This result replicated the findings of van Buchem *et al.* (1998), who had concluded earlier that overall neuropsychological functioning in MS patients depended largely on two factors, brain atrophy and parenchymal MTR values, the latter obtained from a pixel by pixel analysis of the whole brain. Finally, Audoin *et al.* (2005) used MTR and fMRI to explore cerebral correlates of the

PASAT in a group of patients with clinically isolated syndromes. Significant correlations were found between mean MTR values derived from NAWM and poor performance on the PASAT. In addition, increased regional activation on fMRI correlated inversely with mean MTR values obtained from both NAWM and normal appearing gray matter, providing evidence of compensatory brain mechanisms working to offset structural damage in the very earliest phases of the disease. (See p. 199 for a review of fMRI cognition studies in MS.)

Magnetic resonance spectroscopy

The search for brain correlates of cognitive dysfunction using DTI and MTR has much in common with studies that have used NMR spectroscopy. This technique was first developed in the mid 1940s as a method to determine the magnetic properties of atomic nuclei. Initially used in the field of molecular physics and chemistry, it provided valuable information on molecular structure and chemical reaction rates. Biochemists have used NMR spectroscopy to elucidate the structure of cell membranes, nucleic acids, proteins and viruses. The earliest experiments on living systems involved phosphorus (^{31}P) spectroscopy of red blood cells, excised muscle tissue and suspensions of yeast cells. This was followed by studies of systems such as whole animals, perfused organs and cellular suspensions. Other nuclei studied have included hydrogen (^{1}H), fluorine (^{19}F), carbon-13 (^{13}C), sodium (^{23}Na), potassium (^{39}K) and nitrogen (^{15}N and ^{14}N). With respect to medical research, improvements in NMR technology over the last 15–20 years have now enabled the technique to be applied to the in vivo study of the physiology and metabolism of living organizms. Of particular medical interest are in vivo proton, phosphorus and carbon spectra because the three occur in the body in compounds that play an important role in cellular metabolism and in the supply of energy. They are also present in sufficient concentrations to permit detection.

There are a number of ways in which information on biochemistry and physiology can be obtained by NMR spectroscopy. One approach is to measure and compare the levels of metabolites in diseased and healthy tissue. For example, lesions such as tumors or infarcts, demonstrated by other techniques such as MRI or CT, may have their chemical structure clarifed by NMR spectroscopy. The spectra are displayed by expressing the frequencies in relative, not absolute, units. The reason is that frequencies are not constant but increase linearly in relation to field strength. By expressing any given frequency relative to a reference compound, the frequency value becomes constant, allowing for comparisons between measurements obtained on different systems with different field strengths. A commonly used reference compound in brain proton spectroscopy is creatine.

The application of NMR spectroscopy to MS offers new research possibilities such as evaluating a number of interesting metabolites. One example is *N*-acetylaspartate, which is an amino acid found largely in neurones and, therefore, considered a non-specific marker of neuronal integrity. Reduced concentrations of *N*-acetylaspartate in neurones in patients with MS is recognized as a probable measure of axonal loss in chronic lesions, whereas a partial reversal of this concentration loss may occur in acute lesions (Davie *et al.*, 1994). The technique can also detect mobile lipids during periods of myelin breakdown, while a rise in choline concentration (relative to creatine) may relate to changes in membrane viability in association with an inflammatory cell infiltrate. Consequently, serial NMR spectroscopy may play a useful role in studying the natural history of MS in addition to monitoring brain changes during clinical trials (Miller, 1995).

Spectroscopy and cognition

The rationale for applying NMR spectroscopy to a group study of cognitive aspects of MS is compelling. Given the preliminary conclusions from the T_1 relaxation time data (Feinstein *et al.*, 1992b), NMR spectroscopy may provide more substantial evidence of neuronal destruction. A case report illustrates this well (Rozewicz, *et al.* 1996). A 21-year-old patient with MS suffered a relapse that resulted in quadriplegia. This was associated with cognitive deficits affecting primarily left hemisphere function (i.e. the Graded Naming and Token Tests). Given her neurological deficits, a performance IQ score could not be obtained. Gadolinium-enhanced MRI at the time revealed a number of high-signal, often contrast-enhancing, lesions in the white matter and cortex. Proton spectroscopy from an enhancing lesion demonstrated a decrease in the *N*-acetylaspartate/creatine ratio, and a choline/creatine ratio that was not, initially, elevated.

The patient was treated with high-dose intravenous steroids. Seven weeks after admission, her EDSS had decreased from 9.0 to 6.5 and she was able to walk a few yards with assistance. Repeat neuropsychological testing and neuroimaging showed improvement on the Graded Naming and Token Test, and a marked reduction in the size of six of the lesions, with a reduction in some lesion enhancement. Repeat NMR spectroscopy showed a large rise in her choline/creatine ratio and a more modest increase in the *N*-acetylaspartate/creatine ratio. Increased lipid and macromolecule resonances noted in the first examination had decreased at follow-up, but not to the levels found in healthy controls. Given the temporal synchronicity of cognitive, MRI and NMR spectroscopy changes, a more complete picture emerges of the brain changes underlying alterations in mentation.

Although informative, the case report made no mention of any NMR spectroscopic changes in NAWM. If present, this would have supplied more subtle, widespread evidence of cerebral pathology related to cognitive dysfunction.

Tentative evidence to this effect comes from two studies that looked at ratios of N-acetylaspartate (relative to creatine and choline) in bilateral posterior periventricular areas and found correlations with measures of verbal and visual memory and attention (Christodoulou et al., 2003) and verbal learning (Pan et al., 2001). Inconsistencies in laterality data between these two studies have not been adequately explained.

The subtleties of putative brain–behavior relationships were highlighted in a study that reported a reduction in N-acetylaspartate/creatine ratios in frontal NAWM in MS patients rather than healthy controls but failed to elicit correlations with executive dysfunction (Foong et al., 1999). However, when analysis was confined to patients with the most abnormal ratios only, more marked deficits were recorded on a test of spatial working memory. This functional threshold effect may help to explain the clinical scenario occasionally encountered where a cognitively impaired patient has little atrophy or lesion load on brain MRI.

Functional magnetic resonance imaging

In fMRI, changes in blood oxygenation are measured over time. In response to cerebral activity, cerebral blood flow, blood volume and oxygen extraction changes while hemoglobin shifts to its deoxygenated state. The last is associated with a measurable magnetic shift and this forms the basis of the fMRI signal. This technique has many advantages when it comes to detecting brain function. It has excellent temporal (second by second) and spatial (millimeters) localization and it is non-invasive, which means it can be safely repeated many times over (Huettel et al., 2003).

Functional MRI has proved useful in correlating brain activation with neurological function in MS. In particular, it has demonstrated that the brain has the potential to reorganize functionally in an attempt to compensate for the deleterious effects of the disease. This reorganization may take the form of increased levels of activation or additional areas of activation relative to healthy controls and has been observed for motor (Reddy et al., 2000; Filippi et al., 2002a; Pantano et al., 2002), and visual (Werring et al., 2000) function in addition to fatigue (Filippi et al., 2002b).

Functional magnetic resonance imaging and cognition

There is a small, but informative fMRI literature devoted to cognitive function in MS patients. Studies have focussed on three aspects of cognition: sustained attention, working memory and executive function.

A series of studies have used the PASAT or its visual analog, the PVSAT, as an index of attention and working memory. In the earliest report, Staffen et al. (2002)

investigated 21 MS patients with a disease duration of less than three years and compared their cognitive and fMRI results with a healthy control group of the same size and matched for age, sex and years of education. MS patients performed more poorly on the Wechsler Memory Scale, but their performance on the PVSAT did not differ from controls. The fMRI data were acquired during the PVSAT only and showed that MS subjects had a different pattern of cerebral activation, recruiting more brain regions (right prefrontal cortex and left angular gyrus) than the healthy controls. This finding was interpreted as evidence of neuronal plasticity during an early phase of MS, the brain retaining a degree of functional flexibility that allowed it to compensate for the presence of demyelinating pathology.

A similar conclusion was reached using a comparable methodology, albeit in a group of subjects with clinically isolated syndromes (Audoin *et al.*, 2003). Here the average duration of symptoms was just seven months. Performance on the PASAT was similar between 10 patients and 10 matched healthy controls, but once again their fMRI patterns differed, with patients showing more extensive activation (in bilateral lateral prefrontal cortices) and a different topology of activation (right fronto-polar cortex and right cerebellum). These functional changes provided further evidence of a cognition-related compensatory mechanism that begins operating within months of symptom onset.

A third study employed a different methodology and arrived at essentially the same conclusions (Chiaravalloti *et al.*, 2005). Three groups of subjects were tested: six MS patients with working memory impairment, five MS patients without this impairment and five healthy control subjects. Notably, the two MS groups did not differ in regional (right and left frontal, temporal, parietal) lesion loads. The cognitive paradigm used for the fMRI scanning was a modified version of the PASAT. Surprisingly, the performance of the three groups on the modified PASAT did not differ, a finding the authors failed to address adequately. Be that as it may, the fMRI data remain informative. Healthy controls and MS patients without working memory deficits showed a similar pattern of cerebral activation, namely predominantly left prefrontal regions. But the cognitively compromised MS patients showed greater right frontal and right parietal activation.

The PASAT and a memory recall task were the cognitive measures of choice in another fMRI study, which compared imaging findings between 22 MS patients with mild cognitive deficits and 22 matched healthy control subjects (Mainero *et al.*, 2004). A more diffuse pattern of cerebral activation was reported for the PASAT, which included the inferior and middle frontal gyri, inferior parietal cortex and superior and middle temporal gyri (all bilaterally), plus the supplementary motor area and anterior cingulate of the right hemisphere. In all these regions, activation in patients exceeded that of healthy controls. The most interesting finding to emerge was that in 12 of the 22 patients, performance on the PASAT matched that of the controls and it was in this less cognitively affected patient group that the greatest increase in activation was found on fMRI. These data replicate the findings of compensatory activation working to minimize cognitive shortcomings, but with the added caveat that this may only be possible within a more narrowly defined range of brain damage. In other words, the brain's ability to right itself functionally is dependent on the extent of underlying structural damage, a conclusion supported by the correlation found between a measure of regional cerebral activation and matched T_2 weighted lesion load.

The notion that adaptive functional mechanisms are curtailed by the extent of brain pathology was reinforced by the results of a study looking at fMRI responses to attention tasks of varying complexities (Penner *et al.*, 2003). The MS patients with mild attention impairments showed increased cerebral activation in areas utilized by healthy controls, namely motor cortex, inferior temporal and lateral cerebellar regions. The MS patients, but not the healthy controls, also activated additional regions, mainly prefrontal. As the task complexity increased and the degree of impairment became marked, ancillary activation ceased.

Summarizing the fMRI attention (predominantly PASAT) data in MS patients collected so far, the most consistent findings have been as follows. Even if patients do not perform more poorly than healthy controls, they generally still require additional cerebral activation to achieve this result. Compensatory activation may, therefore, restore performance, albeit within a narrower range of milder impairments. It remains unclear, however, if using up additional cerebral resources affects other aspects of cognition, for no study has yet looked at this important question. Furthermore, while there is a broad consensus relating to the presence of limited compensatory mechanisms at work, determining which anatomical regions in which hemisphere are implicated has proven more elusive.

Functional MRI studies of working memory using the *n*-back paradigm have produced results analogous to those of the PASAT studies. In this cognitive test, subjects monitor a series of stimuli and indicate, by pressing a button, whether the current stimulus matches one they have heard previously, be it once or twice or more times back (hence the name *n*-back) in the same series. Whereas a zero-back task requires no more than sustained attention, with subjects responding to a designated stimulus, a one-back task adds to the complexity by demanding subjects respond only to the stimulus if it occurs one back in the series. The task becomes more challenging as the value of *n* increases. Wishart *et al.* (2004) used this paradigm to test 10 patients with mild relapsing–remitting MS and 10 healthy matched controls and found that their performances were similar on the one- and two-back conditions. Patterns of brain activation, however, differed. The MS patients displayed reduced activation of regions known to subserve working memory, including prefrontal and parietal regions, while simultaneously activating regions (bilateral medial frontal and occipital cortices) not typically associated with this aspect of cognition. Furthermore, these anatomical shifts were accentuated in the more demanding (two-back) tasks, where activation in the patients now exceeded that in controls.

A second study using a two-back challenge reported a somewhat different result (Sweet *et al.*, 2004). Both MS patients and healthy matched controls performed similarly, but the MS subjects showed increased activation in certain brain regions (e.g. left primary motor, somatosensory, premotor and dorso lateral prefrontal cortices; anterior cingulate; and bilateral supplementary motor areas) and a reduction in others (e.g. Broca's area, bilateral cerebellum) linked to working memory. However, unlike the study of Wishart *et al.* (2004), MS patients did not show ancillary activation in neural circuits outside those associated with working memory in healthy control subjects.

A third study of working memory employed a modified version of the Sternberg paradigm with the fMRI results from eight MS patients compared with those from five healthy controls (Hilary *et al.*, 2003). Specifically, the study focussed on the ability of MS patients to rehearse or maintain information within working memory. An *a priori* hypothesis that MS patients would show additional activation of the right (non-dominant) prefrontal cortex (in keeping with findings from patients with traumatic brain injuries and the same cognitive deficits) was born out. Two possible explanations were put forward. The first suggested that the cognitive inefficiency noted in MS patients on this task was a reflection of their inability to match healthy controls in shifting activation from an initial right prefrontal focus necessary for the early processing of novel information to a left prefrontal activation required for the manipulation of more routine types of information. A second explanation was that the additional right-sided activations were part of the brain's compensatory attempts at offsetting cognitive difficulties.

Not every fMRI study has, however, noted functional brain plasticity. In an exploration of fMRI correlates of executive function, Lazeron *et al.* (2004) examined 23 MS patients with moderate physical disability and compared the results with those from a sample of 18 healthy controls. The MS patients performed significantly more poorly on the Tower of London test, but did not show additional areas of cerebral activation outside the expected regions of the frontal and parietal lobes bilaterally and the cerebellum. Further, the only significant increase in activation in the MS subjects occurred in the cerebellum. This study, therefore, stands apart from the others cited above, suggesting that not all MS patients have the ability to adapt to the cognitively deleterious effects of cerebral pathology even in the presence of a moderate degree of physical disability.

Finally, Parry *et al.* (2003) have elegantly demonstrated how medication may enhance compensatory mechanisms in the brain. Using the Stroop paradigm, they compared fMRI results in 10 MS patients and 11 healthy controls. No between group differences were present on the Stroop itself, but the patients and controls activated different hemispheres, albeit in the same medial prefrontal regions. The magnitude of these differences correlated with normalized brain parenchymal volume, which was considered an index of disease burden. In the second phase of the study, five MS patients and four healthy controls were given rivastigmine, a central cholinesterase inhibitor that is used primarily as a treatment for memory impairment in Alzheimer's disease. In the five MS patients, treatment resulted in a switch from left- to right-sided medial prefrontal cerebral hemisphere activation. In the controls, no such change occurred, activation remaining in the pretreatment region of the right medial prefrontal cortex. This result raises the intriguing possibility of innate compensatory brain processes, such as dormant neural pathways, being unmasked and modulated by cognitive-enhancing drugs.

Positron emission tomography and single photon emission computed tomography

The paltry number of PET-related behavioral studies is dwarfed by the MRI literature and yet, functional imaging has furnished some interesting insights, not least the demonstration of how anatomical changes, be they discrete lesions or global atrophy, lead to a reduction in cerebral activity and, by extension, cognitive deficits.

In an early CT and PET study, Brooks *et al.* (1984) compared 15 MS patients in remission with 13 healthy controls, looking at regional cerebral oxygen utilization, oxygen extraction, cerebral blood flow and blood volume. A significant global reduction in cerebral oxygen utilization and blood flow were found both in the white and gray matter of the MS patients. These deficits were associated with cortical atrophy on CT and evidence of intellectual decline assessed by the Wechsler Adult Intelligence Scale. No regional abnormalities were found and the authors failed to note a correlation between the functional abnormalities displayed on PET and either disease duration or severity.

Herscovitch *et al.* (1984) described the case of a 24-year-old patient with aphasia, apraxia and left-sided hemiparesis with sensory changes, who had a plaque in the right cerebral white matter on CT while PET showed a reduction in regional cerebral blood flow in the fronto-parietal cortex superficial to the lesion. Subsequent improvement in regional cerebral blood flow was associated with clinical remission. The effects of white matter lesions on cortical perfusion were also demonstrated by Jeffery *et al.* (2000) in three MS patients. A pattern of white matter lesions, cortical hypoperfusion on PET and confluent cognitive deficits considered primarily cortical in origin were recorded in two of three patients.

The functional correlates of memory impairment in MS patients were explored using PET in a three-way comparison between 15 MS patients with memory (verbal and/or visual) impairment, 13 cognitively intact MS patients and 10 healthy controls (Paulesu *et al.*, 1996). The memory-impaired subjects were found to have decreased glucose metabolism in both hippocampi and the dominant hemisphere thalamus. A further comparison was undertaken between those subjects whose cognitive deficits were restricted to memory impairment ($n = 8$) and those who had additional neuropsychological signs of frontal dysfunction ($n = 7$). The latter were noted to have more extensive cerebral hypometabolism, involving bilateral prefrontal cortices, inferior parietal cortex and the basal ganglia.

A wide ranging PET–MRI study was completed by Blinkenberg *et al.* (2000), who looked at measures of cortical cerebral glucose utilization, total lesion area detected by T_2 weighted MRI, cognitive dysfunction and neurological disability in a sample of 23 MS patients. A number of consistent correlations were found: total lesion area with global cortical (glucose) metabolic rate; regional lesion load with regional glucose metabolism; and a composite index of cognitive dysfunction on the one hand and total lesion area and global cerebral metabolism on the other. No significant correlations were noted between any PET index and neurological disability. This replicated an earlier finding from the same research team that suggested serial PET measurements of global cortical metabolism over a two year period were a more sensitive indicator of disease progression than either total lesion area or neurological disability (Blinkenberg *et al.*, 1999).

There is also a single small PET study that reported the results of a cognitive activation paradigm. Scheremata *et al.* (1984) used a word learning activation task in a case–control study involving three MS subjects and three healthy matched controls. They found reduced metabolism in both temporal and, to a lesser extent, frontal lobes of the MS patients during task activation.

Before concluding this section, the results of a SPECT study of behavioral difficulties in MS patients deserves mention. Pozzilli *et al.* (1991a) scanned 17 MS patients and 17 matched, healthy controls using ^{99m}Tc-hexamethylpropylene-amine oxime (HMPAO) SPECT. A ratio of regional to whole brain activity measured by SPECT demonstrated a significant reduction in the frontal lobes and left temporal lobe of the patient sample. Deficits in verbal memory and verbal fluency correlated with the left temporal lobe findings.

Summary

- MRI is considerably more sensitive that CT in detecting MS plaques in the brain. Plaques are typically periventricular in distribution. The use of FLAIR imaging sequences has been helpful in revealing the presence of juxtacortical lesions.

- MRI may also demonstrate abnormalities of the corpus callosum (atrophy or the presence of lesions) and various measures of regional and generalized cerebral atrophy.

- The lesions demonstrated by MRI are not pathognomonic for MS, and vascular disease, in particular, may give rise to a similar picture.

- The use of contrast (gadolinium–DTPA)-enhanced MRI demonstrates the presence of acute MS lesions, with enhancement indicative of breakdown in the blood–brain barrier.

- MRI is a safe procedure and, therefore, ideally suited to longitudinal studies requiring repeated scans.

- Cognitive dysfunction has been linked to many MRI indices of brain pathology, including regional and total lesion load detected by T_1 and T_2 weighted MRI, periventricular and juxtacortical lesions and regional and generalized atrophy.

- Recent data suggest atrophy may be the most important cerebral predictor of impaired cognition.

- Serial MRI and cognitive studies have shown that psychomotor tasks and measures of attention and working memory correlate with a deteriorating brain lesion load. Although MS patients retain the ability to benefit from practice, this can be adversely affected by a worsening MRI picture.

- There are an array of imaging modalities that can furnish information, not only on lesions, but also on normal appearing brain tissue. Here, the use of T_1 relaxation times has given way to newer imaging techniques such as magnetization transfer and diffusion tensor imaging.

- A nascent literature has begun to reveal significant correlations between indices of cognitive dysfunction on the one hand and magnetization transfer and diffusion tensor imaging measures from normal appearing brain tissue on the other.

- The use of magnetic resonance spectroscopy allows in vivo concentrations of important metabolites such as N-acetylaspartate and choline to be measured. Although these are non-specific, their concentrations become abnormal to various degrees in MS depending on the severity of the disease. Changes in concentrations may correlate with cognitive decline and improvement. Spectroscopy, therefore, adds to what is known about MS lesions and normal appearing brain tissue from MRI.

- Functional neuroimaging in MS has undergone a shift in emphasis with the few studies using positron emission tomography and single photon emission computed tomography supplanted by a burgeoning functional MRI (fMRI) literature. The fMRI technique has some important advantages, including excellent spatial and temporal resolution.

- Functional MRI has been used in conjunction with cognitive tests probing attention and working memory. Results reveal that MS patients may retain the ability to compensate, either in part or else completely, for cognitive failings by increasing cerebral activation in brain regions used by healthy controls or by activating additional brain regions not utilized by healthy controls.

- Functional MRI has also shown that cerebral adaptation is limited by the extent of brain pathology. Therefore, compensatory mechanisms are most discernible in association with mild to moderate levels of disease and less-severe cognitive impairment. Adaptation, however, breaks down in the presence of severe disease and a destructive lesion load.
- Preliminary fMRI evidence points towards cognitive-enhancing medications facilitating the brain's compensatory ability.

References

Allen IV, Glover G, Andersen R. (1981) Abnormalities in the macroscopically abnormal white matter in cases of mild or spinal multiple sclerosis. *Acta Neuropathologica* (Berlin) *Supplement* **7**, 176–178.

Amato MP, Bartolozzi ML, Zipoli V, *et al.* (2004) Neocortical volume decrease in relapsing–remitting MS patients with mild cognitive impairment. *Neurology*, **63**, 80–93.

Andrew EE, Bydder G, Griffiths J, Iles R, Styles P. (1990) *Clinical Magnetic Resonance Imaging and Spectroscopy.* Chichester: John Wiley.

Anzola GP, Bevilacqua L, Cappa SF, *et al.* (1990) Neuropsychological assessment in patients with relapsing–remitting multiple sclerosis and mild functional impairment: correlation with magnetic resonance imaging. *Journal of Neurology, Neurosurgery and Psychiatry*, **53**, 142–145.

Arnett PA, Rao SM, Bernardin L, *et al.* (1994) Relationship between frontal lobe lesions and Wisconsin Card Sort Test performance in patients with multiple sclerosis. *Neurology*, **44**, 420–425.

Audoin B, Ibarrola D, Ranjeva J-P, *et al.* (2003) Compensatory cortical activation observed by fMRI during a cognitive task at the earliest stage of MS. *Human Brain Mapping*, **20**, 51–58.

Audoin B, Duong MVA, Ranjeva J-P, *et al.* (2005) Magnetic resonance study of the influence of tissue damage and cortical reorganization on PASAT performance at the earliest stage of multiple sclerosis. *Human Brain Mapping*, **24**, 216–228.

Barkhof F, Filippi M, Miller DH, *et al.* (1997) Comparison of MR imaging criteria at first presentation to predict conversion to clinically definite multiple sclerosis. *Brain*, **120**, 2059–2069.

Benedict RHB, Bakshi R, Simon JH, *et al.* (2002) Frontal cortex atrophy predicts cognitive impairment in multiple sclerosis. *Journal of Neuropsychiatry and Clinical Neurosciences*, **14**, 44–51.

Benedict RHB, Weinstock-Guttman B, Fishman I, Sharma J, Tjoa CW. (2004) Prediction of neuropsychological impairment in multiple sclerosis. Comparison of conventional magnetic resonance imaging measures of atrophy and lesion burden. *Archives of Neurology*, **61**, 226–230.

Berg D, Mathias M, Warmuth-Metz M, Rieckmann P, Becker G. (2000) The correlation between ventricular diameter measured by transcranial sonography and clinical disability and cognitive dysfunction in patients with multiple sclerosis. *Archives of Neurology*, **57**, 1289–1292.

Bermel RA, Bakshi R. (2006) The measurement and clinical relevance of brain atrophy in multiple sclerosis. *Lancet Neurology*, **5**, 158–169.

Bermel RA, Bakshi R, Tjoa C, Puli SR, Jacobs L. (2002) Bicaudate ratio as a magnetic resonance imaging marker of brain atrophy in multiple sclerosis. *Archives of Neurology*, **59**, 275–280.

Besson JAO, Crawford JR, Parker DM, *et al.* (1990) Multimodal imaging in Alzheimer's disease. The relationship between MRI, SPECT, cognitive and pathological changes. *British Journal of Psychiatry*, **157**, 216–220.

Blinkenberg M, Jensen CV, Holm S, Paulsen OB, Sørensen PS. (1999) A longitudinal study of cerebral glucose metabolism. MRI, and disability in patients with MS. *Neurology*, **53**, 149–153.

Blinkenberg M, Rune K, Jensen CV, *et al.* (2000) Cortical cerebral metabolism correlates with MRI lesion load and cognitive dysfunction in MS. *Neurology*, **54**, 558–563.

Brandt-Zawadski M, Fein G, van Dyke C, *et al.* (1985) MR imaging of the aging brain: patchy white matter lesions and dementia. *American Journal of Neuroradiology*, **6**, 675–682.

Brooks DJ, Leenders KL, Head G, *et al.* (1984) Studies on regional cerebral oxygen utilisation and cognitive function in multiple sclerosis. *Journal of Neurology, Neurosurgery and Psychiatry*, **47**, 1182–1191.

Callanan MM, Logsdail SJ, Ron MA, Warrington EK. (1989) Cognitive impairment in patients with clinically isolated lesions of t type seen in multiple sclerosis. *Brain*, **112**, 361–374.

Camp SJ, Stevenson VL, Thompson AJ, *et al.* (1999) Cognitive function in primary progressive and transitional progressive multiple sclerosis. A controlled trial with MRI corelates. (1999) *Brain*, **12**, 1341–1348.

Chamelian L, Bocti C, Gao F-C, Black SE, Feinstein A. (2005) Detecting cognitive dysfunction with a magnetic resonance imaging rating scale: a pilot study. *CNS Spectrums*, **10**, 394–402.

Chiaravalloti ND, Hillary FG, Ricker JH, *et al.* (2005) Cerebral activation patterns during working memory performance in multiple sclerosis using fMRI. *Journal of Clinical and Experimental Neuropsychology*, **27**, 33–54.

Christodoulou C, Krupp LB, Liang Z, *et al.* (2003) Cognitive performance and MTR markers of cerebral injury in cognitively impaired MS patients. *Neurology*, **60**, 1793–1798.

Ciccarelli O, Werring DJ, Wheeler-Kingshott CAM, *et al.* (2001) Investigation of MS normal-appearing brain using diffusion tensor MRI with clinical correlations. *Neurology*, **56**, 926–933.

Clark CM, James G, Li D, Oger J, Paty D, Klonoff H. (1992) Ventricular size, cognitive function and depression in patients with multiple sclerosis. *Canadian Journal of Neurological Sciences*, **19**, 352–356.

Comi G, Filippi M, Martinelli V, *et al.* (1993) Brain magnetic resonance imaging correlates of cognitive impairment in multiple sclerosis. *Journal of the Neurological Sciences*, **115**(Suppl.), 66–73.

Comi G, Filippi M, Martinelli V, *et al.* (1995) Brain MRI correlates of cognitive impairment in primary and secondary progressive multiple sclerosis. *Journal of the Neurological Sciences*, **132**, 222–227.

Davie CA, Hawkins CP, Barker GJ, *et al.* (1994) Serial proton magnetic resonance spectroscopy in acute multiple sclerosis lesions. *Brain*, **117**, 49–58.

DeCarli C, Murphy DGM, Tranh M, *et al.* (1995) The effect of white matter hyperintensity volume on brain structure, cognitive performance and cerebral metabolism of glucose in 51 healthy adults. *Neurology*, **45**, 2077–2084.

De Coene B, Hajnal JV, Gatehouse P, *et al.* (1992) MR of the brain using fluid-attenuated inversion recovery (FLAIR) pulse sequences. *American Journal of Neuroradiology*, **13**, 1555–1564.

de Groot JC, de Leeuw FE, Oudkerk M, *et al.* (2000) Cerebral white matter lesions and cognitive function: the Rotterdam Scan Study. *Annals of Neurology*, **47**, 145–151.

Edwards SGM, Liu C, Blumhardt LC. (2001) Cognitive correlates of supratentorial atrophy on MRI in multiple sclerosis. *Acta Neurologica Scandinavica*, **104**, 214–223.

Feinstein A, Kartsounis LD, Miller DH, Youl BD, Ron MA. (1992a) Clinically isolated lesions of the type seen in multiple sclerosis: a cognitive, psychiatric and MRI follow-up study. *Journal of Neurology, Neurosurgery and Psychiatry*, **55**, 869–876.

Feinstein A, Youl B, Ron MA. (1992b) Acute optic neuritis. A cognitive and magnetic resonance imaging study. *Brain*, **115**, 1403–1415.

Feinstein A, Ron MA, Thompson A. (1993) A serial study of psychometric and magnetic resonance imaging changes in multiple sclerosis. *Brain*, **116**, 569–602.

Filippi M, Campi A, Martinelli V, *et al.* (1995) A brain MRI study of different types of chronic–progressive multiple sclerosis. *Acta Neurologica Scandinavica*, **91**, 231–233.

Filippi M, Capra R, Campi A, *et al.* (1996a) Triple dose of gadolinium–DTPA and delayed MRI in patients with benign multiple sclerosis. *Journal of Neurology, Neurosurgery and Psychiatry*, **60**, 526–530.

Filippi M, Yousry T, Campi A, *et al.* (1996b) Comparison of triple dose versus standard dose gadolinium–DTPA for detection of MRI enhancing lesions in patients with MS. *Neurology*, **46**, 379–384.

Filippi M, Inglese M, Rovaris M, *et al.* (2000) Magnetization transfer imaging to monitor the evolution of MS. A 1 year follow-up study. *Neurology*, **55**, 940–946.

Filippi M, Cerignani M, Inglese M, Horsfield MA, Comi G. (2001) Diffusion tensor magnetic resonance imaging in multiple sclerosis. *Neurology*, **56**, 304–311.

Filippi M, Rocca MA, Falini A, *et al.* (2002a) Correlations between structural CNS damage and functional MRI changes in primary progressive MS. *NeuroImage*, **15**, 537–546.

Filippi M, Rocca MA, Colombo B, *et al.* (2002b) Functional magnetic resonance imaging correlates of fatigue in multiple sclerosis. *NeuroImage*, **15**, 559–567.

Foong J, Rozewicz L, Quaghebeur G, *et al.* (1997) Executive function in multiple sclerosis. The role of frontal lobe pathology. *Brain*, **120**, 15–26.

Foong J, Rozewicz L, Davie CA, *et al.* (1999) Correlates of executive function in multiple sclerosis: the use of magnetic resonance spectroscopy as an index of focal pathology. *Journal of Neuropsychiatry and Clinical Neurosciences*, **11**, 45–50.

Franklin GM, Heaton RK, Nelson LM, Filley CM, Seibert C. (1988) Correlation of neuropsychological and MRI findings in chronic–progressive multiple sclerosis. *Neurology*, **38**, 1826–1829.

Gass A, Barker GJ, Kidd D, *et al.* (1994) Correlation of magnetization transfer ratio with clinical disability in multiple sclerosis. *Annals of Neurology*, **36**, 62–67.

George AE, de Leon MJ, Kalnin A, *et al.* (1986) Leukoencephalopathy in normal and pathological aging: 2. MRI of brain lucencies. *American Journal of Neuroradiology*, **7**, 567–570.

Glydenstedt C. (1976) Computer tomography of the cerebrum in multiple sclerosis. *Neuroradiology*, **12**, 33–42.

Goldberg-Zimring D, Mewes AU, Maddah M, Warfield SK. (2005) Diffusion tensor magnetic resonance imaging in multiple sclerosis. *Journal of Neuroimaging*, **15**(Suppl. 4), 68S–81S.

Goodin DS. (2006) Magnetic resonance imaging as a surrogate outcome measure of disability in multiple sclerosis. *Annals of Neurology*, **59**, 597–605.

Hachinski VC, Potter P, Merskey H. (1987) Leuko-araiosis. *Archives of Neurology*, **44**, 21–23.

Hawkins CP, Munro PMG, Mackenzie F, *et al.* (1990) Duration and selectivity of blood–brain barrier breakdown in chronic relapsing experimental allergic encephalomyelitis studied by gadolinium–DTPA and protein markers. *Brain*, **113**, 365–378.

Herscovitch P, Trotter JL, Lemann W, Raichle ME. (1984) Positron emission tomography (PET) in active MS: demonstration of demyelination and diaschisis. *Neurology*, **34**(Suppl. 1), 78.

Hilary FG, Chiaravalloti ND, Ricker JH, *et al.* (2003) An investigation of working memory rehearsal in multiple sclerosis using fMRI. *Journal of Clinical and Experimental Neuropsychology*, **25**, 965–978.

Hohol MJ, Guttmann CRG, Orav J, *et al.* (1997) Serial neuropsychological assessment and magnetic resonance imaging analysis in multiple sclerosis. *Archives of Neurology*, **54**, 1018–1025.

Horsfield MA. (2005) Magnetization transfer imaging in multiple sclerosis. *Journal of Neuroimaging*, **15**(Suppl. 4), 58S–67S.

Huettel SA, Song AW, McCarthy G. (2003) *Functional Magnetic Resonance Imaging*. Sunderland, MA: Sinauer Associates, pp. 2–25.

Iannucci G, Tortorella C, Rovaris M, *et al.* (2000) Prognostic value of MR and magnetization transfer imaging findings in patients with clinically isolated syndromes suggestive of multiple sclerosis at presentation. *American Journal of Neuroradiology*, **21**, 1034–1038.

Iannucci G, Rovaris M, Giacomotti L, Comi G, Filippi M. (2001) Correlation of multiple sclerosis measures derived from T_2 weighted, T_1 weighted, magnetization transfer and diffusion tensor MR imaging. *American Journal of Neuroradiology*, **22**, 1462–1467.

Isaac C, Li DKB, Genton M, *et al.* (1988) Multiple sclerosis: a serial study using MRI in relapsing patients. *Neurology*, **38**, 1511–1515.

Izquierdo G, Campoy Jr. F, Mir J, Gonzalez M, Martinez-Parra C. (1991) Memory and learning disturbances in multiple sclerosis. MRI lesions and neuropsychological correlation. *European Journal of Radiology*, **13**, 220–224.

Jacobs L, Kinkel WR, Polachini I, Kinkel P. (1986) Correlations of nuclear magnetic resonance imaging, computerised tomography and clinical profiles in multiple sclerosis. *Neurology*, **36**, 27–34.

Jeffery DR, Absher J, Pfeiffer F, Jackson H. (2000) Cortical deficits in multiple sclerosis on the basis of subcortical lesions. *Multiple Sclerosis*, **6**, 50–55.

Kermode AG, Thompson AJ, Tofts P, *et al.* (1990a) Breakdown of the blood–brain barrier precedes symptoms and other MRI signs of new lesions in multiple sclerosis. *Brain*, **113**, 1477–1489.

Kermode AG, Tofts PS, Thompson AJ, *et al.* (1990b) Heterogeneity of blood–brain barrier changes in multiple sclerosis: an MRI study with gadolinium-DTPA enhancement. *Neurology*, **40**, 229–235.

Kidd D, Barkhof F, McDonnell R, *et al.* (1999) Cortical lesions in multiple sclerosis. *Brain*, **122**, 17–26.

Lazeron RHC, Langdon DW, Filippi M, *et al.* (2000) Neuropsychological impairment in multiple sclerosis patients; the role of (juxta)cortical lesion of FLAIR. *Multiple Sclerosis*, **6**, 280–285.

Lazeron RHC, Rombouts S, Scheltens P, Polman CH, Brakhof F. (2004) An fMRI study of planning related brain activity in patients with moderately advanced multiple sclerosis. *Multiple Sclerosis*, **10**, 549–555.

Lazeron RHC, Boringa JB, Schouten M, *et al.* (2005) Brain atrophy and lesion load as explaining parameters for cognitive impairment in multiple sclerosis. *Multiple Sclerosis*, **11**, 524–531.

Locatelli L, Zivadinov R, Grop A, Zorzon M. (2004) Frontal parenchymal atrophy measures in multiple sclerosis. *Multiple Sclerosis*, **10**, 562–568.

Losseff NA, Wang L, Lai HM, *et al.* (1996) Progressive cerebral atrophy in multiple sclerosis. A serial MRI study. *Brain*, **119**, 2009–2019.

Mainero C, Caramina F, Pozzilli C, *et al.* (2004) fMRI evidence of brain reorganization during attention and memory tasks in multiple sclerosis. *NeuroImage*, **21**, 858–867.

Mariani C, Farina E, Cappa SF, *et al.* (1991). Neuropsychological assessment in multiple sclerosis: a follow-up study with magnetic resonance imaging. *Journal of Neurology*, **238**, 395–400.

Martinelli BF, Rovaris M, Comi G, Filippi M. (2004) The use of magnetic resonance imaging in multiple sclerosis: lessons learned from clinical trials. *Multiple Sclerosis*, **10**, 341–347.

Mattioli F, Cappa SF, Cominelli C, *et al.* (1993) Serial study of neuropsychological performance and gadolinium-enhanced MRI in MS. *Acta Neurologica Scandinavica*, **87**, 465–468.

Maurelli M, Marchioni E, Cerretano R, *et al.* (1992) Neuropsychological assessment in MS: clinical, neurophysiological and neuroradiological relationships. *Acta Neurologica Scandinavica*, **86**, 124–128.

McDonald WI, Compston A, Edan G, *et al.* (2001) Recommended diagnostic criteria for multiple sclerosis: guidelines from the international panel on the diagnosis of multiple sclerosis. *Annals of Neurology*, **50**, 121–127.

Medaer R, Nelissen E, Appel B, *et al.* (1987) Magnetic resonance imaging and cognitive functioning in multiple sclerosis. *Journal of Neurology*, **235**, 86–89.

Miller DH. (1995) Magnetic resonance imaging and spectroscopy in multiple sclerosis. *Current Opinion in Neurology*, **8**, 210–215.

Miller DH, Ormerod IEC, Gibson A, *et al.* (1987) MR brain scanning in patients with vasculitis: differentiation from MS. *Neuroradiology*, **29**, 226–231.

Miller DH, Rudge P, Johnson G, Kendall BE, MacManus DG, Moseley IF, *et al.* (1988) Serial gadolinium enhanced MRI in multiple sclerosis. *Brain*, **111**, 927–939.

Miller DH, Johnson G, Tofts PS, MacManus D, McDonald WI. (1989) Precise relaxation time measurements of normal appearing white matter in inflammatory central nervous system disease. *Magnetic Resonance Imaging in Medicine*, **11**, 331–336.

Miller DH, Morrissey SP, McDonald WI. (1992) The prognostic significance of brain MRI at presentation with a single clinical episode of suspected demyelination. A 5 year follow-up study. *Neurology Supplement*, **3**, 427.

Miller DH, Barkhof F, Frank JA, Parker GJM, Thompson AJ. (2002) Measurement of atrophy in multiple sclerosis: pathological basis, methodological aspects and clinical relevance. *Brain*, **125**, 1676–1695.

Moriarty DM, Blackshaw AJ, Talbot PR, *et al.* (1999) Memory dysfunction in multiple sclerosis corresponds to juxtacortical lesion load on fast fluid-attenuated inversion recovery MR images. *American Journal of Neuroradiology*, **20**, 1956–1962.

Mosley TH, Knopman DS, Catellier DJ, *et al.* (2005) Cerebral MRI findings and cognitive dysfunction. The atherosclerosis risk in communities study. *Neurology*, **64**, 2056–2062.

New PFJ, Rosen BR, Brady TJ, *et al.* (1983) Potential hazards and artifacts of ferromagnetic and non-ferromagnetic surgical and dental material and devices in nuclear magnetic resonance imaging. *Radiology*, **147**, 139–148.

Ormerod IEC, Roberts RC, du Boulay EPGH. (1984) NMR in multiple sclerosis and cerebral vascular disease. *Lancet*, **ii**, 1334–1335.

Ormerod IEC, Johnson G, MacManus D, du Boulay EPHG, McDonald WI. (1986) Relaxation times of apparently normal cerebral white matter in multiple sclerosis. *Acta Radiologica Supplement*, **369**, 496.

Ormerod IEC, Miller DH, McDonald WI, *et al.* (1987) The role of NMR imaging in the assessment of multiple sclerosis and isolated neurological lesions. *Brain*, **110**, 1579–1616.

Pan JW, Krupp LB, Elkins LE, Coyle PK. (2001) Cognitive dysfunction lateralizes with NAA in multiple sclerosis. *Applied Neuropsychology*, **8**, 155–160.

Pantano P, Iannetti DI, Caramia F, *et al.* (2002) Cortical motor reorganisation after a single clinical attack of multiple sclerosis. *Brain*, **125**, 1607–1615.

Parry AMM, Scott RB, Palace J, Smith S, Mathews PM. (2003) Potentially adaptive functional changes in cognitive processing for patients with multiple sclerosis and their acute modulation by rivastigmine. *Brain*, **126**, 2750–2760.

Patti F, Failla G, Ciancio MR, L'Episcopo MR, Reggio A. (1998) Neuropsychological, neuroradiological and clinical findings in multiple sclerosis: A 3 year follow-up study. *European Journal of Neurology*, **5**, 283–286.

Paty DW, Hashimoto SA, Hooge J, *et al.* (1988) Magnetic resonance imaging (MRI) in multiple sclerosis: a prospective evaluation of usefulness in diagnosis. *Neurology*, **38**, 180–185.

Paulesu E, Perani D, Fazio F, *et al.* (1996) Functional basis of memory impairment in multiple sclerosis: a [^{18}F]FDG PET study. *NeuroImage*, **4**, 87–96.

Pavlicek W, Geisinger M, Castle L, Borkowski GP, Meaney TF, *et al.* (1983) The effects of nuclear magnetic resonance imaging on patients with cardiac pacemakers. *Radiology*, **147**, 149–153.

Pelletier J, Habib M, Lyon-Caen O, *et al.* (1993) Functional and magnetic resonance imaging correlates of callosal involvement in multiple sclerosis. *Archives of Neurology*, **50**, 1077–1082.

Penner IK, Rausch M, Kappos L, Opwis K, Radü EW. (2003) Analysis of impairment related functional architecture in MS patients during performance of different attention tasks. *Journal of Neurology*, **250**, 461–472.

Piras MR, Magnano I, Canu EDG, *et al.* (2003) Longitudinal study of cognitive dysfunction in multiple sclerosis: neuropsychological, neuroradiological and neurophysiological findings. *Journal of Neurology, Neurosurgery and Psychiatry*, **74**, 878–885.

Polman CH, Reingold SC, Edan G, *et al.* (2005) Diagnostic criteria for multiple sclerosis: 2005 revisions to the "McDonald Criteria." *Annals of Neurology*, **58**, 840–846.

Pozzilli C, Passafiumi D, Bernardi S, *et al.* (1991a) SPECT, MRI and cognitive functions in multiple sclerosis. *Journal of Neurology, Neurosurgery and Psychiatry*, **54**, 110–115.

Pozzilli C, Bastianello S, Padovani A, *et al.* (1991b) Anterior corpus callosum atrophy and verbal fluency in multiple sclerosis. *Cortex*, **27**, 441–445.

Pugnetti L, Mendozzi L, Motta A, *et al.* (1993) MRI and cognitive patterns in relapsing–remitting multiple sclerosis. *Journal of the Neurological Sciences*, **115**(Suppl.) 59–65.

Rabins PV, Brooks BR, O'Donnell P, *et al.* (1986) Structural brain correlates of emotional disorder in multiple sclerosis. *Brain*, **109**, 585–597.

Rao SM. (1990) Neuroimaging correlates of cognitive dysfunction. In *Neurobehavioral Aspects of Multiple Sclerosis*, Ed. SM Rao. New York: Oxford University Press, pp. 118–135.

Rao SM, Glatt S, Hammeke TA, *et al.* (1985) Chronic–progressive multiple sclerosis: relationship between cerebral ventricular size and neuropsychological impairment. *Archives of Neurology*, **42**, 678–682.

Rao SM, Mittenberg W, Bernardin L, Haughton V, Leo GJ. (1989a) Neuropsychological test findings in subjects with leukoaraiosis. *Archives of Neurology*, **46**, 40–44.

Rao SM, Leo GJ, Haughton VM, St. Aubin-Faubert P, Bernardin L. (1989b) Correlation of magnetic resonance imaging with neuropsychological testing in multiple sclerosis. *Neurology*, **39**, 161–166.

Rao SM, Bernardin L, Ellington L, Ryan SB, Burg LS. (1989c) Cerebral disconnection in multiple sclerosis. Relationship to atrophy of the corpus callosum. *Archives of Neurology*, **46**, 918–920.

Rao SM, Leo GJ, Bernardin L, Unverzagt F. (1991) Cognitive dysfunction in multiple sclerosis. 1. Frequency, patterns and prediction. *Neurology*, **41**, 6685–6691.

Reddy H, Narayanan S, Mathews PM, *et al.* (2000) Relating axonal injury to functional recovery in MS. *Neurology*, **54**, 236–239.

Reischies FM, Baum K, Brau H, Hedde JP, Schwindt G. (1988) Cerebral magnetic resonance imaging findings in multiple sclerosis. Relation to disturbance of affect, drive and cognition. *Archives of Neurology*, **45**, 1114–1116.

Ron MA, Callanan MM, Warrington EK. (1991) Cognitive abnormalities in multiple sclerosis: a psychometric and MRI study. *Psychological Medicine*, **21**, 59–68.

Rovaris M, Filippi M, Falautano M, *et al.* (1998) Relation between MR abnormalities and patterns of cognitive impairment in multiple sclerosis. *Neurology*, **50**, 1601–1608.

Rovaris M, Filippi M, Minicucci L, *et al.* (2000) Cortical/subcortical disease burden and cognitive impairment in patients with multiple sclerosis. *American Journal of Neuroradiology*, **21**, 402–408.

Rovaris M, Iannucci G, Falautano M, *et al.* (2002) Cognitive dysfunction in patients with mildly disabling relapsing–remitting multiple sclerosis: an exploratory study with diffusion tensor MR imaging. *Journal of the Neurological Sciences*, **195**, 103–109.

Rovaris M, Gass A, Bammer R, *et al.* (2005) Diffusion MRI in multiple sclerosis. *Neurology*, **65**, 1526–1532.

Rozewicz L, Langdon DW, Davie CA, Thompson AJ, Ron MA. (1996) Resolution of left hemisphere cognitive dysfunction in multiple sclerosis with magnetic resonance correlates: a case report. *Cognitive Neuropsychiatry*, **1**, 17–25.

Ryan L, Clark CM, Klonoff H, Li D, Paty D. (1996) Patterns of cognitive impairment in relapsing–remitting multiple sclerosis and their relationship to neuropathology on magnetic resonance images. *Neuropsychology*, **10**, 176–193.

Santos AC, Narayanan S, de Stefano N, *et al.* (2002) *Journal of Neurology*, **249**, 662–668.

Scheremata WA, Seush S, Knight D, Ziajka P. (1984) Altered cerebral metabolism in multiple sclerosis. *Neurology*, **34**(Suppl. 1), 118.

Sperling RA, Guttmann C, Hohol MJ, *et al.* (2001) Regional magnetic resonance imaging lesion burden and cognitive function in multiple sclerosis: a longitudinal study. *Archives of Neurology*, **58**, 115–121.

Spiegel SM, Vinuela F, Fox AJ, Pelz DM. (1985) CT of multiple sclerosis. Reassessment of delayed scanning with high doses of contrast material. *American Journal of Roentgenology*, **145**, 497–500.

Staffen W, Mair A, Zauner H, *et al.* (2002) Cognitive function and fMRI in patients with multiple sclerosis: evidence for compensatory cortical activation during an attention task. *Brain*, **125**, 1275–1282.

Stone LA, Albert PS, Smith ME, *et al.* (1995) Changes in the amount of diseased white matter over time in patients with relapsing–remitting multiple sclerosis. *Neurology*, **45**, 1808–1814.

Sweet LH, Rao SM, Primeau M, Mayer AR, Cohen RA. (2004) Functional magnetic resonance imaging of working memory among multiple sclerosis patients. *Journal of Neuroimaging*, **14**, 150–157.

Sweetland J, Kertesz A, Prato FS, Nantau K. (1987) The effect of magnetic resonance imaging on human cognition. *Magnetic Resonance Imaging*, **5**, 129–135.

Swirsky-Sacchetti T, Mitchell DR, Seward J, *et al.* (1992) Neuropsychological and structural brain lesions in multiple sclerosis: a regional analysis. *Neurology*, **42**, 1291–1295.

Thompson AJ, Kermode AG, MacManus DG, *et al.* (1990) Patterns of disease activity in multiple sclerosis: clinical and magnetic resonance imaging study. *British Medical Journal*, **300**, 631–634.

Thompson AJ, Kermode AG, Wicks D, *et al.* (1991) Major differences in the dynamics of primary and secondary progressive multiple sclerosis. *Annals of Neurology*, **29**, 53–62.

Thompson AJ, Miller D, Youl B, *et al.* (1992) Serial gadolinium enhanced MRI in relapsing remitting multiple sclerosis of varying disease duration. *Neurology*, **42**, 60–63.

Tintore M, Rovira A, Martinez MJ, *et al.* (2000) Isolated demyelinating syndromes: comparison of different MR imaging criteria to predict conversion to clinically definite MS. *American Journal of Neuroradiology*, **21**, 702–706.

Traboulsee A, Dehmeshki J, Peters KR, *et al.* (2003) Disability in multiple sclerosis is related to normal appearing brain tissue MTR histogram abnormalities. *Multiple Sclerosis*, **9**, 566–573.

Tsolaki M, Drevelegas A, Karachristianou S, *et al.* (1994) Correlation of dementia, neuro-psychological and MRI findings in multiple sclerosis. *Dementia*, **5**, 48–52.

Tupler LA, Coffey CE, Logue PE, Djang WT, Fagan SM. (1992) Neuropsychological importance of subcortical white matter hyperintensity. *Archives of Neurology*, **49**, 1248–1252.

van Buchem MA, Grossman RI, Armstrong C, *et al.* (1998) Correlation of volumetric magnetization transfer imaging with clinical data in MS. *Neurology*, **50**, 1609–1617.

Warren KG, Ball MJ, Paty DW, Banna M. (1976) Computer tomography in disseminated sclerosis. *Canadian Journal of Neurological Science*, **3**, 211–216.

Werring DJ, Bullmore ET, Toosy AT, *et al.* (2000) Recovery from optic neuritis is associated with a change in the distribution of cerebral response to visual stimulation: a functional magnetic resonance imaging study. *Journal of Neurology, Neurosurgery and Psychiatry,* **68**, 441–449.

Willoughby EW, Grochowski E, Li DKB, *et al.* (1989) Serial magnetic resonance scanning in multiple sclerosis: a second prospective study in relapsing patients. *Annals of Neurology,* **25**, 43–49.

Wishart HA, Saykin AJ, McDonald BC, *et al.* (2004) Brain activation patterns associated with working memory in relapsing–remitting MS. *Neurology,* **62**, 234–238.

Young IR, Hall AS, Pallis CA, *et al.* (1981) Nuclear magnetic resonance imaging of the brain in multiple sclerosis. *Lancet,* **ii**, 1063–1066.

Young SW. (1984) *Nuclear Magnetic Resonance Imaging: Basic Principles.* New York: Raven Press.

Zivadinov R, de Masi R, Nasuelli D, *et al.* (2001) MRI techniques and cognitive impairment in the early phase of relapsing–remitting multiple sclerosis. *Neuroradiology,* **43**, 272–278.

11

Multiple sclerosis, disease-modifying treatments and behavioral change

Introduction

There are currently four disease-modifying drugs available: interferon beta-1b, two forms of interferon beta-1a (Rebif, Avonex) and glatiramer acetate (Copaxone). All are injectable, but differ in their route and frequency of administration (Table 11.1). They are usually prescribed for patients with a relapsing–remitting disease course, where their chief benefit is a reduction in the frequency of relapse. A disparate finding is that whereas all treatments significantly reduce the lesion burden as visualized on MRI, this does not necessarily translate into the same degree of clinical improvement (O'Connor, 2000). This chapter will *not* review evidence pertaining to mechanism of action, therapeutic efficacy and general side effects of disease-modifying therapies. Instead, in keeping with the neurobehavioral content of this book, the focus will fall exclusively on the relationship between disease-modifying therapies on the one hand and depression and cognition on the other.

Disease-modifying drugs and depression

Interferon beta-1b

Concerns that treatment with the interferons may trigger depression first surfaced in the initial inteferon beta-1b trial (IFNB Multiple Sclerosis Study Group, 1993, 1995). Adding urgency to the observation was the fact that four subjects attempted, and one completed, suicide over the course of the five year study, in comparison with no such acts in the placebo group. While these differences were not found to be statistically significant, they were a harbinger of future concerns over a possible association between depression and the drug. Subsequently, Neilley *et al.* (1996) reported new or worsened depression as a clinically significant side effect in their sample of 72 MS patients and observed that an interaction between depression and fatigue, symptoms that are often difficult to disentangle, was significantly related to discontinuation of therapy. Indirect evidence supporting these findings came

Table 11.1. Disease-modifying agents

Class	Therapeutic range	Adverse effects
Interferon beta-1a		Influenza-like symptoms
Avonex	Weekly i.m. injection (30 μg)	(fatigue, chills, fever, muscle aches and sweating),
Rebif	Injections s.c. three times a week (22 or 44 μg)	depressive symptoms, injection site reactions (swelling, redness, discoloration or pain), blood abnormalities, elevated liver enzymes
Interferon beta-1b		As for interferon beta-1a
Betaseron	Injections s.c. every other day (250 μg)	
Glatiramir acetate		Flushing, chest pain, weakness,
Copaxone	Once daily s.c. injection (20 mg)	infection, nausea, joint pain, anxiety, muscle stiffness, injection site reactions

i.m., intramuscular, s.c., subcutaneous.

from Mohr *et al.* (1997), who found that 41% of their 85 patients endorsed new or increased depression within six months of starting interferon beta-1b. A second important observation was that patients whose depression was treated with anti-depressant medication or psychotherapy were more likely to remain on interferon beta-1b than patients whose mood was left untreated.

Association does not, however, equate with causality. The source of the reported depression in these studies was unclear and it, therefore, remained to be elucidated whether deterioration in mood was linked to some intrinsic property of the drug or a reaction to unpleasant side effects that include "flu-like" symptoms and inflammation and pain at the injection site. Patients' expectations prior to starting treatment were shown to influence adherence to treatment, in that unrealistic hopes with respect to a reduction in exacerbations and concomitant functional improvement over time increased the drop-out rate (Mohr *et al.*, 1996). Nevertheless, even pretreatment attempts at educating patients about a more realistic set of expectations did not prevent depression emerging as an independent and significant predictor of treatment discontinuation.

These findings contrast with those that failed to find an association between depression and interferon beta-1b. Borras *et al.* (1999), in fact, noted an improvement in mood and anxiety in a sample of 90 patients with relapsing–remitting MS followed serially over 24 months. This supported preliminary results that had failed to find depression as a significant side effect during a 12 month follow-up of 30 patients with relapsing–remitting MS (Dilitz *et al.*, 1998). In a study evaluating the efficacy of interferon beta-1b in patients with secondary progressive MS, depression was found in the placebo but not the treated group (European Study Group, 1998). A study that did not directly address depression, but instead focussed on a related topic, namely quality of life, demonstrated that no discernible change in this outcome variable occurred in the year following instigation of interferon beta-1b treatment (Schwartz *et al.*, 1997). Given the close association between quality of life and depression in MS patients (Vickrey *et al.*, 1997), this result may be construed as indirect evidence that interferon beta-1b does not interfere with patients' moods.

Despite the data suggesting a more promising picture, enough concern persisted about depression as a possible side effect of interferon beta-1b treatment to prompt a consensus report recommending that patients with severe depression and/or suicidal ideation be closely monitored but not necessarily withdrawn from treatment (Lublin *et al.*, 1996). The selective serotonin reuptake inhibitors (SSRI) were proposed as treatment of choice for the patient who either developed a clinically significant depression or whose mood worsened while on the disease-modifying drug. This approach has also been advocated in other studies reviewing the side effect profile of the drug (Munschauer and Kinkel, 1997; Walther and Hohlfield, 1999).

While informative, the focus of most of the above studies was on neurological outcome. Only in passing did the authors comment on the presence or absence of depression as a side effect. One study, however, approached this question head on with the primary emphasis on mood (Feinstein *et al.*, 2002).[1] As such, the results deserve closer inspection and they are discussed in detail below.

Multiple sclerosis, interferon beta-1b and depression: a prospective investigation
Methods
Forty two MS patients with clinically definite MS and a relapsing disease course were followed for one year after starting interferon beta-1b treatment. All subjects were assessed at four time points, namely prior to starting treatment and thereafter

---

[1] By kind permission of Springer Science and Business Media, from Feinstein A, O'Connor P, Feinstein KJ. (2002) Multiple sclerosis, interferon beta-1b and depression: a prospective investigation. *Journal of Neurology*, **249**, 815–820.

at 3, 6 and 12 months. At the initial assessment, demographic and MS-related data were collected. Details of a family history of mental illness were noted and all previous contacts with a mental health worker (psychiatrist, psychologist, thera-pist) recorded. A careful note was also made of all psychotropic medication taken. At each assessment, a detailed neurological examination was undertaken and an Expanded Disability Status Scale (EDSS) score obtained. In addition, a psychiatric interview utilizing the Structured Clinical Interview for DSM-IV axis 1 disorders (mood disorder section; American Psychiatric Association, 1994; First *et al.*, 1994) was completed. Cognizant of the fact that fatigue is endorsed by many MS patients, a diagnosis of major depression was not made if it depended on the inclusion of this symptom. Patients diagnosed with a major depression were referred to a psychiatrist for treatment.

Statistical analysis To investigate the possible influence of past psychiatric history and family history of psychiatric disorders on current mental state and how the mental state may change over time in patient's beginning treatment with interferon beta-1b, the sample was divided in two ways. The first subdivision was into patients with and without a past psychiatric history, while the second was into those with and without a family history of mental illness. The analysis had two primary aims. The first was to analyze group differences in past psychiatric history and family history with regard to current rates of major depression. The second aim was to explore the changes in frequency of depression over time between groups (group $\times$ time effects).

A generalized estimating equation (GEE) was used for analyzing the longitudi-nal data (Liang and Zeger, 1986). The GEE approach directly measures group differences while considering repeated measures of the outcome at different time points. It also incorporates and controls for covariates in the analysis. The advant-age to this method is that it permits a logistic regression analysis with a response or dependent variable that is binary (i.e. depressed versus not depressed). Furthermore, GEE utilizes all available data and does not reduce sample size according to missing data.

In the event of a statistically significant GEE group finding, defined by con-vention as a Z score > 1.96, post-hoc χ^2 analyses were applied to determine at which of the four time points group differences were present.

Results

Demographic and disease-related characteristics of the entire sample Of the 42 subjects, 30 (71.4%) were female. The mean age was 39.8 years (standard deviation [SD], 10.5). Twenty eight (66.7%) subjects were married and 27 (64.3%) were not working. All had relapsing–remitting disease and none were experiencing an exacerbation at their index examination. The mean duration of symptoms was 7.8 years (SD, 6.7) and on average 6.0 years (SD, 6.4) had elapsed since a diagnosis of MS had been made. Their mean EDSS score on entry to the study was 4.2 (SD, 1.7) and at one year was 4.0 (SD, 1.7); this change not proving significant ($t = 1.0$; $p = 0.3$).

Over the course of a year, 10 subjects were lost to study. Of these, two withdrew because they no longer wanted to be part of the research, while eight subjects were withdrawn for other reasons (raised liver enzymes in one, necrosis at injection site in two, deteriorating clinical course in four, loss of funding in one). Consequently, the sample size had decreased to 40, 35 and 32 by the second, third and fourth assessments, respectively. Of the 10 subjects who did not complete the study, six (60%) had a past psychiatric history. Depression was not a reason for any patient leaving the study. At index assessment, 9 (21.4%) of all subjects had a major depression. At 3, 6 and 12 months, this figure had declined to 7 (17.5%), 4 (11.4%) and 2 (6.3%) subjects, respectively.

Psychiatric comparisons between those with and without a past psychiatric history A past history of psychiatric illness was present in 23 (54.8%) subjects and was broken down as follows: mood disorder (42.9%), anxiety disorder (4.8%), substance abuse (2.4%) and comorbid mood and anxiety disorders (4.8%).

There were no demographic nor MS-related differences between those with ($n = 23$) and those without ($n = 19$) a past psychiatric history.

A GEE analysis of major depression found significant group ($Z = 2.1$; $p = 0.04$), but not group $\times$ time interaction ($Z = -0.2$; $p = 0.9$) effects.

Post-hoc χ^2 analyses revealed that subjects with a past psychiatric history were significantly more likely to have a diagnosis of major depression at the first ($x^2 = 5.4$; $p = 0.02$), but not at subsequent assessments. A single patient in the group with no past psychiatric history (5.3% of the sample) had a major depression at index assessment and this percentage remained low throughout the study. In the group with a past history of mental illness, a steady decline in the number of subjects with major depression occurred over the one year follow-up.

This difference between the groups was reflected in the use of psychotropic medication. Subjects with a past psychiatric history were significantly more likely to be using psychotropic medication (in particular anti-depressant drugs) at their index assessment ($x^2 = 38.2$; $p = 0.0001$) and also used more medication during the one year follow-up period ($x^2 = 3.7$; $p = 0.05$).

Psychiatric comparisons between those with and without a family history of mental illness A family history of affective disorder was present in a first-degree relatives of 9 (21.4%) subjects. There were no demographic nor

MS-related differences between subjects with and without a family history of mental illness.

A GEE analysis of major depression found no significant group ($Z = -0.07$: $p = 0.9$), nor group $\times$ time ($Z = -1.7$: $p = 0.09$) effects. In the group without a family history of mental illness, a steady decrease in the percentage of depressed patients over time was noted whereas the group with such a history saw the percentage of subjects with major depression remained constant from the index to the three month assessment, followed by a small increase to six months, before falling to zero at one year.

Post-hoc χ^2 analyses showed there were no between-group differences for depression at all time points. Subjects with a positive family history were not more likely to be taking psychotropic medication at the index assessment ($x^2 = 0.9$; $p = 0.3$) nor during the course of treatment with interferon beta-1b ($x^2 = 2.9$; $p = 0.09$).

Discussion

These findings demonstrate that the treatment of relapsing–remitting MS with interferon beta-1b is not associated with an increase in major depression. Rather, the number of patients with major depression decreased more than threefold over the course of one year. Before examining the data in greater detail, two points need to be made with respect to study design. To assess whether interferon beta-1b is causally linked to depression would have required a different methodology, namely two groups of MS patients followed longitudinally, one on treatment and the other on placebo. The efficacy of interferon beta-1b in treating patients with relapsing–remitting MS, while modest, is still sufficient to make such a design ethically problematic. A second ethical consideration precluded our undertaking a naturalistic study from a mood perspective. Therefore, while it could be postulated that a past psychiatric history or a family history of affective disorder would have left subjects treated with interferon beta-1b at increased risk for developing a mood disorder, from an ethical standpoint all subjects found to be depressed had to be offered treatment, which took the form of a SSRI plus supportive psychotherapy. Anti-depressant treatment is often effective, and so this study could not elucidate whether the presence of one or both putative risk factors (a past psychiatric and/or family history of mental illness) led to a cumulative increase in major depression over time.

Nevertheless, some useful conclusions could be drawn from the data. When the sample was split into those with and without a past psychiatric history, the former were significantly more likely to have a diagnosis of major depression at index assessment. Only one patient without a past psychiatric history had a major depression at index assessment, and this low rate was maintained throughout the follow-up period. The majority of depressed subjects over the course of the one year study were, therefore, found in the group with the past psychiatric history. This is supported by an earlier result from a study of an allied medication, namely interferon beta-1a, which found that depression two months after initiating treatment was linked to pretreatment levels of depression (Mohr *et al.*, 1997). The longitudinal interferon beta-1b study replicates this observation plus demonstrating that when patients on treatment are followed for a longer period, in this case one year, rates of depression decline significantly. Possible reasons for this reduction in depression may be the fact that all patients were treated as the need arose, or the beneficial effects of ongoing interferon beta-1b treatment, or a combination of these two factors.

The interpretation of data with respect to the second putative risk factor for depression (i.e. a family history of major depression) is compromised by small sample size; only nine subjects had a positive family history. However, those subjects with and without a positive family history did not differ in the prevalence of major depression at index assessment and thereafter the percentages tended to fall or remain constant. The absence of any group differences, even at the index assessment, is supported by previous research, which failed to find evidence of a genetic linkage in patients with MS who develop major depression (Joffe *et al.*, 1987a).

The seven subjects who were withdrawn for medical reasons established the drop-out rate at 17.9%, which is comparable with that reported from clinical practice (Vollmer *et al.*, 2000). However, depression, which has been linked to patients dropping out of previous studies (Neilley *et al.*, 1996), was not an issue in our study, possibly because, as others have noted, treating depression enhances compliance with interferon (Mohr *et al.*, 1997).

In summary, the data illustrated that major depression in patients receiving interferon beta-1b was associated, in the majority of cases, with a history of psychiatric illness prior to initiating treatment. Furthermore, providing therapy for depression meant that, even in those patients with a past psychiatric history, instituting and maintaining treatment with interferon beta-1b was associated with a decrease in the prevalence of major depression over time. A family history of an affective disorder was not a harbinger of major depression either before or after treatment with interferon beta-1b. The conclusions to be drawn are clear. The presence of major depression is not a contraindication to treatment with interferon beta-1b. Neurologists must, however, always be alert to the possible development of major depression, as they should in all patients with MS, irrespective of whether disease-modifying treatment is being used or not.

Interferon beta-1a

Interferon beta-1a comes in two commercial forms, Rebif and Avonex. The former is given every second day by subcutaneous injection at doses of either 44 or 22 µg. The latter is given weekly via intramuscular injection, usually at doses of 30 µg.

Rebif

In a two year follow-up study investigating the efficacy and safety of Rebif in patients with *relapsing–remitting* MS, depression did not emerge as a side effect of treatment (PRISMS, 1998). A more detailed analysis of the PRISMS behavioral data was undertaken by Patten and Metz (2001) and is informative. The trial involved 560 subjects from 22 centers, of which 267 participants came from English-speaking centers. Psychiatric symptoms were obtained from the English-speaking subjects at baseline and at 6, 12, 18 and 24 months of treatment, using an array of measures: Center for Epidemiologic Studies Depression Rating Scale, the General Health Questionnaire and the Beck Hopelessness Scale. Subjects were divided into three groups: groups 1 and 2 were treated with Rebif (three injections weekly for both) at 44 and 22 µg, respectively; group 3 received placebo. No significant between-group behavioral differences were found at any of the five assessment points. The incidence of depression in the first six months of the study was 15.6%, confirming that depression is common in MS, but this rate was strongly associated with rates of depression prior to subjects starting interferon beta-1a treatment and not with the treatment itself.

The same methodology (with the same rating scales and drug regimens) was repeated in the SPECTRIMS study, which investigated the efficacy of Rebif in patients with *chronic–progressive* MS (Patten and Metz, 2002). Of the 618 SPECTRIMS participants, 365 (59.1%) were English speaking and their data were analyzed at baseline and after 6, 12, 18, 24, 30 and 36 months of treatment. Once again no group differences emerged on any of the many mood indices recorded.

In the OWINS study, Rebif was given weekly, rather than on alternate days, at doses of either 22 µg or 44 µg (OWINS Study Group, 1999). The aim here was to investigate alternative and potentially more advantageous dosing schedules for patients with relapsing–remitting MS. The depression data replicated that from the PRISMS and SPECTRIMS studies: low mood was not a significant side effect of treatment.

Finally, pooled data from six controlled studies and 17 non-controlled trials have shown that physicians may label patients as depressed despite evidence to the contrary from the patients' self-report rating scales (Patten *et al.*, 2005). This misattribution of symptoms occurs most often within six months of treatment onset. Why this should be is unclear. One possibility is that neurologists may be mislabeling some side effects of treatment, such as fatigue and complaints of physical discomfort, as evidence of mood change.

Encouraging as these results are with respect to the safety of Rebif, there are individual patients who experience, albeit rarely, adverse psychiatric responses to treatment, which may include not only depression but on occasion psychosis as well (Goëb *et al.*, 2003). As these isolated case reports indicate, clinicians should always remain vigilant for adverse psychiatric sequelae and not be lulled into complacency by group data.

Avonex

The depression data with respect to the Avonex formulation of interferon beta-1a is essentially the same as the Rebif findings. A double-blind placebo-controlled trial of Avonex over a two year period did not report differences in depression scores between groups at any time during the study, nor did depression scores in the treated group change from baseline to final outcome. One suicide attempt was noted in the placebo group and none in the Avonex group (Jacobs *et al.*, 1996). Another study specifically explored the relationship with depression in a sample of 106 patients with relapsing–remitting MS (Zephir *et al.*, 2003). Proceeding cautiously, the authors excluded patients with severe depression from enrollment. Assessment took place before treatment onset and at 12 months using the Beck Depression Inventory Revised (Beck *et al.*, 1996). The inventory was used to stratify patients into four categories of depression: minimal, mild, moderate or severe. At baseline, 85% of the subjects fell into the minimum or mild categories, a figure that had hardly changed one year later. These findings were replicated by Zivadinov *et al.* (2003) in a small sample of 27 patients who had been on treatment for a median of 10 months and who were then followed with behavioral assessments for a further 6 and 12 months.

A different picture emerged, however, in a study of patients with a first demyelinating event, that is, a clinically isolated syndrome (Jacobs *et al.*, 2000). A randomized double-blind placebo controlled trial was undertaken in 383 patients presenting with optic neuritis, incomplete transverse myelitis or a brainstem or cerebellar syndrome. All subjects had subclinical evidence of demyelination on brain MRI. During the three year follow-up, patients receiving Avonex rather than placebo were significantly less likely to develop clinically definite MS. They also had a smaller lesion volume in addition to fewer new lesions and gadolinium-enhancing lesions. However, during the first six months of the study, patients in the active treatment arm were also more likely to develop a "flu-like" syndrome and depression. It is unclear, however, whether the label depression applied to a single symptom or the full syndrome of major depression. Whatever the mood state was, it did not affect compliance with treatment, and in the absence of more complete behavioral data the clinical significance of this finding is difficult to interpret.

In general, as with the interferon beta-1b data (Feinstein *et al.*, 2002), rates of depression after starting treatment with Avonex correlate closely with mood state before treatment onset. Mohr *et al.* (1998) assessed 80 patients with relapsing–remitting MS two and four months after starting treatment. A significant increase in depression was noted from baseline to the two month period (p < 0.009), but not from two to four months. Using a different approach that took into account symptoms of low mood up to two weeks preceding onset of interferon beta-1a treatment, increases in depression after beginning treatment were linked with pretreatment levels of depression (Mohr *et al.*, 1999). This finding also fits with research indicating that MS patients who develop mania on steroids are more likely than those who remain euthymic to have a premorbid history of mood disorders or a family history of mood and/or alcohol disorders (Minden *et al.*, 1988). These readily identifiable high-risk factors associated with disease-modifying treatments dictate that physicians should screen patients accordingly and monitor with particular care those who have a premorbid diathesis for mood disorders.

Interferon beta-1a overview

A unique head to head comparison was undertaken of Rebif (44 µg three time a week) and Avonex (30 µg weekly) in 677 MS patients (Panitch *et al.*, 2002). Two endpoints were determined at 24 and 48 weeks: the number of patients relapse free and the number of active lesions on brain MRI. On both indices, patients taking Rebif did better. From a psychiatric perspective, 5% of each group was found to be depressed.

Glatiramer acetate

Unlike the interferons, glatiramer acetate has not been associated with any deterioration in mood. A multicenter placebo-controlled trial in 251 patients over a two year period did not report any mood symptoms, although transient anxiety lasting from 30 seconds to 20 minutes was reported by two patients (Johnson *et al.*, 1995). This result was confirmed in a larger cohort of subjects (Korczyn and Nispeanu, 1996). Isolated cases of psychosis have, however, been noted (Pjrek *et al.*, 2005).

Interferon alpha

Interferon alpha is not a standard treatment for MS. It is instead used for treating chronic hepatitis and a few types of malignancy. Depression has been reported as a side effect in a number of these studies (for reviews see Quesada [1992], Menkes and MacDonald [2000] and Malek-Ahmadi [2001]). In a single, small sample study that used interferon alpha in MS patients, 8% of subjects were diagnosed with depression (Durelli *et al.*, 1996). While the data suggest that depression is more closely related to the alpha variant of interferon, it is unclear why this should be. A putative association between treatment and a reduction in serotonin availability has been suggested, with this effect more pronounced in the alpha rather than the beta variant (Menkes and MacDonald, 2000).

Interpreting the data in the light of methodological limitations

While the weight of evidence suggests that all three interferon beta drugs are not a significant cause of depression in MS patients, there are some important dissenting voices. Here, the contradictory nature of the data is more likely attributable to study design than any intrinsic mood-altering properties of the interferons.

The first potential problem is that few studies utilized a structured, validated clinical interview to diagnose major depression according to DSM-IV criteria. Self-report rating scales were the preferred method of assessing mood, but alone, these cannot define major depression. Expanding on this point, the choice of rating scale also influenced the result. The most commonly used scale was the Beck Depression Inventory, which contains numerous questions linked to somatic complaints (loss of appetite, fatigue, somatic preoccupations, loss of libido, sleep disturbance, work inhibition, to quote directly from the manual; Ch. 2). As injections with the interferon beta drugs are associated with "flu-like" reactions and pain and discomfort at the injection site, it is not surprising that patients experiencing some, if not all, of these physical side effects and endorse certain related responses on a mood questionnaire, thereby spuriously elevating their depression scores.

A second critique, which in part pertains to the method of assessing mood, is that epidemiological evidence has shown that MS alone, without the addition of any disease-modifying treatments, is associated with significant rates of major depression. With a point prevalence of 14% (Joffe et al., 1987b) and with one in three MS patients expected to develop major depression over the course of a year (Minden and Schiffer, 1990), the glatiramer acetate data that failed to find even one case of depression in over 250 patients seen over a two year period confounds the epidemiological evidence. Close scrutiny of the study's methodology fails to reveal how mood was assessed.

A third major critique stems from a series of studies (Mohr et al., 1997, 1999; Feinstein et al., 2002) that demonstrated, inter alia, that mood change post-treatment may be linked to pretreatment depression levels, something that makes intuitive sense and builds on similar findings with respect to steroid-induced mania. In addition, the question of unrealistic expectations of outcome in relation to treatment and how this may influence not only mood but also compliance with treatment has been highlighted.

The above points illustrate that when it comes to teasing out the relationship between depression and the interferons beta-1a and beta-1b, many factors are at play: premorbid mood status; the social mileau within which treatment takes place, including the degree of social support available to the patient; expectations, often unrealistic, on the part of patients with respect to what treatment can accomplish; and, finally, possible serotonin-modulating effects of treatments. A reductionist approach that purports to capture the complexity of these issues with a self-report rating scale helps to explain the conflicting data published to date. It is, therefore, significant that a consistent finding has emerged in the more methodologically sound studies, namely that rates of depression did not increase in patients treated with interferons beta-1a and beta-1b.

Needle anxiety (phobia)

One impediment to patients' compliance with treatment is anxiety that stems from having to self-inject. In some cases, this becomes so intense that the anxiety takes the form of a phobia for needles and behavior turns avoidant. While the prevalence of needle phobia in MS patients with relapsing–remitting MS is not known, the effects on individual patients are: a racheting up of anxiety and an inability to adhere to a potentially helpful treatment.

Two studies have shown that in patients with needle anxiety and phobia respond well to cognitive behavior therapy (CBT). In the first report, eight patients with needle anxiety received six weeks of CBT that focussed on increasing self-efficacy while addressing anxiety. Seven of the eight patients were able to inject after six weeks, while the eighth patient took one week longer to reach the same stage. At three month follow-up, all eight patients were continuing to self-inject (Mohr et al., 2002). In a subsequent study (Mohr et al., 2005), 30 patients with injection-related anxiety or phobia were randomized to receive either six sessions of self-injection anxiety therapy administered by a nurse, or telephone support modelled on a program offered by the drug manufacturer. By six weeks, four patients from the anxiety therapy group and three from the control group (telephone support) had dropped out of the study. Eight of the remaining 11 patients in the therapy group and three from the control group were self-injecting by the end of the study, suggesting this CBT-based method of treatment was potentially useful. A larger clinical trial is, however, needed to provide the statistical power necessary to solidify this conclusion. A further caveat is that both the above studies were undertaken with patients receiving weekly interferon beta-1a (Avonex) via intramuscular injection. It is not known how patients who have to self-inject subcutaneously three times a week with either interferon beta-1a (Rebif) or interferon beta-1b (Betaseron) would respond. While the same CBT principles would still apply, and it is reasonable to assume they would be effective, the greater frequency of self-injection introduces an unknown variable into the equation, one that only a future study can answer.

Disease-modifying drugs and cognitive dysfunction

There is a small literature devoted to this topic with sample sizes generally modest at best. Not surprisingly, results have been mixed.

Interferon beta-1b

Thirty patients who took part in the initial interferon-beta-1b study (IFNB Multiple Sclerosis Study Group, 1993) also completed a brief cognitive battery that included tests of verbal and visuospatial memory, attention, speed of information processing and fine motor speed/coordination. Improvement in delayed visual recall two and four years into treatment was reported (Pliskin *et al.*, 1996). This finding is, however, difficult to interpret. Why only one particular aspect of memory should have responded to interferon-beta-1b is unclear, and was not addressed. The result may have been a statistical artefact, a consequence of multiple uncontrolled comparisons. Alternatively, a more optimiztic view is to invoke a type II error – had the sample size offered greater power, improvement in additional cognitive parameters may have been found.

Evidence supporting the latter comes from an Israeli study, where once again the results are limited by small sample size (Barak and Achiron, 2002). A one year follow-up study of 23 patients taking interferon-beta-1b and a further 23 off treatment revealed that the former had a significantly better cognitive outcome in relation to complex attention, concentration and visual learning and recall. These results must be viewed cautiously because of the unusual cognitive performance of the control group, where the very same psychometric parameters that improved in the treatment group were now found to decline significantly off treatment. Longitudinal studies have demonstrated that this pattern is rarely seen over such a short period (Ch. 8).

A third study that focussed exclusively on the effects of interferon beta-1b on verbal memory failed to find any differences between patients on and off treatment (Selby *et al.*, 1998).

Interferon beta-1a

The most robust evidence attesting to the cognitive benefits of treatment comes from a 104 week study of 276 patients with relapsing–remitting MS who had EDSS scores within the range 1.0 to 3.5 (Fischer *et al.*, 2000). Of the full sample, 166 subjects completed the two year study and it was this group that formed the basis of the subsequent cognitive analysis. Half those who completed the study had received weekly interferon beta-1a (Avonex) 30 μg intramuscularly and the other half had received placebo. A wide array of cognitive tests were administered at baseline and at the 104 week follow-up. The assessments were completed in two three hour sessions over two days. Tests were divided into three broad groups according to the cognitive domains represented, namely set A (information processing, learning and memory); set B (visuospatial abilities and problem solving); and set C (verbal abilities and attention span). Furthermore, to furnish additional cognitive data, a subset of the full cognitive battery of tests was created (visual and verbal learning/recall and information processing speed) and given to patients at 26 week intervals. The brief battery took 90 minutes to administer.

While the treatment ($n = 83$) and placebo ($n = 83$) groups were well matched on all demographic and disease-related variables at the study onset, this was not the case for cognitive function. The Avonex group performed more poorly on set B at baseline, which affected the subsequent serial data analysis. Consequently, the significant treatment effects found with respect to visuospatial abilities and executive functions dissipated when controlled for the baseline differences. This statistical correction should nevertheless not obscure the study's most important finding, namely that subjects receiving active treatment showed greater improvements on measures of information processing speed and memory (set A) compared with the placebo group. No such differences emerged for set C (verbal abilities and attention span). The most notable finding from the secondary analysis involving the brief subset of tests administered more frequently was that the processing rates for the PASAT improved in both groups over time (practice effects). Not all subjects improved, however. When sustained deterioration on the PASAT occurred, this was delayed in subjects taking Avonex.

Whether the improvements noted in the controlled environment of the neuropsychologist's office translates into practical real-life benefits for patients has yet to be determined. However, putting aside questions of ecological validity, which pertain to all the studies discussed here, the study by Fischer *et al.* (2000) with its well thought out methodology and careful analysis provides compelling evidence that, in a disease without cure, treatment with interferon beta-1a offers, at least for some patients, the chance of arresting their impaired cognition.

Glatiramer acetate

The importance of sample selection and how this can influence a study's outcome was demonstrated in a study of 248 MS patients randomized to receive glatiramer acetate or placebo over a two year follow-up period (Weinstein *et al.*, 1999). The cognitive test used was the BRNB (Ch. 9 and Rao *et al.*, 1991). What was surprising about this study was that cognitive scores across both groups in all domains, except for the COWAT, were not impaired at baseline testing. Given the proven sensitivity of the BRNB and the fact that at least 40% of community-living MS patients are cognitively impaired, this sample appeared skewed from inception. The failure to detect any cognitive differences between the glatiramer and placebo groups at the 12 and 24 month follow-ups may, therefore, reflect this bias. Furthermore, both groups showed statistically significant improvements on all but two cognitive measures over the course of the study, an effect attributable to practice. This improvement in a group already largely intact reinforces the impression that subjects enrolled in this study were not representative of MS patients in general.

One of the tests in which no improvement was noted was the COWAT, where performances were impaired at the start. The authors concluded that treatment with glatiramer acetate conferred no cognitive benefits, at least within the first two years of treatment. That may be so, but a better study design is needed to state this conclusion with more certainty.

Summary

- This chapter has presented evidence pertaining to the relationship between behavioral change and disease-modifying treatments, namely the interferons and glatiramer acetate.
- Despite some early concerns that treatment with the interferons, in particular, precipitated significant depressive reactions, the data from the more well-conceived studies have not borne this out. Indeed, there are robust findings highlighting two important clinical observations. The first is that depression post-treatment is most closely linked to depression pretreatment; second, even should a patient develop depression on one of these drugs, treating the depression is frequently successful, thereby allowing the patient to remain on disease-modifying medication that reduces the frequency and severity of relapse.
- The findings in relation to disease-modifying treatments and cognitive benefits are less certain. A meta-analysis comparing all disease-modifying drugs with respect to neurological, inflammatory and cognitive measures makes informative reading (Galetta *et al.*, 2002). Of 21 studies entered into the analysis, only three could furnish useful cognitive data. What few data there are tend to favor Avonex.

References

American Psychiatric Association. (1994) *Diagnostic and Statistical Manual of Mental Disorders*, 4th edn. Washington, DC: American Psychiatric Press.

Barak Y, Achiron A. (2002) Effect of interferon-beta-1b on cognitive functions in multiple sclerosis. *European Neurology*, **47**, 11–14.

Beck AT, Steer RA, Brown GK. (1996) *Beck Depression Inventory (BDI)-II Manual*. San Antonio, TX: Psychological Corporation.

Borras BS, Rio J, Porcel J, *et al.* (1999) Emotional state of patients with relapsing–remitting MS treated with interferon beta-1b. *Neurology*, **52**, 1636–1639.

Dilitz E, Kurz M, Deisenhammer F, Gasse T, Berger T. (1998) Is depression really a side effect of interferon-β therapy in multiple sclerosis? In *ECTRIMS 98. 14th Congress of the European Committee for Treatment and Research in Multiple Sclerosis*, Sweden, (abstract P3058), p. 389.

Durelli L, Bongioanni MR, Ferrero B, *et al.* (1996) Long term recombinant interferon alpha treatment with special emphasis on side effect. *Multiple Sclerosis*, **1**: 366–371.

European Study Group on Interferon B-1b in secondary progressive MS. (1998) Placebo controlled multicentre randomized trial of interferon beta-1b, in treatment of secondary progressive multiple sclerosis. *Lancet*, **352**, 1491–1497.

Feinstein A, O'Connor P, Feinstein KJ. (2002) Multiple sclerosis, interferon beta-1b and depression: a prospective investigation. *Journal of Neurology*, **249**, 815–820.

First MB, Spitzer RL, Gibbon M, Williams JBW. (1994) *Structured Clinical Interview for Axis 1 DSM-IV Disorders*, patient edn (SCID-I/P, version 2.0). New York: Biometrics Research Department, New York State Psychiatric Institute.

Fischer JS, Priore RL, Jacobs LD, *et al.* (2000) Neuropsychological effects of interferon b-1a in relapsing–remitting multiple sclerosis. *Annals of Neurology*, **48**, 885–892.

Galetta SL, Markowitz C, Lee AG. (2002) Immunomodulatory agents for the treatment of relapsing multiple sclerosis: a systematic review. *Archives of Internal Medicine*, **162**, 2161–2169.

Goëb JL, Caileau A, Lainé P, *et al.* (2003) Acute delirium, delusion, and depression during IFN-B-1a therapy for multiple sclerosis. *Clinical Neuropharmacology*, **26**, 5–7.

IFNB Multiple Sclerosis Study Group. (1993) Interferon beta-1b is effective in relapsing–remitting multiple sclerosis. 1. Clinical results of a multi-centre, randomized, double-blind placebo controlled trail. *Neurology*, **43**, 655–661.

IFNB Multiple Sclerosis Study Group and the UBC MS/MRI Analysis Group. (1995) Interferon beta-1b in the treatment of multiple sclerosis: final outcome of the randomized controlled trial. *Neurology*, **45**, 1277–1285.

Jacobs LD, Cookfair DL, Rudick RA, *et al.* (1996) Intramuscular interferon beta-1a for disease progression in relapsing–remitting multiple sclerosis. *Annals of Neurology*, **39**, 285–294.

Jacobs LD, Beck RW, Simon JH, *et al.* (2000) Intramuscular interferon beta-1a therapy initiated during a first demyelination event in multiple sclerosis. *New England Journal of Medicine*, **343**, 898–904.

Joffe RT, Lippert GP, Gray TA, Sawa G, Horvath Z. (1987a) Personal and family history of affective disorder in patients with multiple sclerosis. *Journal of Affective Disorders*, **12**, 63–65.

Joffe RT, Lippert GP, Gray TA, Sawa G, Horvath Z. (1987b) Mood disorder and multiple sclerosis. *Archives of Neurology*, **44**, 376–378.

Johnson KP, Brooks BR, Cohen JA, *et al.* (1995) Copolymer 1 reduces relapse rate and improves disability in relapsing–remitting multiple sclerosis: results of a phase 111 multicentre, double-blind placebo-controlled trial. *Neurology*, **45**, 1268–1276.

Korczyn AD, Nispeanu P. (1996) Safety profile of copolymer 1: analysis of cumulative experience in the United States and Israel. *Journal of Neurology*, **243** (Suppl.1), S23–S26.

Liang KY, Zeger SL. (1986) Longitudinal data analysis for discrete and continuous outcomes. *Biometrics*, **42**, 121–130.

Lublin FD, Whitaker JN, Eidelman BH, *et al.* (1996) Management of patients receiving interferon beta-1b for multiple sclerosis. *Neurology*, **46**, 12–18.

Malek-Ahmadi P. (2001) Mood disorders associated with interferon treatment: theoretical and practical considerations. *Annals of Pharmacotherapy*, **35**, 489–495.

Menkes DB, MacDonald JA. (2000) Interferons, serotonin and neurotoxicity. *Psychological Medicine*, **30**, 259–268.

Minden SL, Schiffer RB. (1990) Affective disorders in multiple sclerosis. Review and recommendations for clinical research. *Archives of Neurology*, **47**, 98–104.

Minden SL, Orav J, Schildkraut JJ. (1988) Hypomanic reactions to ACTH and prednisone treatment for multiple sclerosis. *Neurology*, **38**, 1631–1634.

Mohr DC, Goodkin DE, Likosky W, *et al.* (1996) Therapeutic expectations of patients with multiple sclerosis upon initiating interferon beta-1b: relationship to adherence to treatment. *Multiple Sclerosis*, **2**, 222–226.

Mohr DC, Goodkin DE, Likosky W, *et al.* (1997) Treatment of depression improves adherence to interferon beta-1b therapy for multiple sclerosis. *Archives of Neurology* **54**, 531–533.

Mohr DC, Likosky W, Boudewyn AC, *et al.* (1998) Side effect profile and adherence to in the treatment of multiple sclerosis with interferon beta-1a. *Multiple Sclerosis*, **4**, 487–489.

Mohr DC, Likosky W, Dwyer P, *et al.* (1999) Course of depression during the initiation of interferon beta-1a for multiple sclerosis. *Archives of Neurology*, **56**, 1263–1265.

Mohr D, Cox D, Epstein L, Boudewyn A. (2002) Teaching patients to self-inject: a pilot study of a treatment for injection anxiety and phobia in multiple sclerosis patients prescribed injectable medications. *Journal of Behavior Therapy and Experimental Psychiatry*, **33**, 39–47.

Mohr D, Cox D, Merluzzi N. (2005) Self-injection anxiety training: a treatment for patients unable to self-inject injectable medications. *Multiple Sclerosis*, **11**, 182–185.

Munschauer FE III, Kinkel KP. (1997) Managing side effects of interferon beta in patients with relapsing–remitting multiple sclerosis. *Clinical Therapy*, **19**, 883–893.

Neilley LK, Goodkin DS, Goodkin DE, Mohr DC, Hauser SL. (1996) Side effect profile of interferon beta-1b (Betaseron). *Neurology*, **46**, 552–554.

O'Connor P. (2000) Reason for hope: the advent of disease modifying therapies in multiple sclerosis. *Canadian Medical Association Journal*, **162**, 83–85.

OWINS Study Group. (1999) Evidence of interferon beta-1a dose response in relapsing–remitting MS. *Neurology*, **53**, 679–686.

Panitch H, Goodin DS, Grancis G, *et al.* (2002) Randomized, comparative study of interferon beta-1a treatment regimes in MS. The EVIDENCE trial. *Neurology*, **59**, 1496–1506.

Patten SB, Metz LM. (2001) Interferon beta-1a and depression in relapsing–remitting multiple sclerosis: an analysis of depression data from the PRISMS clinical trial. *Multiple Sclerosis*, **7**, 243–248.

Patten SB, Metz LM. (2002) Interferon beta-1a and depression in secondary progressive MS: Data from the SPECTRIMS trial. *Neurology*, **59**, 744–746.

Patten SB, Francis G, Metz LM, *et al.* (2005) The relationship between depression and interferon beta-1a therapy in patients with multiple sclerosis. *Multiple Sclerosis*, **11**, 175–181.

Pjrek E, Winkler D, Dervic K, Aschauer H, Kasper S. (2005) Psychosis as a possible side-effect of treatment with glatiramer acetate. *International Journal of Neuropsychopharmacology*, **8**, 487–488.

Pliskin NH, Hamer DP, Goldstein MS *et al.* (1996) Improved delayed visual reproduction test performance in multiple sclerosis patients receiving interferon beta-1b. *Neurology*, **47**, 1463–1468.

PRISMS (Prevention of Relapses and Disability by Interferon beta-1a Subcutaneously in Multiple Sclerosis) Study Group. (1998) Randomised double-blind placebo-controlled study of interferon B-1a in relapsing/remitting multiple sclerosis. *Lancet*, **352**, 1498–1504.

Quesada JR. (1992) Toxicity and side effects of interferons. In Baron S, *Interferon: Principles and Medical Applications*, ed. S Baron, DH Coppenhaver, F Dianzani, *et al.* Galveston, TX: University of Texas Medical Branch Department of Microbiology, pp. 427–432.

Rao SM, Leo HJ, Bernardin L, Unverzagt F. (1991) Cognitive dysfunction in multiple sclerosis. 1. Frequency, patterns and prediction. *Neurology*, **41**, 685–691.

Schwartz CE, Coulthard-Morris L, Cole B, Vollmer T. (1997) The quality of life effects of interferon beta-1b in multiple sclerosis. An extended Q-TWIST analysis. *Archives of Neurology*, **54**, 1475–1480.

Selby MJ, Ling N, Williams JM, Dawson A. (1998) Interferon beta-1b in verbal memory functioning of patients with relapsing–remitting multiple sclerosis. *Perceptual Motor Skills*, **86**, 1099–1106.

Vickrey BG, Hays RD, Genovese BJ, Myers LW, Ellison GW. (1997) Comparison of a generic to disease-targeted health related quality of life measures for multiple sclerosis, *Journal of Clinical Epidemiology*, **50**, 557–569.

Vollmer T, Ni W, Hadjimichael O. (2000) MS treatment patterns at the end of the 20th century. [*Consortium of Multiple Sclerosis Centres (CMSC) Annual Meeting*, Halifax, Canada.] *Journal of MS Care*, **2**, 000–000.

Walther EU, Hohlfied R. (1999) Multiple sclerosis. Side effects on interferon beta therapy and their management. *Neurology*, **16**, 22–27.

Weinstein A, Schwid SI, Schiffer RB, *et al.* (1999) Neuropsychologic status in multiple sclerosis after treatment with glatiramer. *Archives of Neurology*, **56**, 319–324.

Zephir H, De Seze J, Stojkovic T, *et al.* (2003) Multiple sclerosis and depression: influence of interferon beta therapy. *Multiple Sclerosis*, **9**, 284–288.

Zivadinov R, Zorzon M, Tommasi MA, *et al.* (2003) A longitudinal study of quality of life and side effects in patients with multiple sclerosis treated with interferon beta-1a. *Journal of the Neurological Sciences*, **216**, 113–118.

12

Multiple sclerosis: a subcortical, white matter dementia?

Medical taxonomy is subject to periodic revision, an inevitable consequence of new information derived from increasingly sophisticated clinical and laboratory investigations. The classification of dementia is a good illustration of this. For much of the past 100 years, the term dementia was considered synonymous with cortical pathology, of which Alzheimer's disease was the most frequent and well-described example. To be sure, Kinnear Wilson had, in 1912, described a distinctive pattern of neurobehavioral disturbance secondary to basal ganglia pathology, but his ideas were not developed in any systematic way for over 60 years. In the last quarter of the twentieth century, the concept of a different form of dementia primarily affecting subcortical structures and with a distinct clinical profile began to gain wider acceptance in psychiatry, neurology and neuropsychology. While some queried the validity of a distinct subcortical syndrome (Hakim and Mathieson, 1979; Whitehouse *et al.*, 1982), their doubts gradually submerged under the weight of current opinion. More recently, however, new data derived from MRI of the brain and neuropathological investigation have opened up the debate anew.

The fourth edition of the Diagnostic and Statistical Manual of the American Psychiatric Association (DSM-IV) (American Psychiatric Association, 1994) has not created a specific category of "subcortical dementia" but has instead approached the issue of the classification of dementia in a more piecemeal fashion, by listing specific causes, many of which are essentially subcortical pathological processes, for example human immunodeficiency virus (HIV) infection, Parkinson's and Huntington's diseases and MS. Dementia according to the DSM-IV requires the presence of four main characteristics: memory loss; one (or more) features of impaired cognition, listed as aphasia, agnosia, apraxia and impaired executive function; the cognitive deficits must lead to significant impairment in occupational or social functioning and represent a significant decline from premorbid levels of functioning; and, finally, the cognitive disturbance cannot be solely

accounted for by a delirium. These basic tenets are regarded as essential prereq-
uisites for the diagnosis, although when it comes to specific causes of dementia, for
example Huntington's disease, descriptive details regarded as characteristic of the
disorder are added to the four cardinal requirements. Inherent in this approach is a
recognition that different causes of dementia are associated with their own particular constellation of signs and symptoms, but the DSM-IV manual stops short of
officially endorsing a cortical–subcortical neurobehavioral divide.

This reticence is understandable, for important questions remain to be answered.
This chapter will review the evidence – clinical, anatomical and physiological –
that underlies the concept of a subcortical dementia. As the term is a broad rubric
encompassing different anatomical areas, the focus will be restricted to pathology
known to appreciably affect the cerebral white matter and will examine whether
this is associated with a recognizable neurobehavioral syndrome. Reference will be
made to MS and other diseases involving the cerebral white matter and similarities
sought in their effects on mentation. These features will be contrasted with those
derived from the cortical and subcortical gray matter dementias. Finally, the
notion of MS as a quintessential white matter subcortical dementia will be
reappraised in light of recent findings from neuropathological and MRI studies,
which have demonstrated more extensive cortical involvement than previously
thought present.

Subcortical dementia

Although Wilson (1912) had noted that patients with hepatolenticular degeneration showed an absence of agnosia and apraxia and had less severe memory
impairment compared with patients with senile dementia, it was Albert and
colleagues (1974) who are generally acknowledged as first giving impetus to the
concept of subcortical dementia. In their report of five cases of supranuclear palsy
and their literature review of a further 42 cases, four characteristic features were
described: forgetfulness, a slowness of thought processes, emotional or personality
changes (summarized as apathy or depression interspersed with irritability) and an
impaired ability to manipulate acquired knowledge. The last referred to difficulties
with calculation or abstraction. The absence of aphasia, agnosia and apraxia was
again strikingly evident. Albert and colleagues were struck by the similarities
in clinical presentation between patients with subcortical dementia and those
with dementia secondary to bilateral frontal lobe pathology, and they noted that
patients in both groups may also display signs of pseudobulbar palsy including
pseudobulbar affect (forced laughing or crying). This overlap was considered a
natural consequence of the extensive neural connections linking subcortical structures to the frontal cortex, a theme that will be expanded on later in this chapter.

McHugh and Folstein (1975) added to the emergent concept by demonstrating that patients with Huntington's disease demonstrated many of the same behavioral characteristics as those with pseudobulbar palsy, which, in turn, were distinct from those with Alzheimer's disease and the Wernicke–Korsakoff syndrome. The cortical–subcortical dichotomy was further validated by the results from studies of patients with pathology in the substantia nigra and thalamus. The emphasis in these early studies was, however, focussed almost exclusively on disorders affecting the deep gray matter. Consequently, a decade after the landmark paper of Albert *et al.* (1974), Cummings (1986), in reviewing a burgeoning literature, took Huntington's and Parkinson's diseases as the prototypical subcortical conditions against which the findings from cortical dementias, predominantly Alzheimer's disease, were compared.

Neuropsychological features

Early descriptions of subcortical dementia emphasised that a reduction in cognitive speed, or a slowness in information processing (also termed bradyphrenia), was a cardinal feature. This occurred in excess of any motor difficulties. Patients with cortical dementias are largely spared these difficulties. While both groups suffer from memory impairment, the patients with subcortical dysfunction are better at encoding new information but have trouble retrieving it, whereas the patients with predominantly cortical involvement struggle with encoding and are not aided by cues or recognition prompts. Language is usually less affected, apart from dysarthria and mild anomia, in the subcortical dementias, which contrasts with the expressive and non-expressive difficulties experienced by patients with predominantly cortical involvement. Different aspects of visuospatial and abstracting difficulties are present in both groups. Cortical involvement is more likely to lead to poor copying skills, while subcortical involvement is associated with problems manipulating egocentric space (e.g. map reading). Deficits in abstracting and categorization generally appear earlier and with greater severity in the cortical dementias. Attention and vigilance may be affected in both groups.

Psychiatric features

The cortical–subcortical division is harder to sustain if based on psychiatric instead of cognitive discriminators. This reflects the more diffuse nature of psychiatric symptomatology in general and explains why particular syndromes and symptoms have defied easy localization. There are many reports of depression, personality change, mania and psychosis occurring in subcortical conditions, but the same may be applied to dementias that are cortical in origin and it would be incorrect to suggest that one group is predominantly affected. An additional problem is how one defines the various terms. For example, depression may refer to a transient symptom or an enduring, disabling syndrome, and equating the two, or a failure to distinguish how studies have dealt with this question, will lead to comparisons that lack validity. Similarly, psychosis is a broad term that, depending on definition, may refer to delusions, hallucinations, thought disorder, catatonia or various combinations of these symptoms. Definitions of psychosis have been subject to periodic revision but the criteria for including or excluding psychotic patients from studies has generally been arbitrary, for example the distinction made between psychotic patients with or without delirium or dementia. If one takes a working definition of psychosis as the presence of delusions and/or hallucinations in the presence of clear consciousness, then there are strong data demonstrating that psychosis is a frequent concomitant of subcortical conditions such as Huntington's disease (Dewhurst *et al.*, 1969; Caine and Shoulson, 1983) and metachromatic leukodystrophy (Hyde *et al.*, 1992). This finding does not, of course, reduce the etiological significance of the cortex in psychosis. After all, the most common and disabling of all psychotic illnesses, namely schizophrenia, has long been attributed primarily to cortical involvement (Suddath *et al.*, 1990; Harvey *et al.*, 1993). And yet even here, opinions are shifting, driven by new technologies that allow for more detailed in vivo and postmortem exploration of brain pathology. Diffusion tensor imaging (DTI), MRI voxel-based morphometry and histopathological studies exploring neuronal distribution and oligodendro- cyte number, density and function have revealed a hitherto unrecognized disrup- tion in white matter integrity in patients with schizophrenia (Kubicki *et al.*, 2005).

In light of these new developments, it is, therefore, not surprising that attempts at qualitatively differentiating subcortical from cortical-based psychotic features have met with mixed results. Neither Davison and Bagley (1969) nor Feinstein and Ron (1990) noted differences, although Cummings (1986) reported that patients with Alzheimer's disease generally had more severe dementia and delusions with a simpler content than patients with subcortical dementias, whose intellectual impairment was less marked and whose delusional thought content was consequently more complex.

Summarizing the cognitive and psychiatric findings with respect to subcortical dementia, there is firmer evidence of a discrete cognitive as opposed to a psychi- atric profile. However, "subcortical dementia" refers to a syndrome encompassing both cognitive and emotional/behavioral changes, and a closer inspection of the relevant neuroanatomy and neurophysiology explains why a degree of overlap with the predominantly cortical dementias is inevitable.

Subcortical neuroanatomy

Fronto-subcortical circuits and behavior

There is a rich network of bidirectional white matter tracts that connect the frontal lobes to other areas of the brain. While there is no lobe that does not have frontal connections, of particular interest are those fronto-subcortical circuits that are known to subserve discrete behavioral syndromes. Five fronto-subcortical circuits have been demonstrated (Alexander *et al.*, 1986; Alexander and Crutcher, 1990) and their neuroanatomy and functional characteristics summarized (Cummings, 1993). All begin in the frontal lobes, project to the striatum (caudate, putamen and ventral striatum) and thereafter to the globus pallidus and substantia nigra, from where they relay with specific thalamic nuclei before completing the circuit by returning to the frontal area of origin. Although this overall pattern of connections is followed by all five circuits, each circuit is discrete and within each anatomical area will relay with circuit-specific nuclei. Of the five circuits, three originate in separate prefrontal cortical areas, namely dorso lateral prefrontal cortex, lateral orbital cortex and anterior cingulate cortex. The remaining two circuits begin in the supplementary motor area and frontal eye fields, respectively. The three prefrontal circuits have subsidiary pathways at various stages throughout their course and send and receive connections to and from related limbic structures. As the circuit progresses from cortex to subcortex, so the neurones funnel into increasingly smaller areas, all the while maintaining their parallel and distinct anatomical integrity. This "squeezing" of the circuits helps to explain how lesions situated at various points along the pathways give rise to differing clinical presentations.

Each prefrontal circuit is associated with a specific behavioral syndrome. Lesions located in the dorso lateral prefrontal cortex produce deficits with executive function, namely planning, organizing, sequencing and abstracting. Lesions in the orbito frontal area produce a syndrome characterized by changes in personality, typically of the labile, disinhibited, impulsive and aggressive type. Patients may appear irritable, euphoric, overtalkative and display a lack of social tact. They differ from individuals with pathology of the dorso lateral prefrontal cortex, by performing better on tests that challenge executive function. Anterior cingulate pathology typically produces abnormalities of motivation, and individuals may present as profoundly apathetic or abulic.

Lesions affecting the striatal structures may produce clinical states similar to those described above, depending on the extent to which the pathological process remains localized. This becomes increasingly less likely as the circuit projects postero-inferiorly, so lesions involving the globus pallidus or thalamus may not produce a discrete syndrome but rather a mixture of signs and symptoms. The clinical picture, therefore may be a combination of disinhibition and irritability (orbito frontal syndrome), reduced motivation and interest (medial fronto-anterior cingulate syndrome) and neuropsychological deficits (dorso lateral prefrontal cortex syndrome). These circuits subserve not only personality attributes, but mood as well. While mania and obsessive–compulsive behavior have been linked to dysfunction of the orbito frontal circuits, depression may arise from lesions affecting the orbito frontal and dorso lateral prefrontal cortex circuits.

Cerebral white matter

Separating the cerebral cortices from the ventricular system, the cerebral white matter comprises three main types of fibers. The projection fibers reciprocally link the cortex to more distant structures such as the brainstem; association fibres connect regions in the same hemisphere, and commissural fibers link the two hemispheres. This widespread neural network subserves many functions ranging from maintaining alertness (the reticular activating system) to facilitating more complex aspects of mentation such as mood and memory. The major neurotransmitter systems (norepinephrine from the locus ceruleus, serotonin from the raphe nuclei, dopamine from the tegmentum, acetylcholine from the nucleus basalis of Meynert) are dependent on the integrity of the white matter tracts, chiefly the medial forebrain bundle as they traverse from brainstem and midbrain to the cortex. Release of neurotransmitters is, however, dependent on axonal conduction and the latter is, in turn, dependent on myelin. Consequently, in demyelinating disorders such as MS, impaired neural conduction may vary from slowing to a complete interruption of transmission. It is, however, unclear whether in vivo evidence of altered neurotransmitter metabolism in a white matter disease such as MS (Johansson and Roos, 1974; Markianos and Sfagos, 1988) is directly attributable to demyelination or an epiphenomenon (i.e. secondary to mood change, a response to stress).

Pathogenesis of subcortical dementia

One conceptual distinction has been to regard cortical functions as *instrumental* and subcortical as *fundamental* (Albert, 1978). Instrumental functions refer to discrete aspects of cognition such as language, reading, calculation, memory and praxis, which are all primarily dependent on neocortical areas. Fundamental functions include less highly evolved activities such as attention, arousal, motivation and mood, which is reflected in their more diffuse neural networks, spanning subcortical nuclei that connect with the cortex via the white matter.

Although early descriptions stressed that subcortical dementia was a clinical, not an anatomical, concept, by focussing largely on the deep gray matter, almost 50% of the total cerebral volume was overlooked (Cummings and Benson, 1984). The functional importance of the cerebral white matter is well illustrated in a brief description of the neural circuitry subserving attention. Attention, defined as the ability of a subject to attend to a specific stimulus without being distracted by extraneous environmental stimuli, is one of the basic building blocks of cognition underpinning other aspects of cognitive function. Impaired attention occurs often in demyelinating disease (Filley *et al.*, 1989a; Feinstein *et al.*, 1993; Kujala *et al.*, 1995). Mesulam (1981) has identified four distinct contributions (sensory, motor, limbic and reticular activation) to the overall organization of one aspect of attention, namely spatially directed attention. All are richly interconnected. Spatially directed attention is thus a balance between ascending (reticulo-cortical) activation and cortical (cortico-reticular) modulation, the limbic system adding emotional importance to the object of attention and conscious voluntary effort supplied by the frontal lobes. A pivotal cortical area in integrating sensory input is the dorso lateral portion of the posterior parietal cortex. This area contains an elaborate sensory representation of extrapersonal space, a prerequisite for distributing attention. The frontal cortex, particularly the frontal eye fields, and surrounding regions assist in initiating or inhibiting motor mechanisms involved in attentive behavior. Damage to this area manifests as failure to orientate, manipulate and explore perceptual representations. The anatomical separation of sensory and motor components is not, however, complete. Some sensory representation occurs in the frontal cortex and vice versa, an arrangement shown to improve functional efficiency (Mesulam, 1981). The cingulate region, with extensive limbic connections, gives motivational relevance to sensory events, which may then receive more extensive representation in the dorso lateral prefrontal cortex, thereby enhancing activation of frontal mechanisms. Finally, an intact reticular formation is essential in maintaining arousal, without which attention and vigilance become impaired.

For object-specific attention, additional components are required. Examples include the association areas in regions such as the inferior temporal cortex, which are responsible for attention to an object's attributes such as color, texture and shape (Wise and Demisone, 1988).

A single lesion occurring anywhere within this extensive network may disrupt functional integrity through a process of disconnection (Geschwind, 1995). The same holds for any of the myriad neural networks underpinning all aspects of behavior. The cerebral white matter is particularly important in this regard, for it fulfills an essential integrative function reciprocally linking cortical to other cortical and subcortical areas. It has long been recognized that a cerebral lesion may produce more distant cerebral effects, a process termed diaschisis. In conditions that diffusely affect the white matter, such as MS, the concept has been demonstrated through a combination of structural (computed tomography [CT]) and functional (positron emission tomography [PET]) neuroimaging (Brooks *et al.*, 1984), with primarily white matter lesions producing a reduction in cortical cerebral perfusion.

White matter neurobehavioral syndromes

In trying to ascertain whether there is a specific behavioral syndrome pertinent to white matter pathology, the researcher confronts the same dilemmas that first challenged those defining the behavioral characteristics of the basal ganglia disorders three decades back. During the intervening years, improved technology has demonstrated, in vivo, that to understand cerebral function is to understand the role of neural networks. With neural networks spanning the cortical, subcortical gray and white matter, it is even more relevant today to repeat the assertion of Cummings and Benson (1984) that the term subcortical should be regarded more as a clinical than an anatomical entity.

Disorders of the cerebral white matter

A comprehensive list of disorders affecting the cerebral white matter has been provided by Filley (1996) (Table 12.1), who has noted the paucity of associated neurobehavioral data compared with cortically based conditions. A distinction is made between adult and childhood disorders, although it is recognized that some may apply to both age groups. The childhood disorders will not be considered here, the exception being metachromatic leukodystrophy.

Most of the neurobehavioral research in this area has been undertaken in patients with MS. Therefore, taking MS as a central reference point, a MEDLINE search was undertaken looking for neuropsychiatric studies that compared MS with the following: (a) white matter disorders, (b) deep gray matter disorders and (c) cortical disorders. The yield was small. With respect to the white matter search, only two conditions were found: the acquired immunodeficiency syndrome

Table 12.1. Adult cerebral white matter disorders

Type	Disorder
Demyelinating	Multiple sclerosis
Vascular	Binswanger's disease, stroke
Toxic	Alcoholic dementia, toluene dementia, radiation, chemotherapy
Infectious	Acquired immuno deficiency syndrome, progressive multifocal leukoencephalopathy
Metabolic	Hypoxia, cobalamin deficiency, Marchiafava–Bignami disease, central pontine myelinosis
Traumatic	Traumatic brain injury, corpus callosotomy
Neoplastic	Tumors, gliomatosis cerebri

(AIDS) and traumatic brain injury. Both are discussed below. In addition, two other predominantly white matter disorders will be briefly reviewed, even though there are no studies that directly contrast their clinical features with those found in MS. They are Binswanger's subcortical encephalopathy and metachromatic leuko-dystrophy. Before concluding, this section will discuss the few neuropsychological studies comparing MS with Alzheimer's and Huntington's diseases.

Traumatic brain injury

Over thee million people in the USA suffer a traumatic brain injury each year (Collins, 1990), making it by far the most frequent cause of acquired brain injury. While evidence of cortical damage is often readily discernible, even to the naked eye (subdural and intracerebral bleeds), it is also recognized that the cerebral white matter may be adversely affected. Extensive white matter degeneration was noted by Strich (1961) at postmortem in patients who had survived for months in a comatose state. She proposed that lesions resulted from a direct tearing of nerve fibers at the time of impact, although others argued they were secondary to raised intracranial pressure (Jellinger and Seitelberg, 1970). The argument has since been resolved; it is now accepted that diffuse axonal injury, primarily affecting the white matter, can occur following a closed (non-penetrating) head injury and in the absence of raised intracranial pressure (Adams *et al.*, 1977).

In vivo evidence of cerebral involvement has come from neuroimaging and neuropsychological studies of patients with mild to moderate closed head injuries. Levin *et al.* (1987) showed that at least 80% of patients had cerebral lesions visible on CT or MRI within days of sustaining the injury. The majority of lesions were localized to frontal and temporal regions and were associated with neuropsychological deficits pertaining to frontal lobe and memory tasks. Of the 39 parenchymal lesions demonstrated by MRI, 27 involved both the gray and white matter, while fewer were confined either to the white or the gray matter alone. Serial MRI follow-up of a similar sample (Levin *et al.*, 1992) demonstrated substantial lesion resolution by three months post trauma, with a concomitant improvement in neuropsychological deficits. Nevertheless, some patients whose lesions had resolved by one month continued to perform poorly on tests of executive function and memory. The reason for this was provided by functional neuroimaging (PET), which demonstrated reduced glucose metabolism in brain regions deemed normal on structural neuroimaging (Humayun *et al.*, 1989; Ruff *et al.*, 1994), abnormalities correlating with deficits in attention and memory. Significantly, some of the patients with neuropsychological and PET deficits had not lost consciousness but rather had experienced an alteration in consciousness at the time of injury, demonstrating that mild traumatic brain injury may lead to clearly demonstrable deficits in cerebral function.

As with MS patients, magnetization transfer imaging has been used in patients with traumatic brain injury, where it has helped to elucidate the functional significance of normal appearing white matter (NAWM). In a study of 28 patients with traumatic brain injury and 15 healthy controls, magnetization transfer ratios (MTR) were calculated for areas of shearing injury and NAWM in regions usually subjected to diffuse axonal injury (Bagley *et al.*, 2000). The results were mixed: abnormal MTR values were detected in eight patients who had neurological deficits and cognitive dysfunction and normal MTR values were found in seven patients with traumatic brain injury who had no neurological or cognitive problems. However, these promising results were offset by normal MTR values in 13 patients with persisting neurological dysfunction, a finding that leaves a question mark over the sensitivity of this imaging technique in patients with traumatic brain injury. Magnetization transfer imaging has, however, been able to differentiate brain lesions secondary to MS and traumatic brain injury. In a study that directly compared the imaging data from 30 patients with MS and 10 patients with traumatic brain injury, clear MTR differences emerged (Bagley *et al.*, 1999). Contour plots for the MTR data were constructed around lesions and in MS subjects revealed a gradual increase in MTR as the region of interest shifted away from the center of the lesion. In patients with a traumatic brain injury, however, the gradations were replaced by an abrupt transition in MTR values between lesion and the surrounding NAWM.

Finding from DTI complement the magnetization transfer data in patients with traumatic brain injury. Even in patients with a mild injury, a reduction in fractional anisotropy has been noted in the corpus callosum, internal capsule and centrum semiovale (Inglese *et al.*, 2005). The presence of DTI changes soon after injury and years later suggest this imaging technique may have prognostic value in the assessment of patients with a traumatic brain injury.

Acquired immuno deficiency syndrome

The acquired immunodeficiency syndrome (AIDS) results from infection with the human immunodeficiency virus (HIV). Neuropsychiatric sequelae may result from the direct effect of HIV on the CNS or from the many secondary diseases associated with the AIDS syndrome. The term aids dementia complex was put forward by physicians to describe changes in mentation and motor function that were not attributable to CNS tumors, opportunistic infections and systemic diseases (Navia *et al.*, 1986). AIDS has been regarded as primarily a subcortical disease because the virus has a predilection for the central white matter and structures such as the basal ganglia, thalamus and brainstem, leaving the cortex relatively unaffected. White *et al.* (1995) have reviewed the literature from 57 studies that compared the presence or absence of cognitive deficits in asymptomatic HIV-seropositive and HIV-seronegative subjects. The median rate of

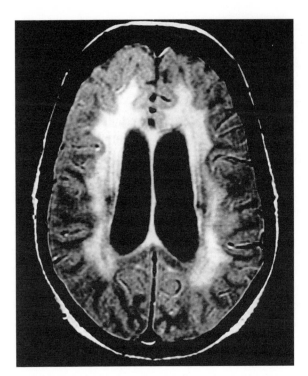

Fig. 12.1.   An axial proton density magnetic resonance image in a 25-year-old male with HIV dementia. The cerebrospinal fluid appears hypointense and offsets the extensive periventricular, confluent white matter lesions.

neuropsychological impairment for the seropositive group was 35%, compared with 12% for the seronegative group. Therefore, changes in mentation may precede physical signs and symptoms of HIV infection. Deficits such as cognitive slowing, impaired learning efficiency, apathy and avoidance of complex tasks (Markowitz and Perry, 1992) suggest a subcortical dementing process. There is also evidence that cognitive impairment may increase as the disease progresses, with abnormalities attributable to cerebral involvement (mainly white matter atrophy), rather than mood changes, substance abuse or constitutional symptoms (Heaton *et al.*, 1995).

The typical MRI picture is one of diffuse white matter lesions of high signal intensity (Olsen *et al.*, 1988; Fig. 12.1) and lesion detection may be improved with the use of contrast enhancement (Tuite *et al.*, 1993). Multifocal as opposed to diffuse white matter lesions are more typical of progressive multifocal leuko-encephalopathy, a papova virus infection that may occur together with AIDS (Fig. 12.2). Rarely, HIV-positive patients can present with a fulminating MS-like leukoencephalopathy, the typical histological features of MS confirmed at post-mortem (Gray *et al.*, 1991). Whether this association represents chance occurrences or a possible etiological link remains uncertain.

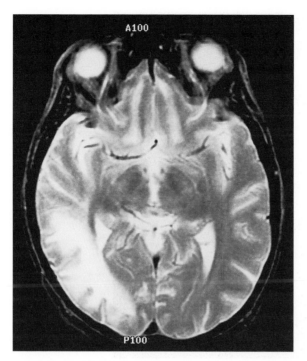

Fig. 12.2.   An axial T_2 weighted magnetic resonance image in a 27-year-old male with progressive multifocal leukoencephalopathy.

The use of DTI to examine NAWM in HIV-positive patients can provide indices of disease severity, response to treatment and cognitive status. For example, high diffusion constant elevations and large anisotropy decreases correlate with advanced HIV disease. Conversely, highly active antiretroviral therapy and low viral load levels are associated with normal anisotropy and diffusion constants (Fillippi *et al.*, 2001). A reduction in whole-brain fractional anisotropy is indicative of significant cognitive deficits (Ragin *et al.*, 2004a). A similar relationship pertains to a whole brain reduction in MTR (Ragin *et al.*, 2004b).

Vascular disorders: Binswanger's disease

Binswanger's disease has also been termed subcortical arteriosclerotic encephalopathy (Babikian and Ropper, 1987) and is thought to arise from chronic cerebral ischemia, primarily affecting the white matter. Hypertension is frequently implicated (Babikian and Popper, 1987), cerebral amyloid angiopathy less so (Gray *et al.*, 1985). The relationship of the disorder to asymptomatic white matter lesions viewed on MRI in asymptomatic elderly (Filley *et al.*, 1989b) or middle-aged (Rao *et al.*, 1989) subjects is open to debate (Ch. 10). The clinical presentation is compatible with that of subcortical dementia and the confluent, periventricular

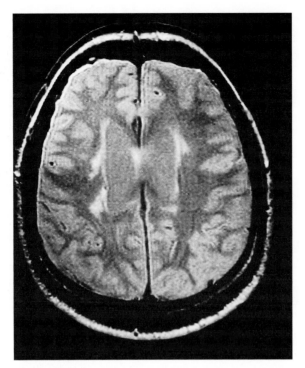

Fig. 12.3.   An axial magnetic resonance image in a 44-year-old male with Binswanger's subcortical encephalopathy, demonstrating periventricular confluent white matter lesions.

white matter lesions seen on T_2 weighted MRI may be indistinguishable from MS (Fig. 12.3). Although Binswanger's disease is considered a separate clinical entity from other vascular causes of dementia such as multi-infarct dementia and stroke, more recently recognized causes of vascular-mediated white matter change, such as the genetic variant "cerebral autosomal dominant arteriopathy with subcortical infarcts and leukoencephalopathy" (CADASIL; Stevens *et al.*, 1977; Salloway, 1996), should also be part of any differential diagnosis.

Metachromatic leukodystrophy

First described by Alzheimer (1910), metachromatic leukodystrophy is a familial disease with an autosomal recessive mode of inheritance and is caused by a deficiency or absence in the enzyme arylsulfatase A, which catalyzes the hydrolysis of sulfate groups. As a result, cerebroside sulfate accumulates and this is toxic to nerve cells, causing demyelination of axons and peripheral nerves. The age of presentation, which may vary from infancy to adulthood, is dependent on the degree of enzyme deficiency, less severe diminutions associated with a later onset (Polten *et al.*, 1991). Neuroimaging reveals that demyelination usually starts in the frontal lobes, affecting the periventricular white matter and corpus callosum before spreading more posteriorly.

A feature of metachromatic leukodystrophy with onset in adolescents and young adults is the high prevalence of psychosis, estimated to be in excess of 50% (Hyde *et al.*, 1992). The clinical presentation is frequently indistinguishable from schizophrenia, with patients displaying prominent and bizarre delusions and hallucinations. The occurrence of psychosis is age related, giving way to dementia as the patient ages. Thus, psychosis appears dependent on intact, albeit pathologically functioning, neural circuitry, which is predominantly located in frontal white matter. With the progression of demyelination, frontal subcortical circuits are presumably ablated with a subsequent resolution of psychosis.

Hyde *et al.* (1992), in their comprehensive review of all published reports of metachromatic leukodystrophy, have concluded that the prevalence of psychosis far exceeds that found in other neurological disorders that have been historically linked to elevated rates of psychosis, such as temporal lobe epilepsy (Roberts *et al.*, 1990) and Huntington's disease (Dewhurst *et al.*, 1969). This suggests that white matter tracts, particularly those connected to the frontal lobes, play a pivotal role in the pathogenesis of psychosis, presumably by disconnecting the region from the medial temporal lobe, basal ganglia and diencephalon (Davison and Bagley, 1969). The data on metachromatic leukodystrophy thus negate theories that regard psychosis as predominantly cortical in origin (Filley and Gross, 1992).

Neurobehavioral comparisons between multiple sclerosis and other disorders affecting white matter, deep gray matter and cortical areas

Comparisons of this nature are beset by methodological difficulties. Controlling for different demographic features and varying degrees of cerebral involvement, physical disability, disease severity and disease course will always be, at best, an imprecise exercise. Consequently, caution should be adopted in interpreting the findings. Nevertheless, looking for similarities and differences according to the anatomical substrate affected allows the researcher to test *a priori* assumptions with respect to descriptive and construct validity.

Multiple sclerosis and traumatic brain injury

The only study directly to compare neuropsychological abnormalities in patients with MS and with those in patients with traumatic brain injury failed to demonstrate common areas of deficit (Horton and Siegel, 1990). Instead, the profile to emerge in the patients with traumatic brain injury was one of predominantly cortical deficits, which contrasted with the abnormalities noted in the MS patients. However, the very small sample size, limited psychometric battery and the absence of any data describing the type or site of the brain injury effectively negated the significance of the results. Nevertheless, the study is worth citing if for no other reason than it remains a good example of the problems that may arise when comparing different disorders.

Multiple sclerosis and acquired immunodeficiency disease

A comparison between three groups of 20 patients each, namely MS, with AIDS and HIV-seronegative subjects (the last used as a control group), illustrates some of the hazards mentioned above (Morriss *et al.*, 1992). The subjects with AIDS were homosexual males and, to achieve a demographic match, the MS sample was limited to males as well, an atypical situation in a disorder with a female preponderance. In addition, the MS sample was significantly older than the other two groups, which was controlled for using analysis of covariance, a method considered problematic when dealing with demographic mismatch (Adams *et al.*, 1985).

The cognitive findings demonstrated a three-way split in that patients with AIDS occupied an intermediate position between the MS group and the HIV-seronegative group. The MS patients had the greatest cognitive impairment, but when the demographic confounders were eliminated, this difference was only apparent for performance on the Symbol–Digit Modalities Test (SDMT). Regarding psychopathology, MS patients were significantly more likely to develop an affective disorder following the onset of their neurological symptoms, whereas the AIDS group had a higher prevalence of premorbid mental illness and current mental illness (anxiety disorders, psychosis, adjustment disorders) with the exception of affective disorder. Although the authors concluded that major differences in mentation were present between the two patient groups, a contrary opinion can also be extracted from the data. For example, the limited psychometric battery concentrated on speed of information processing, verbal fluency and some indices of motor sequencing (Luria three-step procedure; go no-go tests). Performances between patients with MS or AIDS were similar on all measures except the SDMT, although even here, the patients with AIDS performed worse than their matched HIV-seronegative control group, indicating they too had difficulties with attention and processing speed. As for the psychiatric differences, these were hard to interpret because of biased sample selection. Viewed from this perspective, the study offered some tentative evidence of symptom overlap, at least in the cognitive domain. Larger, more representative sample selection and an expanded psychometric battery are needed before more definite conclusions can be reached.

Multiple sclerosis and Alzheimer's disease

Many studies have upheld the cortical–subcortical behavioral dichotomy by directly comparing the neuropsychological profiles of patients with Alzheimer's disease on the one hand and those with Huntington's disease (Brandt *et al.*, 1988; Salmon *et al.*, 1989; Tröster *et al.*, 1989; Rouleau *et al.*, 1992; Paulsen *et al.*, 1995) and Parkinson's disease (Pillon *et al.*, 1991; Bancher *et al.*, 1993) on the other. Only a single study has, however, contrasted the cognitive performances of patients with Alzheimer's disease with those in MS patients (Filley *et al.*, 1989c). Controlling for the effects of age, sex and education mismatch, the patients with Alzheimer's disease were found to be more globally demented with greater deficits in verbal skills, memory, learning and visuospatial function also noted. The MS patients, by contrast, were relatively more impaired on psychomotor tasks and particular emphasis was placed on disturbances in attention as a principal mental state abnormality in MS. The results supported a distinct subcortical cognitive profile, but the authors acknowledged the heterogeneous nature of the brain pathology and suggested a further subcortical split into white and gray matter disorders.

Multiple sclerosis and Huntington's disease

Neuropsychological examination revealed that the overall pattern of deficits in MS patients was similar to those seen in Huntington's disease, although some individual differences were still discernible (Caine *et al.*, 1986). The study was methodologically robust because globally demented patients and those on psychoactive medication were excluded, a comprehensive battery of tests was utilized and attempts were made to match the groups with respect to functional disability. In addition, the inclusion of a normal control group illustrated that although MS patients were less impaired than the Huntington's disease group, in relation to healthy subjects both subcortical diseases were associated with widespread cognitive deficits.

The patients with Huntington's disease had more pronounced difficulties with language, calculations and visuospatial tasks. While both groups showed memory deficits, these were more marked in those with Huntington's disease, who had problems both with retrieval and verbal recognition. The MS patients, by comparison, did relatively well with verbal recognition tasks, and their difficulties were largely retrieval based. The latter could explain the mild naming deficits found in MS patients, which occurred in the absence of other language abnormalities. Speed of cognition in MS was noted to be slow. The importance of this study lay in the fact that it was the first to tease out the more subtle cognitive differences that characterize white matter and subcortical gray matter disease, thereby adding impetus to the notion not only of a subcortical dementia but also, more specifically, of a subcortical white matter dementia.

Of note is that neither of the studies comparing MS patients with those with Huntington's disease (Caine *et al.*, 1986) or Alzheimer's disease (Filley *et al.*, 1989c) made mention of implicit (procedural) memory. This refers to motor skills (driving, playing a musical instrument), classical conditioning and priming. Patients with Huntington's disease show deficits in motor skill learning (Heindel *et al.*, 1988) but have intact priming (Shinamura *et al.*, 1987), whereas patients with Alzheimer's disease have the reverse: difficulty with priming tasks (Salmon *et al.*, 1988) but intact motor learning skills (Heindel *et al.*, 1988). As MS patients do not have problems with either priming (Beatty and Monson, 1990) or motor learning skills (Beatty *et al.*, 1990), this suggests a further discriminating cognitive feature.

The review has, until now, focussed on studies that involved two-way comparisons of behavioral differences between MS and another disorder. However, there is also a report of a four-way comparison: MS versus Alzheimer's versus Huntington's versus Parkinson's diseases, the last further divided into cognitively intact and impaired groups. Tröster *et al.* (1998) undertook a series of separate studies across these four diseases probing verbal fluency as a means of assessing patients' lexical (phonemic) and semantic memories. Prior research of verbal fluency had indicated that healthy subjects usually generated words in semantic clusters on semantic fluency tasks and in phonemic clusters on phonemic fluency tasks. In this study, all subject groups completed three cognitive tests, often as part of a larger cognitive battery. The tests were the Dementia Rating Scale, the Boston Naming Test and measures of verbal fluency (the FAS test as a measure of phonemic fluency, and a semantic fluency test, in which subjects were given 60 seconds to name animals). In the first experiment, patients with Alzheimer's disease were compared with the two groups of patients with Parkinson's disease, those with and without dementia. In the second experiment, the three tests were given to a group of 133 MS patients and 63 healthy controls. In the third experiment, 24 patients with Huntington's disease were given the same three tests.

Bringing together the data from the three studies (and five study groups), the authors discerned some clear group differences. Patients with Alzheimer's disease, Parkinson's disease with dementia, Huntington's disease and MS all produced fewer words and fewer switching responses, but the MS patients, unlike those from the other three groups, were the only ones to have a normal semantic cluster size. (The patients with Parkinson's disease without dementia performed normally on all the tests.) These data were interpreted as evidence that MS patients were more efficient in accessing lexical and semantic memory stores and provided evidence for a distinct profile of cognitive deficits associated with MS.

Recovery of function

There is evidence that the cerebral white, but not gray, matter may show varying degrees of recovery from insult. Serial MRI has demonstrated the waning of white matter plaques in MS patients (Miller *et al.*, 1988), which occasionally may be accompanied by improvements in mentation (Rozewicz *et al.*, 1996). The ability of myelin to regenerate spontaneously, although limited, has been pursued as a potential treatment option in MS (ffrench-Constant, 1994). Other therapeutic possibilities for an array of white matter disorders have been reviewed by Filley (1996) and range from surgical correction of normal pressure hydrocephalus to the reversal of cognitive decline in abstinent alcoholics. Irrespective of the disorder, the point to be made is that a similar recovery is not possible after cortical destruction.

A fresh challenge to the concept of a subcortical white matter dementia

Over the past few years, data have emerged from different sources implicating significant cortical gray matter involvement in MS.[1] Neuropathological findings (Kutzelnigg and Lassmann, 2005; Kutzelnigg et al., 2005) to this effect have been complemented by neuroimaging results from multiple modalities, including conventional spin echo voxel-based morphometry (Prinster et al., 2006), diffusion tensor (Vrenken et al., 2006) and magnetization transfer (Dehmeshki et al., 2003) imaging, magnetic resonance spectroscopy (Kapeller et al., 2001; Sharma et al., 2001) and PET (Blinkenberg et al., 2000). The importance of this shift in knowledge is underscored by the fact that from a behavioral viewpoint cortical pathology may be a more robust marker of cognitive decline than lesion volume measurement.

All this begs the question whether MS can still be considered the archetypal white matter subcortical dementia? And here an interesting paradox is found, one that the existing literature has yet to address. On the one hand, there are the imaging data that increasingly reveal cortical pathology and on the otherhand, a cognitive profile that is distinct from that seen in disorders such as Alzheimer's disease. How can theory reconcile the relative absence of aphasia, agnosia, apraxia and Alzheimer-type memory deficits with the newfound MS cortical data? For it remains a striking observation that the most widely cited arbiter of cognitive dysfunction, the Mini-Mental State Examination (still the standard bearer in diseases such as Alzheimer's disease), is singularly insensitive in patients with MS.

In defining the characteristics of a dementia, what assumes primacy: the cognitive profile, the imaging data or the postmortem findings? Ideally of course, all three march in tandem and the confluence of facts assert a tight diagnostic validity. In MS, the discordance has yet to be resolved. If one takes the DSM-IV as the final diagnostic arbiter, then the debate is bypassed, because the DSM is primarily a descriptive document, shying away from etiology. Even in the absence of a distinct subcortical category, one can still quite comfortably invoke a substitute, namely

---

[1] An analogous situation, albeit working in the opposite direction, has now begun implicating white matter changes in diseases such as schizophrenia.

"dementia due to a general medical condition" and total up the various cognitive deficits. But new and compelling brain imaging findings cannot be downplayed. They must be incorporated into a schema that at least bridges, if it cannot as yet resolve, these tensions.

One theoretical way of doing this is to reexamine the relationship between cognition and brain changes. Earlier research from the 1980s and 1990s reported modest correlations (in the order of $r = 0.3$–0.5) between disease burden (usually measures of T_2 weighted total lesion volume) and various aspects of cognition. Over the past few years, cortical lesions/atrophy have emerged from regression analyses as an important – and on occasions, preeminent – predictor of cognitive decline. This finding does not invalidate the T_2 lesion burden data. It simply suggests that, statistically, cortical pathology may be more important. Our reliance, as researchers, on the power of statistics and the attainment of an acceptable p value may, therefore, be throwing us off the clinical scent. White matter pathology cannot suddenly just fade from our theoretical constructs.

A better interpretation of the data is to attribute the pathogenesis of cognitive deficits to many factors, cortical and subcortical, with demyelination per se influencing the *content* or *type* of deficits seen. And here we need to return to a point made earlier in this chapter, namely that the cortical–subcortical distinction is essentially an artificial one because the two regions are intimately joined and functionally integrated. Revisiting the neuroimaging data of Christodoulou *et al.* (2003) provides good empirical support for this assertion. The study reported that central cerebral atrophy (i.e. the percentage of central CSF to total cranial volume [gray and white matter, lesion and CSF volumes]) was the most robust predictor of neuropsychological deficits in MS patients, accounting for more than half the variance in cognitive performance. Furthermore, it was a delay in information processing speed (as recorded by the SDMT) that correlated most strongly with the MRI findings. Essentially, what this implies is that it is an amalgam of various aspects of brain pathology that not only best predicts cognitive decline in MS patients but also determines the particular nature of that decline, with its tell-tale subcortical stamp.

Summary

- The a demyelinating disorder MS has long been regarded as the quintessential white matter disease. As such, cognitive dysfunction associated with MS has been termed a subcortical dementia.
- The hallmarks of a subcortical dementia are forgetfulness, a slowness of thought processes, emotional or personality changes (summarized as apathy or depression interspersed with irritability), and an impaired ability to manipulate acquired knowledge.

- Aphasia, apraxia, and agnosia, all characteristic of a cortical dementia, are found less frequently in patients with a subcortical dementing process.
- The early descriptions of subcortical dementia were limited to patients with basal ganglia disease, which begs the question to what degree do the neuro-behavioral aspects of MS differ from these disorders?
- Unlike the basal ganglia disorders, MS is not associated with movement disorders nor deficits in implicit memory. There are also qualitative differences in explicit memory. The Mini-Mental State Examination lacks sensitivity in cognitively compromised MS patients.
- There is evidence that the cerebral white matter, unlike the gray, may show varying degrees of recovery from insult, thereby establishing an important difference between these two substrates.
- Recent data from neuroimaging and neuropathology studies have demonstrated more extensive gray matter involvement in MS than formerly recognized. In addition, cerebral atrophy has emerged as a more important correlate of cognitive dysfunction than lesion volume.
- Whether the concept of MS as a white matter dementia will endure in the face of these brain imaging findings is unclear. What is clear, however, is that white matter disease, even in the presence of cortical atrophy, can influence the *type* of cognitive deficits elicited.

References

Adams JH, Mitchell DE, Graham DI, Doyle D. (1977) Diffuse brain damage of immediate impact type. *Brain*, **100**, 489–502.

Adams KM, Brown GG, Grant I. (1985) Analysis of covariance as a remedy for demographic mismatch of research subject groups: some sobering simulations. *Journal of Clinical and Experimental Neuropsychology*, **7**, 445–462.

Albert ML. (1978) Subcortical dementia. In *Alzheimer's Disease: Senile Dementia and Related Disorders*, ed. R Katzman, RD Terry, KL Bick. New York: Raven Press, pp. 173–180.

Albert ML, Feldman RG, Willis AL. (1974) The "subcortical dementia" of progressive supranuclear palsy. *Journal of Neurology, Neurosurgery and Psychiatry*, **37**, 121–130.

Alexander GE, Crutcher MD. (1990) Functional architecture of basal ganglia circuits: neural substrates of parallel processing. *Trends in Neuroscience*, **13**, 266–271.

Alexander GE, DeLong MR, Strick PL. (1986) Parallel organisation of functionally segregated circuits linking basal ganglia and cortex. *Annual Reviews in Neuroscience*, **9**, 357–381.

Alzheimer A. (1910) Beitrag zur Kenntnis der pathologischen Neuroglis und ihrer Beziehungen zu Abbauvorgangen Nervengewebe. In *Histologische und histopathologische Arbeiten uber die Grosshirnrinde*, ed. F Nissl, A Alzheimer. Jena, Germany: Gustsav Fischer, pp. 401–404.

American Psychiatric Association. (1994) *The Diagnostic and Statistical Manual of Mental Disorders*, 4th edn. Washington, DC: American Psychiatric Press.

Babikian V, Ropper AH. (1987) Binswanger's disease: a review. *Stroke*, **18**, 2–12.

Bagley LL, Grossman RI, Galetta SL, *et al.* (1999) Characterization of white matter lesions in multiple sclerosis and traumatic brain injury as revealed by magnetization transfer contour plots. *American Journal of Neuroradiology*, **20**, 977–981.

Bagley LL, McGowan JC, Grossman RI, *et al.* (2000) Magnetization transfer imaging in traumatic brain injury. *Journal of Magnetic Resonance Imaging*, **11**, 1–8.

Bancher C, Braak H, Fischer P, Jellinger KA. (1993) Neuropsychological staging of Alzheimer lesions and intellectual status in Alzheimer's and Parkinson's disease patients. *Neuroscience Letters*, **162**, 179–182.

Beatty WW, Monson N. (1990) Semantic priming in multiple sclerosis. *Bulletin of the Psychonomic Society*, **28**, 397–400.

Beatty WW, Goodkin DE, Monson N, Beatty PA. (1990) Implicit learning in patients with chronic–progressive multiple sclerosis. *International Journal of Clinical Neuropsychology*, **12**, 166–172.

Blinkenberg M, Rune K, Jensen CV, *et al.* (2000) Cortical cerebral metabolism correlates with MRI lesion load and cognitive dysfunction in MS. *Neurology*, **54**, 558–563.

Brandt J, Folstein SE, Folstein MF. (1988) Differential cognitive impairment in Alzheimer's disease and Huntington's disease. *Annals of Neurology*, **23**, 555–561.

Brooks DJ, Leenders KL, Head G, *et al.* (1984) Studies on regional cerebral oxygen utilisation and cognitive function in multiple sclerosis. *Journal of Neurology, Neurosurgery and Psychiatry*, **47**, 1182–1191.

Caine ED, Shoulson I. (1983) Psychiatric syndromes in Huntington's disease. *American Journal of Psychiatry*, **140**, 728–733.

Caine ED, Bamford KA, Schiffer RB, Shoulson I, Levy S. (1986) A controlled neuropsychological comparison of Huntington's disease and multiple sclerosis. *Archives of Neurology*, **43**, 249–254.

Christodoulou C, Krupp LB, Liang Z, *et al.* (2003) Cognitive performance and MTR markers of cerebral injury in cognitively impaired MS patients. *Neurology*, **60**, 1793–1798.

Collins JG. (1990) Types of injuries by selected characteristics: United States, 1985–1987. In *Vital and Health Statistics*, Series 10: *Data from the National Health Survey*, No. 175. [DHHS Publication No [PHS]91-1503.] Hyattsville, MD: US Department of Health and Human Services.

Cummings JL. (1986) Subcortical dementia: neuropsychology, neuropsychiatry, and pathophysiology. *British Journal of Psychiatry*, **149**, 682–697.

Cummings JL. (1993) Frontal-subcortical circuits and human behavior. *Archives of Neurology*, **50**, 873–880.

Cummings JL, Benson F. (1984) Subcortical dementia. Review of an emerging concept. *Archives of Neurology*, **41**, 874–879.

Davison K, Bagley CR. (1969) Schizophrenia-like psychoses associated with organic disorders of the central nervous system: a review of the literature. In *Current Problems in Neuropsychiatry*, ed. RN Harrington. Ashford, UK: Headley, pp. 113–184.

Dehmeshki J, Chard DT, Leary SM, *et al.* (2003) The normal appearing grey matter in primary progessive multiple sclerosis: a magnetisation transfer imaging study. *Journal of Neurology*, **250**, 67–74.

Dewhurst K, Oliver J, Trick KLK, McKnight AL. (1969) Neuropsychiatric aspects of Huntington's disease. *Confina Neurologica*, **31**, 258–268.

Feinstein A, Ron MA (1990) Psychosis associated with demonstrable brain disease. *Psychological Medicine*, **20**, 793–803.

Feinstein A, Ron MA, Thompson A. (1993) A serial study of psychometric and magnetic resonance imaging changes in multiple sclerosis. *Brain*, **116**, 569–602.

ffrench-Constant C (1994) Pathogenesis of multiple sclerosis. *Lancet*, **343**, 271–274.

Filley CM. (1996) Neurobehavioral aspects of cerebral white matter disorders. In *Neuropsychiatry*, ed. BS Fogel, RB Schiffer, SM Rao. Baltimore, MD: Williams and Wilkins, pp. 913–934.

Filley CM, Gross KF. (1992) Psychosis with cerebral white matter. *Neuropsychiatry, Neuropsychology and Behavioral Neurology*, **5**, 119–125.

Filley CM, Franklin GM, Heaton RK, Rodenberg NL. (1989a) White matter dementia. Clinical disorders and implications. *Neuropsychiatry, Neuropsychology and Behavioral Neurology*, **1**, 239–254.

Filley CM, Davis KA, Schmitz SP, *et al.* (1989b) Neuropsychological performance and magnetic resonance imaging in Alzheimer's disease and normal aging. *Neuropsychiatry, Neuropsychology, and Behavioral Neurology*, **2**, 81–91.

Filley CM, Heaton RK, Nelson LM, Burks JS, Franklin GM. (1989c) A comparison of dementia in Alzheimer's disease and multiple sclerosis. *Archives of Neurology*, **46**, 157–161.

Fillippi CG, Ulug AM, Ryan E, Ferrando SJ, van Gorp W. (2001) Diffusion tensor imaging of patients with HIV and normal appearing white matter on MR images of the brain. *American Journal of Neuroradiology*, **22**, 277–283.

Geschwind N. (1965) Disconnection syndromes in animals and man. *Brain*, **88**, 237–94.

Gray F, Dubas F, Roullet E, Escourolle R. (1985) Leukoencephalopathy in diffuse haemorrhagic cerebral amyloid angiopathy. *Annals of Neurology*, **18**, 54–59.

Gray F, Chimelli L, Mohr M, *et al.* (1991) Fulminating multiple sclerosis-like leukoencephalopathy revealing human immunodeficiency virus infection. *Neurology*, **41**, 105–109.

Hakim AM, Mathieson G. (1979) Dementia in Parkinson's disease. A neuropathologic study. *Neurology*, **29**, 1209–1214.

Harvey I, Ron MA, du Boulay GE, *et al.* (1993) Reduction in cortical volume in schizophrenia on magnetic resonance imaging. *Psychological Medicine*, **23**, 591–604.

Heaton RK, Grant I, Butters N, *et al.* (1995) The HNRC 500: neuropsychology of HIV infection at different disease stages. HIV Neurobehavioral Research Centre. *Journal of the International Neuropsychological Society*, **1**, 231–251.

Heindel WC, Butters N, Salmon DP. (1988) Impaired learning of a motor skill in patients with Huntington's disease. Behavioral Neuroscience, **102**, 141–147.

Horton AM, Siegel E. (1990) Comparison of multiple sclerosis and head trauma patients: a neuropsychological pilot study. *International Journal of Neuroscience*, **53**, 213–215.

Humayun MS, Presty SK, Lafrance ND, *et al.* (1989) Local cerebral glucose abnormalities in mild closed head injured patients with cognitive impairment. *Nuclear Medicine Communications*, **10**, 335–344.

Hyde TM, Ziegler JC, Weinberger DR. (1992) Psychiatric disturbances in metachromatic leukodystrophy. Insights into the neurobiology of psychosis. *Archives of Neurology*, **49**, 401–406.

Inglese M, Makani S, Johnson G, *et al.* (2005) Diffuse axonal injury in mild traumatic brain injury: a diffusion tensor imaging study. *Journal of Neurosurgery*, **103**, 298–303.

Jellinger K, Seitelberg G. (1970) Protracted post-traumatic encephalopathy: pathology, pathogenesis and clinical implications. *Journal of the Neurological Sciences*, **10**, 51–94.

Johansson B, Roos B-E. (1974) 5-Hydroxyindoleacetic acid and homovanillic acid in cerebrospinal fluid of patients with neurological disease. *European Neurology*, **11**, 37–45.

Kapeller P, McLean MA, Griffin CM, *et al.* (2001) Preliminary evidence for neuronal damage in cortical grey matter and normal appearing white matter in short duration relapsing–remitting multiple sclerosis. A quatitative MR spectroscopic imaging study. *Journal of Neurology*, **248**, 131–138.

Kubicki M, McCarley RW, Shenton ME. (2005) Evidence for white matter abnormalities in schizophrenai. *Current Opinion in Psychiatry*, **18**, 121–134.

Kujala P, Portin R, Revonsuo A, Ruutiainen J. (1995) Attention related performance in two cognitively different subgroups of patients with multiple sclerosis. *Journal of Neurology, Neurosurgery and Psychiatry*, **59**, 77–82.

Kutzelnigg A, Lassmann H. (2005) Cortical lesions and brain atrophy in MS. *Journal of the Neurological Sciences*, **233**, 55–59.

Kutzelnigg A, Lucchinetti CF, Stadelman C, *et al.* (2005) Cortical demyelination and diffuse white matter injury in multiple sclerosis. *Brain*, **128**, 2705–2712.

Levin HS, Amparo E, Eisenberg HM, *et al.* (1987) Magnetic resonance imaging and computerised tomography in relation to the neurobehavioral sequelae of mild and moderate head injuries. *Journal of Neurosurgery*, **66**, 706–713.

Levin HS, Williams DH, Eisenberg HM, High WM, Guinto FC. (1992) Serial MRI and neurobehavioral findings after mild to moderate closed head injury. *Journal of Neurology, Neurosurgery and Psychiatry*, **55**, 255–262.

Markianos M, Sfagos C. (1988) Altered serotonin uptake kinetics in multiple sclerosis. *Journal of Neurology*, **235**, 236–237.

Markowitz JC, Perry SW. (1992) Effects of the human immunodeficiency virus on the central nervous system. In *The American Psychiatric Press Textbook of Neuropsychiatry*, ed. SC Yudowsky, RE Hales. Washington DC: American Psychiatric Press, Ch. 21, pp. 499–518.

McHugh PR, Folstein MF. (1975) Psychiatric syndromes of Huntington's chorea: a clinical and phenomenologic study. In *Psychiatric Aspects of Neurological Disease*, ed. DF Benson, D Blumer New York: Grune and Stratton, pp. 265–286.

Mesulam M-M. (1981) Large scale neurocognitive networks and distributed processing for attention, language and memory. *Annals of Neurology*, **28**, 597–613.

Miller DH, Rudge P, Johnson G, *et al.* (1988) Serial gadolinium enhanced MRI in multiple sclerosis. *Brain*, **111**, 927–939.

Morriss R, Schaerf F, Brandt J, McArthur J, Folstein M. (1992) AIDS and multiple sclerosis: neural and mental features. *Acta Psychiatrica Scandinavica*, **85**, 331–336.

Navia BA, Jordan BD, Price RW. (1986) The AIDS dementia complex, I: clinical features. *Annals of Neurology*, **19**, 517–524.

Olsen WL, Longo FM, Mills CM, Norman D. (1988) White matter disease in AIDS: findings at MR imaging. *Neuroradiology*, **169**, 445–448.

Paulsen JS, Butters N, Sadek JR, *et al.* (1995) Distinct cognitive profiles of cortical and subcortical dementia in advanced illness. *Neurology*, **45**, 951–956.

Pillon B, Dubois B, Ploska A, Agid Y. (1991) Severity and specificity of cognitive impairment in Alzheimer's, Huntington's, and Parkinson's diseases and progressive supranuclear palsy. *Neurology*, **41**, 634–643.

Polten A, Fluharty AL, Fluharty CB, *et al.* (1991) Molecular basis of different forms of meta-chromatic leukodystrophy. *New England Journal of Medicine*, **324**, 18–22.

Prinster A, Quarantelli M, Orefice G, *et al.* (2006) Grey matter loss in relapsing–remitting multiple sclerosis: a voxel based morphometry study. *NeuroImage*, **29**, 859–867.

Ragin AB, Storey P Cohen BA, Epstein LG, Edelman RR. (2004a) Whole brain diffusion tensor imaging in HIV-associated cognitive impairment. *American Journal of Neuroradiology*, **25**, 195–200.

Ragin AB, Storey P Cohen BA, Edelman RR, Epstein LG. (2004b) Disease burden in HIV-associated cognitive impairment: a study of whole brain measures. *Neurology*, **63**, 2293–2297.

Rao SM, Mittenberg W, Bernardin L, Haughton V, Leo GJ. (1989) Neuropsychological test findings in subjects with leukoaraiosis. *Archives of Neurology*, **46**, 40–44.

Roberts GW, Done DJ, Bruton C, Crow TJ. (1990). A "mock-up" of schizophrenia: temporal lobe epilepsy and schizophrenia-like psychoses. *Biological Psychiatry*, **28**, 127–143.

Rouleau I, Salmon DP, Butters N, Kennedy C, McGuire K. (1992) Quantitative and qualitative analyses of clock drawings in Alzheimer's and Huntington's disease. *Brain and Cognition*, **18**, 70–87.

Rozewicz L, Langdon DW, Davie CA, Thompson AJ, Ron MA (1996) Resolution of left hemisphere cognitive dysfunction in multiple sclerosis with magnetic resonance correlates: a case report. *Cognitive Neuropsychiatry*, **1**, 17–25.

Ruff RM, Crouch JA, Troster AI, *et al.* (1994) Selected cases of poor outcome following minor brain trauma: comparing neuropsychological and positron emission tomography assessment. *Brain Injury*, **8**, 297–308.

Salloway S. (1996) Clinico-pathologic case conference: depression, behavior change and subcortical dementia in a 57 year old woman. *Journal of Neuropsychiatry and Clinical Neurosciences*, **8**, 215–221.

Salmon DP, Shinamura AP, Butter N, Smith S. (1988) Lexical and semantic priming deficits in patients with Alzheimer's disease. *Journal of Clinical and Experimental Neuropsychology*, **10**, 477–494.

Salmon DP, Kwo-on-Yen PF, Heindel WC, Butters N, Thal LJ. (1989) Differentiation of Alzheimer's disease and Huntington's disease with the dementia rating scale. *Archives of Neurology*, **46**, 1204–1208.

Sharma R, Narayana PA, Wolinsky JS. (2001) Grey matter abnormalities in multiple sclerosis: proton magnetic resonance spectroscopic imaging. *Multiple Sclerosis*, **7**, 221–226.

Shinamura AP, Salmon DP, Squire LR, Butters N. (1987) Memory dysfunction and word priming in dementia and amnesia. *Behavioral Neuroscience*, **101**, 347–351.

Stevens, DL, Hewlett RH, Brownell B. (1977) Chronic-familial vascular encephalopathy. *Lancet*, **i**, 1364–1365.

Strich SJ. (1961) Shearing of nerve fibres as a cause of brain damage due to head injury. *Lancet*, **ii**, 443–468.

Suddath RL, Christison GW, Torrey EF, Casanova MF, Weinberger DR. (1990) Anatomical abnormalities in the brains of monozygotic twins discordant for schizophrenia. *New England Journal of Medicine*, **322**, 789–794.

Tröster AI, Salmon DP, McCullough D, Butters N. (1989) A comparison of the category fluency deficits associated with Alzheimer's and Huntington's disease. *Brain and Language*, **37**, 500–513.

Tröster AI, Fields JA, Testa JA, *et al.* (1998) Cortical and subcortical influences on clustering and switching in the performance of verbal fluency tasks. *Neuropsychologia*, **36**, 295–304.

Tuite M, Ketonenen L, Kieburtz K, Handy B. Efficacy of gadolinium in MR brain imaging of HIV-infected patients. (1993) *American Journal of Neuroradiology*, **14**, 257–263.

Vrenken H, Pouwels PJ, Geurts JJ, *et al.* (2006) Altered diffusion tensor in multiple sclerosis normal appearing brain tissue: cortical diffusion changes seem related to clinical deterioration. *Journal of Magnetic Resonance Imaging*, **23**, 628–636.

White DA, Heaton RK, Monsch AU, and the HNRC Group. (1995) Neuropsychological studies of asymptomatic human immunodeficiency virus-type-1 infected individuals. *Journal of the International Neuropsychological Society*, **1**, 304–315.

Whitehouse PJ, Price DL, Struble RG, *et al.* (1982) Alzheimer's disease and senile dementia: loss of neurons in the basal forebrain. *Science*, **215**, 1237–1239.

Wilson SAK. (1912) Progressive lenticular degeneration: a familial nervous disease associated with cirrhosis of the liver. *Brain*, **34**, 295–307.

Wise SP, Demisone R. (1988) Behavioral neurophysiology: insights into seeing and grasping. *Science*, **242**, 736–741.

Index